I0055202

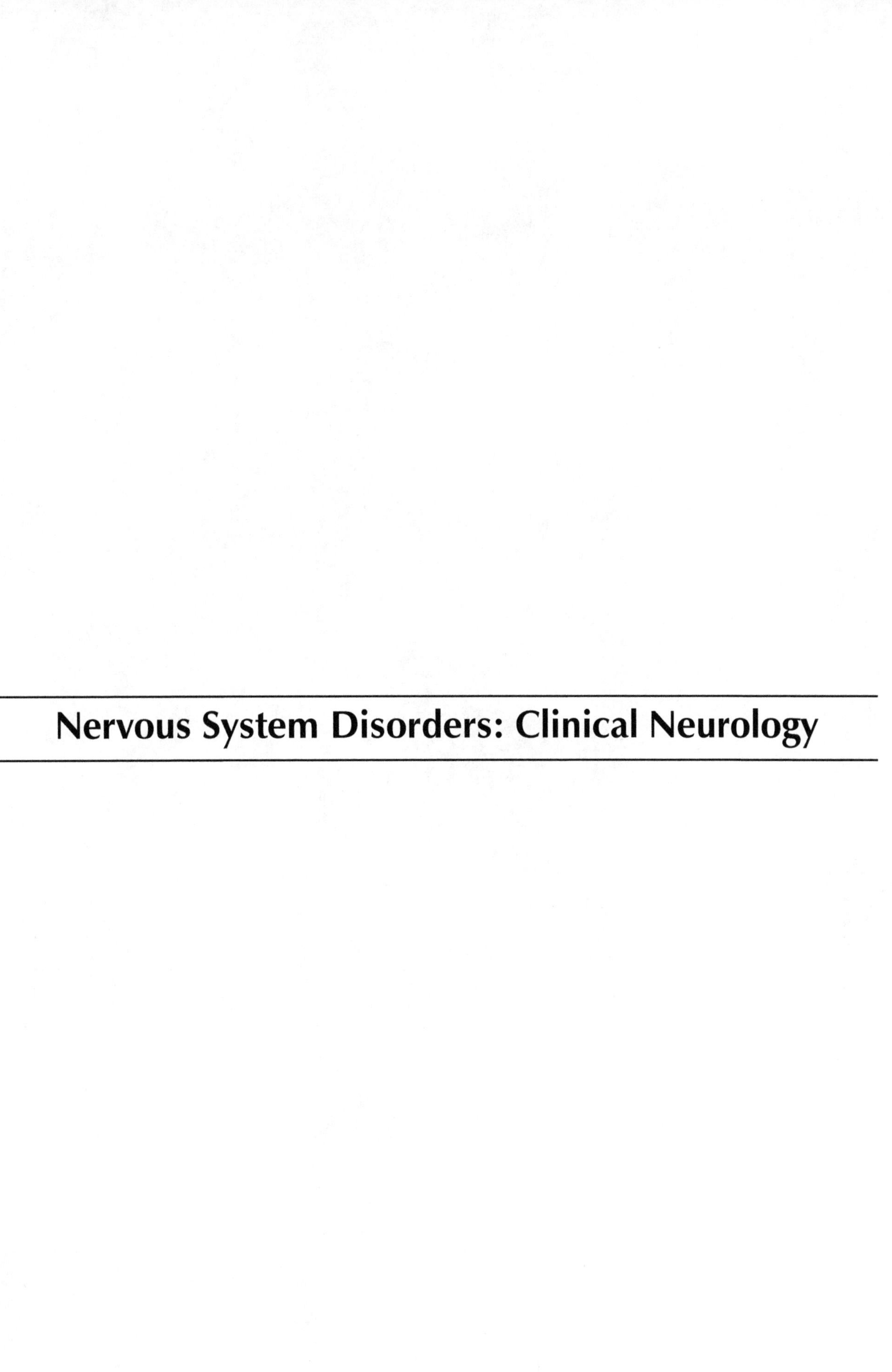

Nervous System Disorders: Clinical Neurology

Nervous System Disorders: Clinical Neurology

Editor: Erica McGregor

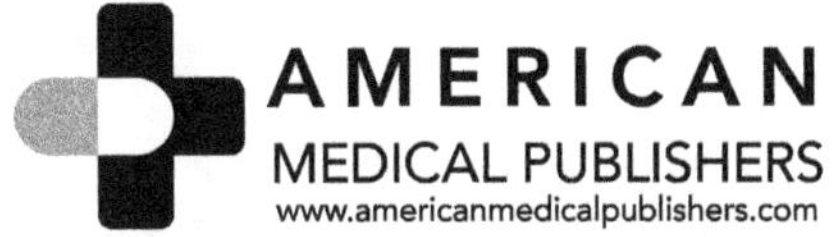

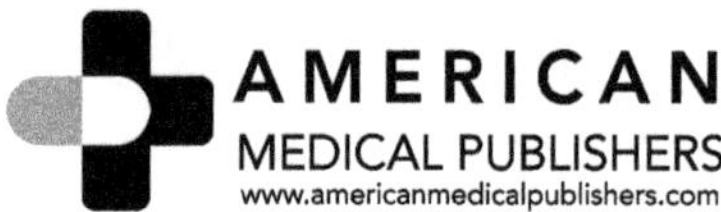

Cataloging-in-Publication Data

Nervous system disorders : clinical neurology / edited by Erica McGregor.
p. cm.
Includes bibliographical references and index.
ISBN 978-1-63927-308-9
1. Nervous system--Diseases. 2. Neurology. 3. Nervous system--Diseases--Treatment. I. McGregor, Erica.
RC346 .N47 2022
616.8--dc23

© American Medical Publishers, 2022

American Medical Publishers,
41 Flatbush Avenue,
1st Floor, New York,
NY 11217, USA

ISBN 978-1-63927-308-9 (Hardback)

This book contains information obtained from authentic and highly regarded sources. Copyright for all individual chapters remain with the respective authors as indicated. All chapters are published with permission under the Creative Commons Attribution License or equivalent. A wide variety of references are listed. Permission and sources are indicated; for detailed attributions, please refer to the permissions page and list of contributors. Reasonable efforts have been made to publish reliable data and information, but the authors, editors and publisher cannot assume any responsibility for the validity of all materials or the consequences of their use.

Trademark Notice: Registered trademark of products or corporate names are used only for explanation and identification without intent to infringe.

Contents

Preface

The main aim of this book is to educate learners and enhance their research focus by presenting diverse topics covering this vast field. This is an advanced book which compiles significant studies by distinguished experts in the area of analysis. This book addresses successive solutions to the challenges arising in the area of application, along with it; the book provides scope for future developments.

The improper functioning of the central and peripheral nervous system is known as nervous system disorders. The most common symptoms of nervous disorders include lack of concentration, loss of feeling, paralysis, memory loss, seizures, tremors, relaxed pronunciation, confusion, pain and increased reflexes. The causes of nervous system disorders include tumor, brain injury, spinal cord injury, metal poisoning and infections. The diagnosis of nervous system disorders is done on the basis of the neurological examination. It evaluates the effects of neurological damage on the brain functioning in terms of behavior and cognition. The preventions for nervous system disorders include physiotherapy, neurorehabilitation, pain management, operations and medications. The book presents researches and studies performed by experts across the globe. This book presents the complex subject of nervous system disorders in the most comprehensible and easy to understand language. Those in search of information to further their knowledge will be greatly assisted by this book.

It was a great honour to edit this book, though there were challenges, as it involved a lot of communication and networking between me and the editorial team. However, the end result was this all-inclusive book covering diverse themes in the field.

Finally, it is important to acknowledge the efforts of the contributors for their excellent chapters, through which a wide variety of issues have been addressed. I would also like to thank my colleagues for their valuable feedback during the making of this book.

Editor

1

Syncope and Epilepsy coexist in 'possible' and 'drug-resistant' epilepsy (Overlap between Epilepsy and Syncope Study -OESYS)

Andrea Ungar[1], Alice Ceccofiglio[1], Francesca Pescini[2], Chiara Mussi[3], Gianni Tava[4], Martina Rafanelli[1], Assunta Langellotto[5], Niccolò Marchionni[1], J. Gert van Dijk[6], Gianlugi Galizia[7], Domenico Bonaduce[8] and Pasquale Abete[8*]

Abstract

Background: Differential diagnosis between syncope and epilepsy in patients with transient loss of consciousness of uncertain etiology is still unclear. Thus, the aim of the present work is to evaluate the prevalence of syncope in patients with "possible" or "drug-resistant" epilepsy.

Methods: The Overlap between Epilepsy and SYncope Study (OESYS) is a multicenter prospective observational study designed to estimate the prevalence of syncope in patients followed in Epilepsy Centers for "possible" or "drug-resistant" epilepsy and assessed according the European Society of Cardiology (ESC) guidelines of syncope diagnosis.

Results: One hundred seven patients were evaluated; 63 (58.9%) had possible and 44 (41.1%) drug-resistant epilepsy. A final diagnosis of isolated syncope was in 45 patients (42.1%), all with possible epilepsy (45/63, 71.4%). Isolated epilepsy was found in 21 patients (19.6%) and it was more frequent in the drug-resistant than in the possible epilepsy group (34.1% vs. 9.5%, $p = 0.002$). More importantly, syncope and epilepsy coexisted in 37.4% of all patients but the coexistence was more frequent among patients with drug-resistant than possible epilepsy (65.9% vs. 17.5%, $p < 0.001$).

Conclusions: Isolated syncope was diagnosed in ≈ 70% of patients with possible epilepsy. Syncope and epilepsy coexisted in ≈ 20% of patients with possible and in ≈ 60% of patients with drug-resistant epilepsy. These findings highlight the need of ESC guidelines of syncope approach in patients with possible and drug-resistant epilepsy.

Background

As many as 20–40% of patients diagnosed as having epilepsy may not actually have epilepsy [1]. In such patients, antiepileptic drugs (AEDs) are harmful because they have adverse effects, are ineffective, unnecessary, and reanalysis is postponed until their efficacy is judged, usually after a very long time [1, 2]. Syncope is the most frequent cause of misdiagnosis in epilepsy [2]. In patients defined as having "drug-resistant epilepsy", attacks persist because the underlying disorder (i.e., syncope) has not been correctly diagnosed [3]. There are several reasons why syncope may be erroneous considered as epileptic seizures. Firstly, syncope affects up to 40% of the population [4], so even a small proportion of cases may contaminate "epilepsy" cohorts. Secondly, syncope is frequently associated with abnormal movements such as myoclonic jerks, oral automatism, head-turning and, more rarely, urinary incontinence, thus mimicking the clinical presentation of epileptic seizures [2, 5–7]. Thirdly, syncope and seizures may coexist in a patient, either by pure chance or by pathophysiology mechanism. Temporal seizure may, on rare occasions cause asystole, and therefore, syncope by cardiac mechanism [8–10]. Conversely, syncope may provoke a true epileptic seizure [11, 12]. More specifically, an epileptic-anoxic seizure arising usually from a temporal lobe is seen in epilepsy;

* Correspondence: p.abete@unina.it
[8]Department of Translational Medical Sciences, University of Naples Federico II, Via S. Pansini, 80131 Naples, Italy

whereas an anoxic-epileptic seizure (an epileptic seizure triggered by syncope, typically during recovery) is seen in syncope in patients without necessarily having epilepsy.

Thus, the rate of coexistence of epileptic seizures and syncope appears complex and needs to be better defined.

The Overlap of Epilepsy and SYncope Study (OESYS) is multicenter prospective observational study designed to estimate the prevalence of syncope according to the European Society of Cardiology (ESC) guidelines [4] in patients followed in Epilepsy Centers for possible or drug-resistant epilepsy.

Methods

This study was carried out on consecutive patients followed in Epilepsy Centers for possible or drug-resistant epilepsy and evaluated in 4 different Italian Syncope Units (Florence, Modena, Trento and Naples) between November 2009 and June 2012.

Inclusion and exclusion criteria

Patients were selected in the Epilepsy Centers by neurologists if they had a diagnosis of either possible or drug-resistant epilepsy and presented recurrent episodes of non-convulsive transient loss of consciousness (T-LOC) followed or not followed by jerks or involuntary movements, whose origin remained unknown after the neurological clinical and diagnostic evaluations. All episodes of functional T-LOC (non-epileptic T-LOC with normal blood pressure and heart rate) were classified as Psychogenic Non-Epileptic Seizures (PNES).

Thus, the inclusion criteria were age ≥ 18 years, recurrent T-LOC (≥2 episodes) of unknown cause and:

a) drug-resistant epilepsy, defined according to the International League Against Epilepsy (ILAE) Commission as "failure of adequate trials of two tolerated and appropriately chosen and used AED schedules (whether as mono-therapy or in combination) to achieve sustained seizure freedom". Seizure-free duration that is at least three times the longest interseizure interval prior to starting a new intervention would need to be observed or at least 12 months [13].

or

b) possible epilepsy, defined as "seizure with an alternative explanation for the attack and insufficient evidence to support a confident diagnosis of epilepsy" [14].

The exclusion criteria were the presence of generalized tonic-clonic seizure (GTCS) and the inability or unwillingness to give informed consent.

Management strategy

In the Epilepsy Centers the evaluation of the patients included: i) history, mainly focused on past and current AEDs treatment, comorbidity with neurological and non neurological diseases, clinical aspects of described and/or witnessed episodes (i.e. number, type, predisposing circumstances, prodromes, etc); ii) physical examination; iii) instrumental tests, including electroencephalogram (EEG) and computed tomography (CT) or magnetic resonance imaging (MRI) of the brain.

Selected patients, who fulfilled the inclusion criteria were referred to the Syncope Unit and managed according to the ESC guidelines for diagnosis and management of syncope[12]. The initial evaluation consisted of a careful history, focused on cardiovascular diseases and drugs, and patient tests that included a 12-lead electrocardiogram, orthostatic blood pressure measurements, Head-Up Tilt testing (HUT) with sublingual nitroglycerin according to the Italian protocol [15], and Carotid Sinus Massage (CSM), performed according to the symptoms method [16]: when associated with reproduction of spontaneous symptoms by patients or relatives, HUT and CSM were defined as diagnostic of syncope. Possible cardiac causes of syncope were evaluated using previous medical history, drug use and standardized cardiovascular evaluation when indicated. In patients with unexplained syncope, a loop recorder (ILR) was implanted for diagnosis at the end of an otherwise negative work-up.

The final diagnosis was made though consensus between a syncope expert and an epileptologist at the end of evaluation and confirmed during follow-up, conforming to the ESC classification[12]. In particular, a) patients "positive" to syncope algorithm were considered as "isolated syncope", b) patients "negative" to syncope algorithm were considered as "isolated epilepsy" after a careful consensus between a syncope expert and an epileptologist, and c) in patients "positive" to syncope algorithm and with suggestive clinical evidences of epilepsy, the coexistence of syncope and epilepsy was considered. New findings were treated appropriately.

Follow-up

Follow-up visits were planned at 3, 6 and 12 months during which data was collected based on a predefined structured questionnaire...

Statistical analysis

The sample size of the study ($n = 100$) was calculated by assuming prevalence of coexistence of syncope and epilepsy equal to 40% in a population of possible and drug-resistant epilepsy (95% confidence interval of 30–50%). Statistical analysis was performed using Statistica version 8.0 (Stat Soft Italia, Padova, Italy). Student's t-test for unpaired data was used to compare differences in continuous data between groups. The chi-square test was used for dichotomous variables. Anova and Bonferroni's post-hoc test were performed to compare mean in more than two groups. A value of $p < 0.05$ was considered significant. Data was reported as mean ± standard deviation or as percentages.

Results

Out of 4800 consecutive patients followed in the Epilepsy Centers 107 (2.2%) (46 men, 61 women, mean age 56 ± 21 years) presented recurrent T-LOC of unknown cause and a diagnosis of possible or drug-resistant epilepsy 63 patients (58.9%) had possible epilepsy and 44 (41.1%) drug-resistant epilepsy (Table 1). Patients with drug-resistant epilepsy had a significantly higher frequency of heart disease and intake of cardiovascular drugs than those with possible epilepsy (50 vs. 20.6% and 56.8 vs 33.3, respectively). Seventy-seven patients (72.0%) used AEDs distributed as follows: all patients with drug-resistant epilepsy and more than half patients with possible epilepsy (Table 1). The median number of T-LOC episodes for patient in the last year was 4 ± 4 (range 2–20) and 66 patients had pre-syncopal symptoms (61.7%). After T-LOC, involuntary movements, including myoclonic jerks, were present in half of the patients (54.2%). The most frequent after T-LOC event was mental confusion (24.3%) and half the number of patients (51.4%) had suffered physical injury during the episode (Table 1).

EEG and neuro-imaging results are shown in Table 2. Normal or non-epileptiform abnormalities were common and more frequent in the possible epilepsy group than in the drug-resistant group. Interictal epileptiform activity was present in more than 70% of the patients with drug- resistant epilepsy. Brain CT/MRI did not show abnormalities in 58 patients (54.2%), leukoencephalopathy was present in 24 (22.4%) and cortical atrophy in 9 (8.4%) patients.

Orthostatic hypotension was present in 33 patients (30.8%) (Table 3). HUT reproduced vasovagal syncope in 52 patients (48.6%), of which 18 patients had myoclonic jerks that resulted frequent in patients with possible than in drug-resistant epilepsy (25.4% vs. 4.5%). Carotid Sinus message was diagnostic for carotid sinus syndrome in 7 patients (6.5%). Based on suspicion of a cardiac syncope, 43 patients (40.2%) underwent second-level cardiac examinations (echocardiography, 24 h Holter monitoring, and exercise test) that revealed pathological conditions in 3 cases (n.1 bradycardia/tachycardia syndrome, n. 1 advanced second-degree atrio-ventricular block, n.1 severe aortic stenosis). Thirteen patients (12.1%) received an ILR that lead 3 diagnoses during follow-up (n.1 ventricular tachycardia and n.2 asystolic pauses) (Table 3).

Table 1 Baseline characteristics of patients

	Total population (*n* = 107)	Possible Epilepsy (*n* = 63, 58.9%)	Drug- resistant Epilepsy (*n* = 44, 41.1%)
Mean age, years (mean ± SD, range)	56 ± 21 (18–88)	52 ± 21 (18–88)	62 ± 18 (29–88)
Male gender, n (%)	46 (43.0)	28 (44.4)	18 (40.9)
Heart diseases[a], n (%)	35 (32.7)	13 (20.6)	22 (50.0)
Neurological diseases[b], n (%)	32 (29.9)	22 (34.9)	10 (22.7)
Cardiovascular drugs[c], n (%)	46 (43.0)	21 (33.3)	25 (56.8)
Antiepileptic drugs[d], n (%)	77 (72.0)	33 (52.4)	44 (100.0)
T-LOC/patient/year (mean ± SD, range)	4 ± 4 (2–20)	3 ± 4 (2–20)	4 ± 4 (2–20)
T-LOC Prodromal symptoms	66 (61.7)	40 (63.5)	26 (59.1)
After T-LOC characteristics			
Involuntary movements	58 (54.2)	37 (58.7)	21 (47.7)
Mental contusion, n (%)	26 (24.3)	26 (41.3)	12 (27.3)
Physical injury, n (%)	55 (51.4)	31 (49.2)	24 (54.6)
Comorbidities, n (%)			
Hypertension, n (%)	41 (38.3)	20 (31.7)	21 (47.7)
Diabetes, n (%)	10 (9.3)	6 (9.5)	4 (9.1)
Dyslipidemia, n (%)	18 (16.8)	9 (14.3)	9 (20.5)

T-LOC transient loss of consciousness

[a]Ischemic cardiomyopathy, atrial fibrillation, pulmonary embolism, heart failure

[b]Stroke, Parkinson's disease, dementia, limbic encephalitis, normal pressure hydrocephalus

[c]Diuretics, angiotensin-converting enzyme inhibitors, angiotensin II receptor blockers, calcium channel blockers, nitrate, alpha-blockers, beta-blockers, antiarrhythmics, cardiac glycosides

[d]Phenobarbital, phenytoin, lamotrigine, valproate, levetiracetam, carbamazepine, gabapentin, pregabalin, topiramate, primidone, vigabatrin

Table 2 EEG and neuroradiological (CT/MRI) findings

	Total population ($n = 107$)	Possible Epilepsy ($n = 63$, 58.9%)	Drug-resistant Epilepsy ($n = 44$, 41.1%)
EEG: normal pattern[a], n (%)	12 (11.2)	12 (19.0)	0 (0)
EEG: abnormal not epileptiform[b], n (%)	61 (57.0)	51 (81.0)	10 (22.7)
EEG: epileptiform[c], n (%)	34 (31.8)	0 (0.0)	34 (77.3)
Temporal lobe spike activity, n (%)	27 (25.2)	0 (0.0)	27 (61.4)
Neuro-imaging (CT/MRI)			
Normal, n (%)	58 (54.2)	40 (63.5)	18 (40.9)
Tumors, n (%)	4 (3.7)	3 (4.8)	1 (2.3)
Cortical Atrophy, n (%)	9 (8.4)	5 (7.9)	4 (9.1)
Leukoaraiosis, n (%)	24 (22.4)	14 (22.2)	10 (22.7)
Neurosurgery findings, n (%)	7 (6.5)	0 (0.0)	7 (15.9)
Cortico-subcortical infarcts, n (%)	2 (1.9)	0 (0.0)	2 (4.5)
Limbic Encephalitis findings, n (%)	1 (0.9)	0 (0.0)	1 (2.3)
Cortical malformations, n (%)	2 (1.9)	1 (1.6)	1 (2.3)

CT computed tomography, *EEG* electroencephalogram, *MRI* magnetic resonance imaging
[a]Background activity generally characterized by alpha rhythm (with a frequency of 8–13 Hz), reacting to the opening and closing of the eyes, and a typical posterior representation; morphology mostly regular
[b]Slow activity (theta activity) focal or diffuse, non-paroxysmal and/or non-dominant
[c]Epileptiform activity (spikes; polyspikes, sharp waves, spikes and waves or polyspike-waves complexes) both generalized and focal

The diagnoses at the end of the work-up in the syncope unit are shown in Table 4. Isolated syncope was diagnosed in 45 patients (42.1%), all of them being patients enrolled for possible epilepsy (71.4% of the group). The most frequent cause of isolated syncope was neurally-mediated (28.0%), while cardiac syncope was rare (1.9%). In 2 patients (2.8%) the episodes were strongly suggestive of syncope, but the etiology remained unexplained (Table 4). Isolated epilepsy was diagnosed in 21 patients (19.6%), of which 15 presented with drug-resistant epilepsy (34.1%) and only 6 with possible epilepsy (Fig. 1). Isolated epilepsy was classified as idiopathic in 14 patients (13.1%), symptomatic in 6 patients (5.6%) and probably symptomatic only in 1 patient (0.9%) (Table 4).

Syncope and epilepsy coexisted in 37.4% of all patients but the coexistence was more prevalent in drug-resistant than in possible epilepsy (65.9% vs. 17.5%) (Table 4). In Fig. 1, the frequency of the different types of syncope

Table 3 Cardiovascular and neurally-mediated diagnostic tests

	Total population ($n = 107$)	Possible Epilepsy ($n = 63$)	Drug-resistant Epilepsy ($n = 44$)
Abnormal ECG[a], n (%)	9 (8.4)	6 (9.5)	3 (6.8)
Orthostatic Hypotension, n (%)	33 (30.8)	17 (27.0)	16 (36.4)
Head-up Tilt testing			
Performed, n (%)	92 (86.0)	55 (87.3)	37 (84.1)
Diagnostic, n (%)	52 (48.6)	35 (55.6)	17 (38.6)
Myoclonic jerks, n (%)	18 (16.8)	16 (25.4)	2 (4.5)
Carotid Sinus Massage			
Performed, n (%)	104 (97.2)	60 (95.2)	44 (100.0)
Diagnostic, n (%)	7 (6.5)	5 (7.9)	2 (4.5)
Echocardiography performed [b], n (%)	43 (40.2)	27 (42.9)	16 (36.4)
24 h Holter monitoring performed[c], n (%)	43 (40.2)	20 (31.7)	23 (52.3)
Exercise test performed, n (%)	13 (12.1)	10 (15.9)	3 (6.8)
Electrophysiological study performed, n (%)	3 (2.8)	2 (3.2)	1 (2.3)
ILR implanted [d], n (%)	13 (12.1)	6 (9.5)	7 (15.9)

ECG electrocardiogram, *ILR* intermittent loop recorder
[a]Left bundle-branch block, bifascicular block, previous myocardial infarction, atrial fibrillation
[b]Revealed 1 severe aortic stenosis
[c]Revealed 1 bradycardia/tachycardia syndrome and 1 advanced second-degree AV block
[d]Revealed 1 ventricular tachycardia and 2 asystolic pauses

Table 4 Diagnosis at the end of work-up in the Syncope Unit

	Total population (*n* = 107)	Possible Epilepsy (*n* = 63)	Drug-resistant Epilepsy (*n* = 44)
Isolated Syncope, n (%)	45 (42.1)	45 (71.4)	0 (0.0)
Neurally-mediated, n (%)	30 (28.0)	30 (47.6)	0 (0.0)
Vasovagal, n (%)	24 (22.4)	24 (38.1)	0 (0.0)
Carotid Sinus Syndrome, n (%)	5 (4.7)	5 (7.9)	0 (0.0)
Situational, n (%)	1 (0.9)	1 (1.6)	0 (0.0)
Orthostatic hypotension, n (%)	10 (9.3)	10 (15.9)	0 (0.0)
Cardiac, n (%)	2 (1.9)	2 (3.2)	0 (0.0)
Unexplained syncope, n (%)	3 (2.8)	3 (4.8)	0 (0.0)
Isolated Epilepsy, n (%)	21 (19.6)	6 (9.5)	15 (34.1)
Idiopathic, n (%)	14 (13.1)	5 (7.9)	9 (20.5)[a]
Symptomatic, n (%)	6 (5.6)	1 (1.6)	5 (11.4)
Probably symptomatic, n (%)	1 (0.9)	0 (0.0)	1 (2.3)
Syncope & Epilepsy	40 (37.4)	11 (17.5)	29 (65.9)
Psychogenic non-epileptic seizures	1 (0.9)	1 (1.6)	0 (0.0)

[a]In 2 of 9 patients with idiopathic isolated epilepsy, psychogenic non-epileptic seizures are also present

and epilepsy is shown in patients with coexistence of syncope and epilepsy. Patients showing idiopathic epilepsy presented the highest percentage of neurally-mediated syncope (76.9%).

PNES have been diagnosed in only 1 patient with possible diagnosis of epilepsy and coexisted in 2 of 9 patients with idiopathic isolated epilepsy.

Follow-up

Forty-seven patients with an initial diagnosis of possible epilepsy and 38 with drug-resistant epilepsy were available for follow-up analysis (85 of the enrolled patients, 79.4%) (Mean follow-up duration was 390 days, range 3 months–3.5 years). Forty patients (47.0%) had a recurrence of T-LOC (mean number of episodes was 4 ± 3, range 1–20); of these, 13 had recurrence of syncope (32.5%), 22 of epileptic seizures (55.0%) and 5 of both (12.5%). Regarding AEDs, 32 patients with possible epilepsy were on AEDs before enrolment (32/47, 68%), in 21 patients syncope was diagnosed and AEDs were discontinued (21/38, 55.2%). In 11 patients with possible epilepsy at enrollment and in whom the diagnosis of epilepsy was confirmed, AEDs was continued in 11 (11/47, 23.4%), and started in 8 (8/47, 17.0%).

Discussion

A group of highly selected patients (2.2% of the full amount of patients followed in the Epilepsy Centers) who presented recurrent T-LOC of unknown cause

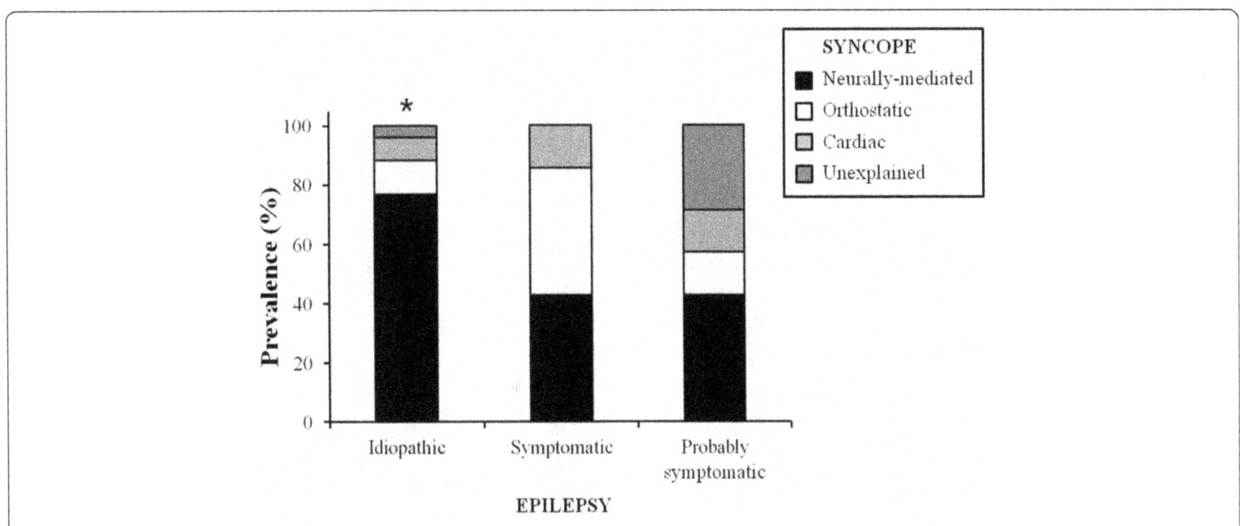

Fig. 1 Prevalence of different type of syncope and epilepsy in patients with coexistence of syncope and epilepsy. (*$p < 0.01$ neurally-mediated vs. patients with symptomatic and probably symptomatic epilepsy)

when evaluated by the neurologists. Patients with a diagnosis of possible or drug-resistant epilepsy were enrolled and referred to the syncope Units. Isolated syncope was diagnosed in the 42.1% of all cases, being more frequent among patients affected by possible epilepsy (≈70%). Interestingly, syncope and epilepsy coexisted in ≈ 40% of patients. In the follow-up, T-LOC recurrence was ≈ 50%. More importantly, in patients with possible epilepsy taking AEDs before enrolment (≈50%) the administration was discontinued, confirmed, and started according to epilepsy diagnosis confirmation. These results involve important implications for the management of T-LOC patients with possible or drug-resistant epilepsy.

Overlap of syncope and epilepsy

Few studies addressed the overlap between syncope and epilepsy [1, 17, 18]. Although the selection of patients was very restrictive (2.2% of consecutive patients followed in the Epilepsy Centers) OESYS shows a very high occurrence of syncope, i.e. ≈70% of patients with possible epilepsy in the absence of witnessed and/or epileptiform EEG abnormalities. Previous studies included patients with either recurrent "seizure-like" episodes [1] or presented "episodes of loss of consciousness, falls and seizures" [16]. In contrast, in OESYS, the main selection symptom was the "T-LOC". In some forms of epilepsy, postural control remains intact, and therefore, they do not determine T-LOC and are not confused with syncope [19]. Consequently, in selected patients a probability of having syncope is very high. Moreover, the inclusion of patients with "suspected epilepsy" might have also caused the enrolment of patients without epilepsy. In OESYS, only 52% of patients with possible epilepsy were on AEDs treatment. These patients were selected by neurologists, highly experienced in the management of epilepsy and trained in the diagnosis of syncope, and therefore, with clinical features poorly suggestive of epilepsy. Another aspect to consider is that patients in our study had a higher mean age in comparison with previous series (56 vs. 39 and 41 years) [1, 17]. Our patients presented a high comorbidity for heart diseases and most of them were on therapy with cardiovascular drugs (no data available in the previous studies). Considering the high prevalence of syncope in subjects over 65 years (from 35 to 39%) [1, 17], and the higher recurrence of syncope among patients with cardiovascular comorbidity [20, 21], the high frequency of syncope in our sample could, in part, be due to these demographic and clinical characteristics.

Coexistence of syncope and epilepsy

In our study, the coexistence of syncope and epilepsy was found in ≈ 40% of patients and in more than 60% of patient with drug-resistant epilepsy. Differently from the "possible epilepsy" group, no patient with drug resistant epilepsy was found with isolated syncope. This could implicitly confirm the presence of epilepsy in this group, in some cases, coexisting with syncope. Rangel et al. showed the coexistence of syncope and epilepsy only in 21% of the patients with refractory epilepsy [18]. As suggested before, the higher prevalence observed in our study may be due to a higher mean age with respect to those patients studied by Rangel et al. [18]. In addition, neurally-mediated syncope together with idiopathic epilepsy represents the more frequent association (50%). However, idiopathic epilepsy is a young person condition. Neurally mediated syncope has onset in adolescence, with a second incidence peak in the advancing age [22]. Similarly, idiopathic epilepsy is a young person condition but it may have also "a late onset" because of a genetic predisposition triggered by acquired epileptogenic factors [23]. Interestingly, it has been suggested that autonomic seizures may depend on age-dependent epileptogenic susceptibility (Panayiotopoulos syndrome) [24]. Nevertheless, neurally-mediated syncope is the more frequent syncope observed in a geriatric sample (66%) [25]. Thus, it should be hypothesized that the higher frequency of coexistence of syncope and epilepsy observed in our study may have the same autonomic dysfunction origin.

Epilepsy misdiagnosis

It should be underlined that at the end of the diagnostic work-up, the presumptive diagnosis of epilepsy was confirmed only in 10% of patients for possible epilepsy without epileptiform EEG abnormalities. For our sample the inter-ictal EEG was used even if its sensitivity is limited, ranging between 26 and 59% [26]. This tool was chosen in order to allow a high number of epileptic patients referred to the Epilepsy Centers including false positive patients in whom a final diagnosis of epilepsy was not confirmed. Moreover, these patients had T-LOC episodes often not recalled and/or occurred in the absence of witnesses leading to an increase of the possibility of the clinical diagnosis. Rodrigues et al. excluded patients with brain lesions [17] while in OESYS secondary forms of epilepsy were not excluded. Thus, abnormalities on neuro-imaging, occurring in about half of patients with possible epilepsy, might have influenced the neurologists to consider epilepsy more than the non-specific clinical presentation and normal EEG features would otherwise suggest.

Many authors have assessed the importance of the clinical presentation of T-LOC in distinguishing syncope from epilepsy [27, 28]. In our study, involuntary movements during the T-LOC were referred in almost half of patients with possible epilepsy and, more importantly, myoclonic jerks occurred in a high proportion of patients with possible epilepsy during the HUT-evocated T-LOCs. Accordingly, "convulsive syncope" is often characterized by involuntary movements, mostly myoclonic jerks [29]. The high frequency of myoclonic jerks may have also contributed to a selection bias, and epileptic phenomena might be misdiagnosed at the initial evaluation. Interestingly, in this group, T-LOC episodes manifested with the same stereotyped features while T-LOC differed from the usual seizures in the group of patients with drug-resistant epilepsy. The data supports the high frequency of coexisting epilepsy and syncope in the group with drug-resistant epilepsy (65.9%), and highlight the importance of a careful clinical characterization of T-LOC episode that requires a careful knowledge of signs and symptoms of syncope and epilepsy.

Finally, PNES represent a serious diagnostic challenge for physicians, especially in drug-resistant epilepsy. Video–electroencephalography studies have provided detailed knowledge of the spectrum of visible PNES manifestations. Unfortunately, in our study video-electroencephalography was not performed. Moreover, findings based on the self-report of patients with well-characterized PNES and witnesses of their seizures demonstrate a large intra- and inter-individual variability of reported PNES manifestations that may lead to incorrect diagnoses [6]. PNES accounts for 20 to 30% of patients seen in epileptic clinics [30–32]. Differently, in our sample PNES has been found only in 1 patient with possible diagnosis of epilepsy and coexisted in 2 of of 9 patients with idiopathic isolated epilepsy. However, we should consider that our sample is made up by patients with T-LOC of unknown cause, selected among 4800 subjects followed in the Epilepsy Center. Thus, patients with PNES could have been likely diagnosed and not carried out for our study because their cause of T-LOC was already clear. Moreover, our HUT procedure did not include scalp EEG, as this is the best way to identify functional T-LOC.

Diagnostic and therapeutic implications

In more than 70% of patients with possible epilepsy, the final diagnosis of epilepsy was not confirmed. It should be underlined that pharmacological treatment with AEDs was undertaken only in half of these patients because of the possibility of the initial diagnosis. At the end of the evaluation, AEDs were discontinued in more than 30% of patients suggesting a high percentage of true misdiagnosis of epilepsy in our study. This data also confirms that in clinical practice AEDs should be started when the diagnosis is definite [2]. Our diagnostic protocol provided the ILR implantation for selected patients with a high suspicion of cardiogenic and/or unknown syncope. It has been reported the use of ILR in a small cohort of syncopal patients able to identify an arrhythmogenic cause at the origin of seizure-like manifestations [33].

Finally, is "OESYS" approach helpful to define the presence of syncope in patients with possible or drug-resistant epilepsy? Angus-Leppan described that in 158 patients with loss of consciousness or possible epilepsy, the neurologist reached a diagnosis in 87% of the cases (43% epilepsy, 25% syncope, 12% non-epileptic seizures and in 7% other diagnoses). Unfortunately, in 13% of the cases the diagnosis remained unknown [5]. In this subset of patients, the "OESYS" approach may be particularly helpful.

Limitation of the study

The main limitation of OESYS study is the absence of the data regarding patients with "definite" epilepsy. This lack is clearly related to the inclusion criteria of the study. Only patients with "possible or "drug-resistant" epilepsy followed in the Epilepsy Centers were enrolled. Of course, the retrospective recovery of this data is unreliable especially for the mix of clinical centers, and the vagueness of the groups' composition. Thus, although patients with clear diagnosis of epilepsy (not enrolled in our study) may be easier recognized, the detection of syncope in patients with "possible" or "drug resistant" epilepsy diagnosis may be extremely difficult. In his regard, OESYS' protocol should be extremely helpful especially in patients with uncertain epilepsy in whom the clinical scenario is unclear. A further limitation is the lack of video-EEG monitoring especially in the diagnosis of PNES. However, as our sample has been selected from a population deeply studied in the Epilepsy Centers, we could expect that from this group, already diagnosed as PNES, only a very low percentage was enrolled in our study.

Conclusions

Syncope was diagnosed in $\approx 70\%$ of patients initially identified with "possible" epilepsy. It means that through diagnostic algorithm a clear diagnosis of syncope was found out despite of the initial suspect of "possible epilepsy". Syncope and epilepsy coexisted in $\approx 40\%$ of patients with "possible" and "drug-resistant" epilepsy. Syncope recurrence was $\approx 50\%$ in the follow-up. AEDs administration in patients with "possible" epilepsy was started, stopped or continued, according to syncope diagnosis. Thus, diagnostic protocol for syncope plays a key role in the management of T-LOC patients with "possible" or "drug-resistant" epilepsy.

Abbreviations

AEDs: Antiepileptic drugs; CSM: Carotid Sinus Massage; CT: Computed tomography; EEG: Electroencephalogram; ESC: European Society of Cardiology; HUT: Head-Up Tilt testing; ILR: Implantable loop recorder; MRI: Magnetic resonance imaging; OESYS: Epilepsy and SYncope Study; PNES: Psychogenic Non-Epileptic Seizures; T-LOC: Transient loss of consciousness

Acknowledgments

We would like to thank prof. Salvatore Striano (Department of Neurosciences, University of Naples Federico II, Italy) for his help in defining inclusion and exclusion criteria of the study.

There are no financial or other relationships with industry that might lead to conflict of interest.

Funding

None.

Authors' contributions

All authors conceived and participated in the design of the study. AC, FP, CM, GT, MR, AG collected the data. AU, NM, DB and PA carried out the analyses and drafted the manuscript. JGVN supported the analyses and interpretation of the study results. GG carried out the revision of the manuscript. All authors read and approved the final manuscript.

Competing interests

The authors declare that they have no competing interests.

Author details

[1]Department of Clinical and Experimental Medicine, Syncope Unit, Geriatric Cardiology and Medicine, University of Florence, Florence, Italy. [2]Department of Neurological and Psychiatric Sciences, Epilepsy Center, University of Florence, Florence, Italy. [3]Geriatric and Gerontology Institute, University of Modena, Modena, Italy. [4]Geriatric Unit, Santa Chiara Hospital, Trento, Italy. [5]Division of Geriatrics, Ospedale "S. Maria di Ca' Foncello", Treviso, Italy. [6]Department of Neurology, Leiden University Medical Centre, Leiden, The Netherlands. [7]Istituti Clinici Scientifici Maugeri- Syncope unit – UOC Cure sub-acute, Milan, Italy. [8]Department of Translational Medical Sciences, University of Naples Federico II, Via S. Pansini, 80131 Naples, Italy.

References

1. Zaidi A, Clough P, Cooper P, Scheepers B, Fitzpatrick AP. Misdiagnosis of epilepsy: many seizure-like attacks have a cardiovascular cause. J Am Coll Cardiol. 2000;36(1):181–4.
2. Chowdhury FA, Nashef L, Elwes RD. Misdiagnosis in epilepsy: a review and recognition of diagnostic possiblety. Eur J Neurol. 2008;15(10):1034–42.
3. Kwan P, Schachter SC, Brodie MJ. Drug-Resistant Epilepsy. New Engl J Med. 2011;365(10):919–26.
4. Task Force for the Diagnosis and Management of Syncope; European Society of Cardiology (ESC); European Heart Rhythm Association (EHRA); Heart Failure Association (HFA); Heart Rhythm Society (HRS), Moya A, Sutton R, Ammirati F, Blanc JJ, Brignole M, Dahm JB, Deharo JC, Gajek J, Gjesdal K, Krahn A, Massin M, Pepi M, Pezawas T, Ruiz Granell R, Sarasin F, Ungar A, van Dijk JG, Walma EP, Wieling W. Guidelines for the diagnosis and management of syncope (version 2009). Eur Heart J. 2009;30(21):2631–71.
5. Angus-Leppan H. Diagnosing epilepsy in neurology clinics: a prospective study. Seizure. 2008;17(5):431–6.
6. Lempert T, Bauer M, Schmidt D. Syncope: a videometric analysis of 56 episodes of transient cerebral hypoxia. Ann Neurol. 1994;36(2):233–7.
7. Sander JW, O'Donoghue MF. Epilepsy: getting the diagnosis right. BMJ. 1997;314(7075):158–9.
8. Rocamora R, Kurthen M, Lickfett L, Von Oertzen J, Elger CE. Cardiac asystole in epilepsy: clinical and neurophysiologic features. Epilepsia. 2003;44(2):179–85.
9. Rugg-Runn FJ, Simister RJ, Squirrell M, Holdright DR, Duncan JS. Cardiac arrhythmias in focal epilepsy: a prospective long-term study. Lancet. 2004;364(9452):2212–9.
10. Schuele SU, Bermeo AC, Alexopoulos AV, Locatelli ER, Burgess RC, Dinner DS, Foldvary-Schaefer N. Video-electrographic and clinical features in patients with ictal asystole. Neurology. 2007;69(5):434–41.
11. Horrocks IA, Nechay A, Stephenson JBP, Zuberi SM. Anoxic-epileptic seizures: observational study of epileptic seizures induced by syncopes. Arch Dis Childhood. 2005;90(12):1283–7.
12. Stephenson J, Breningstall G, Steer C, Kirkpatrick M, Horrocks I, Nechay A, Zuberi S. Anoxic-epileptic seizures: home video recordings of epileptic seizures induced by syncopes. Epileptic Disord. 2004;6(1):15–9.
13. Téllez-Zenteno JF, Hernández-Ronquillo L, Buckley S, Zahagun R, Rizvi S. A validation of the new definition of drug-resistant epilepsy by the International League Against Epilepsy. Epilepsia. 2014;55(6):829–34.
14. Leach JP, Lauder R, Nicolson A, Smith DF. Epilepsy in the UK: misdiagnosis, mistreatment, and undertreatment? The Wrexham area epilepsy project. Seizure. 2005;14(7):514–20.
15. Bartoletti A, Alboni P, Ammirati F, Brignole M, Del Rosso A, Foglia Manzillo G, Menozzi C, Raviele A, Sutton R. 'The Italian Protocol': a simplified head-up tilt testing potentiated with oral nitroglycerin to assess patients with unexplained syncope. Europace. 2000;2(4):339–42.
16. Puggioni E, Guiducci V, Brignole M, Menozzi C, Oddone D, Donateo P, Croci F, Solano A, Lolli G, Tomasi C, Bottoni N. Results and complications of the carotid sinus massage performed according to the "method of symptoms". Am J Cardiol. 2002;89(5):599–601.
17. Rodrigues Tda R, Sternick EB, Moreira Mda C. Epilepsy or Syncope? An analysis of 55 consecutive patients with loss of consciousness, convulsion, falls, and no EEG abnormalities. PACE. 2010;33(7):804–11.
18. Rangel I, Freitas J, Correia AS, et al. The usefulness of the head-up tilt test in patients with suspected epilepsy. Seizure. 2014;23(5):367–70.
19. Olde Nordkamp LR, van Dijk N, Ganzeboom KS, Reitsma JB, Luitse JS, Dekker LR, Shen WK, Wieling W. Syncope prevalence in the ED compared to general practice and population: a strong selection process. Am J Emerg Med. 2009;27(3):271–9.
20. van Dijk JG, Thijs RD, Benditt DG, Wieling W. A guide to disorders causing transient loss of consciousness: focus on syncope. Nat Rev Neurol. 2009;5(8):438–48.
21. Sun BC, Hoffman JR, Mangione CM, Mower WR. Older Age Predicts Short-Term, Serious Events After Syncope. J Am Geriatr Soc. 2007;55(6):907–12.
22. Driscoll DJ, Jacobsen SJ, Porter CJ, Wollan PC. Syncope in children and adolescents. J Am Coll Cardiol. 1997;29(5):1039–45.
23. Marini C, King MA, Archer JS, Newton MR, Berkovic SF. Idiopathic generalized epilepsy of adult onset: clinical syndromes and genetics. J Neurol Neurosurg Psychiatry. 2003;74(2):192–6.
24. Panayiotopoulos CP. Autonomic seizures and autonomic status epilepticus peculiar to childhood: diagnosis and management. Epilepsy Behav. 2004;5(3):286–95.
25. Ungar A, Mussi C, Del Rosso A, Noro G, Abete P, Ghirelli L, Cellai T, Landi A, Salvioli G, Rengo F, Marchionni N, Masotti G, Italian Group for the Study of Syncope in the Elderly. Diagnosis and characteristics of syncope in older patients referred to geriatric departments. J Am Geriatr Soc. 2006;54(10): 1531–6.
26. King MA, Newton MR, Jackson GD, Fitt GJ, Mitchell LA, Silvapulle MJ, Berkovic SF. Epileptology of the first-seizure presentation: a clinical, electroencephalographic, and magnetic resonance imaging study of 300 consecutive patients. Lancet. 1998;352(9133):1007–11.
27. McKeon A, Vaughan C, Delanty N. Seizure versus syncope. Lancet Neurol. 2006;5(2):171–80.
28. Sheldon R, Rose S, Ritchie D, Connolly SJ, Koshman ML, Lee MA, Frenneaux M, Fisher M, Murphy W. Historical criteria that distinguish syncope from seizures. J Am Coll Cardiol. 2002;40(1):142–8.
29. van Dijk JG, Thijs RD, van Zwet E, Tannemaat MR, van Niekerk J, Benditt DG, Wieling W. The semiology of tilt-induced reflex syncope in relation to electroencephalographic changes. Brain. 2014;137(Pt 2):576–85.
30. Sahaya K, Dholakia SA, Sahota PK. Psychogenic non-epileptic seizures: a challenging entity. J Clin Neurosci. 2011;18:1602–7.
31. Lesser RP. Psychogenic seizures. Neurology. 1996;46:1499–507.
32. Benbadis SR, Chichkova R. Psychogenic pseudosyncope: an underestimated and provable diagnosis. Epilepsy Behav. 2006;9:106–10.
33. Maggi R, Rafanelli M, Ceccofiglio A, Solari D, Brignole M, Ungar A. Additional diagnostic value of implantable loop recorder in patients with initial diagnosis of real or apparent transient loss of consciousness of uncertain origin. Europace. 2015;16(8):1226–30.

2

Late-onset jaw and teeth pain mimicking trigeminal neuralgia associated with chronic vagal nerve stimulation

Gabriela Timarova[1*] and Andrej Šteňo[2]

Abstract

Background: Vagal nerve stimulation (VNS) for refractory epilepsy is well established. Trigeminal neuralgia itself is a common disease in adults, and thus, late-onset pain in the trigeminal region under VNS, which is extremely rare, may not be recognized as caused by VNS.

Case presentation: Two patients with drug-resistant symptomatic epilepsy treated with chronic VNS experienced stimulation-related pain in the lower and upper jaw and teeth on the side of stimulation. No evidence of local spread of the stimulation current was present. The pain started with a delay of years after device implantation and weeks after the last increase in the pacing parameters. At the time of onset, the pain was not recognized as VNS-related, leading to extensive examinations. The trigeminal neuralgia-like pain resolved after adjustment of the stimulation current intensity. In one of the patients, the pain disappeared within one to two days following every epileptic seizure. To our knowledge, this is the first case report of late-onset trigeminal pain under VNS revealing a direct link between epileptogenic and pain processes.

Conclusion: A painless interval between the last change of the pacing parameters and trigeminal pain can lead to the erroneous interpretation that this is a typical trigeminal neuralgia. The lack of its recognition as a side effect of VNS can lead to unnecessary examinations and delayed adjustment of stimulation parameters. In patients with signs of late-onset trigeminal pain under VNS with normal electrode impedance and no evidence of local current spread, the replacement of the VNS lead does not seem to be beneficial. A review of the literature on VNS side effects including pain and device malfunctions was undertaken.

Keywords: VNS, Epilepsy, Trigeminal pain, Side effects, Pain, Case report

Background

Vagal nerve stimulation (VNS), delivered by the NCP System (Cyberonics, Houston, TX, USA) for treatment of drug-resistant epilepsy is approved as an add-on therapy in adults and children for partial and generalized epileptic seizures. New, noninvasive stimulation devices are under development [1, 2]. The VNS efficacy has been established, showing a 50% reduction in epileptic seizure rate in approximately 30% of patients after one year with an increase to approximately 50-70% after three years, with relatively few patients (less than 10%) becoming seizure free [3–5]. Despite more than 20 years of VNS accessibility, the discussion of its safety and efficacy is ongoing. The evidence-based guidelines from the American Academy of Neurology in 2013 [6] emphasized the need for further safety information.

The adverse events (AE) of VNS are of two types: implantation procedure-related and stimulation-related. Surgery-related AE have been reported in 3-22% of VNS implantations. The most often reported surgery-related AE are hardware failure in 3.7-16.8%, lead fracture or disconnection in 3.7-13.7%, wound infections in 1.7-

* Correspondence: gtimarova@gmail.com; gabriela.timarova@kr.unb.sk; https://www.fmed.uniba.sk/
[1]2nd Department of Neurology, Faculty of Medicine, Comenius University, Dérer's University Hospital, Limbova str.5, 83305 Bratislava, Slovak Republic

7.1%, wound hematoma in 0.7-1.9%, transient asystole/ bradycardia up to 1%, left vocal cord palsy, mostly transient, in 1.4-5.1%, and lower facial weakness in 0.2-1.2% [7–14]. Stimulation-related AE in different studies have been reported to occur in up to 68% of patients, with 97.8% of the AE reported as mild to moderate. The AE usually appeared immediately after VNS adjustments and disappeared spontaneously over some time or after the adjustment of the stimulation current to the previous level of stimulation [7, 15–17]. Most often reported stimulation-related AE were voice alterations (6-66%), hoarseness (1.4-64%), cough (7-45%), dyspnea (2-25%), throat pain (4.7-22%), neck pain and/or tingling and twitching in the neck muscles (0.5–22%), dysphagia (13-17.9%), headache (7-30%) and chest pain (up to 13%). Cases with some pain were reported in 6-30% of implantations [7, 18–23]. In addition to the VNS side effects reported in population studies, there are rare cases or case series reports of unusual or late-onset stimulation-related AE such as parkinsonism [24], late-onset bradyarrhythmia/asystole [25–28], sleep apnea [29, 30], psychosis or mania [31], glossopharyngeal tonsillar pain [32] and pharyngeal dysesthesia [33]. Cases of late-onset trigeminal pain associated with VNS, considering the large number of VNS implantations performed worldwide, are an extremely rare and unexpected event [34, 35] (Table 1).

Case presentation

At the University Hospital Bratislava, Slovakia, we implanted VNS systems in 54 patients with drug-resistant epilepsy not amenable to resection epilepsy surgery between April 2009 and December 2016. Forty-seven of the patients were followed for a long time (one to eight years). The VNS systems were implanted on the left side, and patients had regular follow-up visits with a stepwise increase in stimulation current by 0.25 mA in 4-8 weeks. The target range of the stimulation current intensity, if tolerated, was between 1.25 and 2.00 mA with a stimulation frequency 25-30 Hz, pulse width of 250-500 µsec and a duty cycle of 30-21 s on and 5 to 1.1 min off, as recommended by the manufacturer.

Two of our patients perceived stimulation-related pain in the upper and lower jaw and teeth ipsilateral to the side of stimulation with a delay of years after device implantation and weeks after last augmentation of the stimulation current intensity, thus mimicking coincidental trigeminal neuralgia to the VNS (Table 2). Both were treated with antiepileptic drugs (AED), which are usually effective in pain treatment (see below), but the AED were not effective in the prevention and control of the pain associated with VNS stimulation.

Case 1

A 46-year-old man with intractable symptomatic bitemporal epilepsy lasting 33 years, with MRI-verified right temporooccipital periventricular heterotopy, was implanted with VNS in November 2012. His seizure frequency before implantation was up to 10 motor seizures with impaired awareness per month and sporadic bilateral tonic-clonic seizures. After implantation, the stimulation current was increased stepwise in 4-8 weeks. He achieved a 50% reduction in seizures with 2.0-mA stimulation current, 30-Hz frequency, 500-µsec pulse width, and 30-s on-time and 1.8-min off-time. Eighteen months after initiation of VNS stimulation, two months since the last increase in the stimulation current, the patient began to complain of sharp, shooting pain in the upper and lower jaw and teeth on the left side, without trigger points or a sensory deficit. The patient underwent CT scans and detailed dental examination, but no pathological processes were discovered. It was the patient who first noticed that the painful shootings were regular, lasting for tens of seconds with the stimulation on, and that the painless intervals lasted minutes with the stimulation off. The consequent analysis, when we checked the painful and pain-free intervals, ascertained that the pain was associated with the stimulation period of VNS. When the device was off,

Table 1 Characteristics of late-onset trigeminal pain under VNS in reported patients

Author	Type of disease	Time to pain onset from implantation	Time to pain onset from last augmentation	SC (mA)	Pain localisation
Shih [35]	Epilepsy-Tuberous sclerosis	9 months	2 months	1.25[a]	Left cheek, mentally retarded child with unprecise description of the pain
Carius and Schulze-Bonhage [34]	Cryptogenic epilepsy, focal seizures	5 months	few days	1.5[a]	The lower jaw, left
	Epilepsy-right frontotemporal	2 months	1 month	0.5[a]	The lower jaw and occipital headache, left
	Epilepsy- bitemporal	11 months	2 weeks	1.75[a]	The lower jaw and throat, left

SC stimulation current intensity at the time of pain onset

[a] In all patients was stimulation frequency 30 Hz, pulse width 500usec, duty cycle 30s on and 5 min off

Table 2 Characteristics of late-onset trigeminal pain under VNS in the current case series patients

Sex (age, years)	Type of epilepsy	Time to pain onset from implantation	Time to pain onset from last augmentation	SC (mA)	Pain localisation
Man (46)	Bitemporal-periventricular heterotopy	18 months	2 months	2,0[a]	The upper and lower jaw and teeth, left
Woman (50)	Bitemporal- bilateral cystic hippocampal malformations	4,5 years	2 weeks	1,25[b]	The upper and lower jaw and teeth, left

SC stimulation current intensity at the time of pain onset
[a] Stimulation frequency 30 Hz, pulse width 500 µsec, duty cycle 30s on/ 1,8 min off
[b] Stimulation frequency 30 Hz, pulse width 250 µsec, duty cycle 30s on/ 1,8 min off

he was pain-free. The impedance of the electrode was normal. The intensity of the pain was evaluated as 10 on a visual analogous 10-point scale (VAS). The patient had no signs of local current spread to the surrounding tissues (breathing and voice problems, muscle tingling or twitching, no pain in the head, chest or neck). The pain mimicked trigeminal neuralgia type 1 according to Burchiel's classification [36]. According to the seizure diary, where the patient recorded all seizures and painful days, there was a discontinuous course of pain attacks. He was pain-free for 1-2 days following every epileptic seizure, with reoccurrence of the pain in the following days. His antiepileptic treatment that time was a combination of lacosamide at 400 mg/day, lamotrigine at 200 mg/day and pregabaline at 300 mg/day. He was treated for concomitant hypertension with perindopril at 4 mg/day, moxonidine at 0.2 mg/day and rilmenidine at 1 mg/day and for anxiety with alprazolam at 1 mg/day. We started adjustments of the stimulation parameters of VNS with a three-month delay due to diagnostic work-up. The patient reported pain relief at a stimulation current of 1,5 mA and complete resolution at a stimulation current of 0.5 mA. At that time, the frequency of the seizures increased to the original level with a loss of responsivity. At that time, the patient preferred to switch off the device. Six months later, the system was retested. He tolerated a stimulation current up to 1.5 mA without painful sensations.

Case 2

A 50-year-old woman with intractable symptomatic bitemporal epilepsy lasting 37 years, with MRI-verified bilateral cystic malformations of mesial temporal lobe structures, was implanted with VNS in April 2011. Her seizure frequency was up to 6 motor seizures with impaired awareness per month and sporadic bilateral tonic-clonic seizures. After VNS implantation, the stimulation current was increased stepwise in 4-8 week intervals up to a 1.0-mA stimulation current intensity, 30-Hz frequency, 250-µsec pulse width, 30-s on-time and 3-min off-time. At these stimulation parameters, she was a 50% responder. Four years later, she overcame status epilepticus. The stimulation current was increased to 1.25 mA and the duty cycle to 30 s on and 1.8 min off. Two weeks later, she began to complain of shooting, sharp pain in the upper and lower jaw and teeth on the left side, without a trigger point or sensory deficit. The intensity of the pain was evaluated as an 8 on the VAS. The pain mimicked trigeminal neuralgia type 1 according to Burchiel's classification [36]. The patient had no signs of local current spread to surrounding tissues. At that time, she was treated with anti-epileptic drugs levetiracetam at 2000 mg/day, lamotrigine at 300 mg/day and carbamazepine at 1200 mg/day. She did not use any other drugs or treatments. The impedance of the electrode was normal. Because of the experience with patient 1, we immediately checked the relation of the shooting pain to the stimulation period of the VNS and the relation of the pain-free intervals to the off period of the VNS. The pain was recognized as stimulation-related, and we immediately began the adjustments. The patient reported complete pain resolution at a 1.0-mA stimulation current and continued the VNS.

Discussion and conclusions

Carius and Schulze-Bonhage [34] reported late-onset trigeminal pain in 3 out of 27 implanted patients (11.1%), whereas we found it in 2 out of 47 implanted patients longer than one year after implantation (4.3%). Carius and Schulze-Bonhage proposed mechanisms of central sensitization as the probable cause of the reported pain [34]. Later, Spitz et al. [37] reported a case with a small discontinuity in the lead silicone insulation that led to vocal cord paralysis, impaired breathing and cervical, mandibular, pharyngeal and dental pain. The electrode impedance was normal. The problems started in the early titration period, and the maximum tolerated stimulation current intensity was low (0.5 mA maximum). Spitz et al. [37] postulated that the aberrant spread of current through the disrupted insulation likely accounted for other reports of stimulation-related pain (referred trigeminal pain, tonsillar pain, sometimes delayed onset). In other cases, where device malfunction was confirmed, clinical signs of the spread of the stimulation current to surrounding tissues were described (hoarseness, vocal cord palsy, distorted breathing, pharyngeal and neck pain, tingling or twitching in the neck muscles and diaphragm dysfunction). The problems typically started after an accident (trauma, puncture, traction, excessive manipulations, tight electrode). In most cases of device malfunctions, the lead impedance is too high or too low [38–41].

In our patients with late-onset jaw and dental pain, the gradual increase in the stimulation current intensity up to 1 mA and more was uncomplicated. The pain appeared after a pain-free interval from the last adjustment without any accident or trauma and no signs of local current spread. After a 6-month stimulation-free period, patient 1 regained the tolerance for stimulating current up to 1.5 mA, thus pointing to possible desensitization. A unique, intermittent course of stimulation related pain was documented in him with pain relief for 24-48 h following every epileptic seizure. Mechanisms of activity-dependent central sensitization are likely explanations [42]. The nucleus of the solitary tract is the recipient of most afferent sensory fibers of the vagal nerve, but the vagal nerve also sends ipsilateral projections to the spinal trigeminal nucleus (STN). Animal studies have revealed an interesting pattern of trigeminal nociceptive neuronal activation and somatic-visceral trigemino- vagal integration that is mediated by vagal afferents to STN. Central sensitization has been described in the dorsal horn of the spinal cord, as well as in the STN pars caudalis (Vc) and the transition zone (Vi/Vc) [43]. In an animal experiment, activation of vagal C-fibers was confirmed to not be required to obtain VNS-induced seizure suppression; activation of A- and/or B-fibers seems to be sufficient. These data are clinically important since A- and B-fibers have a much lower activation threshold than C-fibers, thus reducing the amount of current necessary to produce the antiepileptic effects of VNS. Lack of C-fiber recruitment is also important since activation of these fibers would produce central sensitization and undesirable side effects that are not seen in most patients and may have rendered the therapy intolerable in some [44]. The modulatory effects of vagal nerve stimulation on nociception have been studied in animal studies, including the effects in the STN. Both facilitatory and inhibitory effects on neuronal responses to noxious stimuli were observed [45, 46]. The stimulation parameters favoring pro- or antinociceptive effects of VNS in man are not known [42]. Postictal pain relief was observed in one of our cases. To the best of our knowledge, this is the first case report of late-onset trigeminal pain under VNS revealing a direct link between epileptogenic and pain processing. The postictal state is generally followed by antinociception. Intrinsic neural circuits between dorsal midbrain neurons control seizure activity and the nuclei of the pain inhibitory system elaborating postictal antinociceptive processes. Endogenous opioid-, acetylcholine-, serotonin-, and norepinephrine-mediated systems have been implicated in the organization of tonic-clonic seizure-induced anti-nociception [47]. The locus coeruleus represents a key structure in the organization of epilepsy-induced norepinephrine-mediated hypoalgesia, and its lesions suppress the seizure-attenuating effects of VNS [48–50].

With reference to the data accumulated in previous years, late-onset trigeminal pain under VNS stimulation in our patients and patients reported previously can be explained by mechanisms of activity-dependent central sensitization, lead revisions in cases with normal electrode impedance and no signs of local spread of the current seem not to be beneficial. It has to be recognized by physicians, so immediately began to reduce the stimulation current intensity.

Abbreviations

AE: Adverse events; AED: Antiepileptic drug/drugs; CT: Computed tomography; MRI: Magnetic resonance imaging; STN Vc: Spinal trigeminal nucleus pars caudalis; STN Vi/Vc: Spinal trigeminal nucleus transition zone; STN: Spinal trigeminal nucleus; VAS: Visual analogous scale; VNS: Vagal nerve stimulation

Acknowledgements

The authors would like to thank Professor Juraj Šteňo, DSc, Chair of the Dept. of Neurosurgery, Faculty of Medicine Comenius University, Dérer's University Hospital Bratislava, Slovakia, for his valuable advice on interpreting the case findings and literature data.

Funding

No funding was obtained.

Authors' contributions

Both authors, GT and AS conducted the follow-up of patients, data analysis and interpretation. GT prepared the manuscript, which was revised by AS. Both authors approved the final manuscript.

Competing interests

The authors declare that they have no competing interests.

Author details

[1]2nd Department of Neurology, Faculty of Medicine, Comenius University, Dérer's University Hospital, Limbova str.5, 83305 Bratislava, Slovak Republic. [2]Department of Neurosurgery, Faculty of Medicine, Comenius University, Dérer's University Hospital, Bratislava, Slovak Republic.

References

1. Howland RH. Vagus nerve stimulation. Curr Behav Neurosci Rep. 2014;1:64–73.
2. Ben-Menachem E, Revesz D, Simon J, Silberstein S. Surgically implanted and non-invasive vagus nerve stimulation: a review of efficacy, safety and tolerability. Eur J Neurol. 2015;22:1260–8.
3. Uthman BM, Reichl AM, Dean JC, Eisenschenk S, Gilmore R, Reid S, et al. Effectiveness of vagus nerve stimulation in epilepsy patients. A 12-year observation. Neurology. 2004;63:1124–6.
4. Elliott RE, Rodgers SD, Bassani L, Morsi A, Geller EB, Carlson C, et al. Vagus nerve stimulation for children with treatment-resistant epilepsy: a consecutive series of 141 cases. J Neurosurg Pediatr. 2011;7:491–500.
5. Van Straten AF, Jobst BC. Future of epilepsy treatment: integration of devices. Future Neurol. 2014;9:587–96.

6. Morris GL III, Gloss D, Buchhalter J, Mack KJ, Nickels K, Harden C. Evidence-based guideline update: Vagus nerve stimulation for the treatment of epilepsy. Epilepsy Currents. 2013;13(6):297–303.
7. Ben-Menachem E. Vagus-nerve stimulation for the treatment of epilepsy. Lancet Neurol. 2002;1:477–82.
8. Kahlow H, Olivecrona M. Complications of vagal nerve stimulation for drug-resistant epilepsy. A single center longitudinal study of 143 patients. Seizure. 2013;22:227–33.
9. Horowitz G, Amit M, Fried I, Neufeld MY, Sharf L, Kramer U, et al. Vagal nerve stimulation for refractory epilepsy: the surgical procedure and complications in 100 implantations by a single medical center. Eur Arch Otorhinolaryngol. 2013;270:355–8.
10. Orosz I, McCormick D, Zamponi N, Varadkar S, Feucht M, Parain D, et al. Vagus nerve stimulation for drug-resistant epilepsy: a European long-term study up to 24 months in 347 children. Epilepsia. 2014;55(10):1576–84.
11. Yu C, Ramgopal S, Libenson M, Abdelmoumen I, Powell C, Remy K, et al. Outcomes of vagal nerve stimulation in a pediatric population: a single center experience. Seizure. 2014;23:105–11.
12. Galbarriatu L, Pomposo I, Aurrecoechea J, Marinas A, Agúndez M, Gómez JC, et al. Vagus nerve stimulation therapy for treatment-resistant epilepsy: a 15-year experience at a single institution. Clin Neurology and Neurosurgery. 2015;137:89–93.
13. Ghani S, Vilensky J, Turner JB, Tubbs RS, Loukas M. Meta-analysis of vagus nerve stimulation treatment for epilepsy: correlation between device setting parameters and acute response. Childs Nerv Syst. 2015;31:2291–304.
14. Révész D, Rydenhag B, Ben-Menachem E. Complications and safety of vagus nerve stimulation: 25 years of experience at a single center(article). J Neurosurg Pediatrics. 2016;18(1):97–104.
15. Handforth A, De Giorgio CM, Schachter SC, Uthman BM, Naritoku DK, Tecoma ES, et al. Vagus nerve stimulation therapy for partial-onset seizures: a randomized active-control trial. Neurology. 1998;51(1):48–55.
16. Frost M, Gates J, Helmers SL, Wheless JW, Levisohn P, Tardo C, et al. Vagus nerve stimulation in children with refractory seizures associated with Lennox–Gastaut syndrome. Epilepsia. 2001;42(9):1148–52.
17. Rychlicki F, Zamponi N, Trignani R, Ricciuti RA, Iacoangeli M, Scerrati M. Vagus nerve stimulation: clinical experience in drug-resistant pediatric epileptic patients. Seizure. 2006;15:483–90.
18. Schachter SC, Saper CB. Vagus nerve stimulation. Epilepsia. 1998;39(7):677–86.
19. Rush AJ, George MS, Sackeim HA, Marangell LB, Husain MM, Giller C, et al. Vagus nerve stimulation (VNS) for treatment-resistant depressions: a multicenter study. Biol Psychiatry. 2000;47(4):276–86.
20. De Giorgio CM, Schachter SC, Handforth A, Salinsky M, Thompson J, Uthman B, et al. Prospective long-term study of vagus nerve stimulation for the treatment of refractory seizures. Epilepsia. 2000;41:1195–200.
21. Liporace J, Hucko D, Morrow R, Barolat G, Nie M, Schnur J, et al. Vagal nerve stimulation: adjustments to reduce painful side effects. Neurology. 2001;11:885–6.
22. Milby AH, Halpern CH, Baltuch GH. Vagus nerve stimulation in the treatment of refractory epilepsy. Neurotherapeutics. 2009;6(2):228–37.
23. Ramsey RE, Uthman BM, Augustinsson LE, Upton ARM, Naritoku D, Willis J, et al. Vagus nerve stimulation for treatment of partial seizures: 2. Safety, side effects, and tolerability. Epilepsia. 1994;35(3):627–36.
24. Cukiert A, Mariani PP, Burattini JA, Cukiert CM, Forster C, Baise C. Parkinsonism induced by VNS in a child with double-cortex syndrome. Epilepsia. 2009;50(12):2667–9.
25. Amark P, Stödberg T, Wallstedt L. Late onset bradyarrhythmia during vagus nerve stimulation. Epilepsia. 2007;48(5):1023–4.
26. Iriarte J, Urrestarazu E, Alegre M, Macias A, Gomez A, Amaro P, et al. Late-onset periodic asystolia during vagus nerve stimulation. Epilepsia. 2009;50(4):928–32.
27. Cantarín-Extremera V, Ruíz-Falcó-Rojas ML, Tamaríz-Martel-Moreno A, García-Fernández M, Duat-Rodriguez A, Rivero-Martín B. Late-onset periodic bradycardia during vagus nerve stimulation in a pediatric patient. A new case and review of the literature. Eur J Paediatr Neurol. 2016;20(4):678–83.
28. Singleton AH, Rosenquist PB, Kimball J, McCall WV. Cardiac rhythm disturbance in a depressed patient after implantation with a vagus nerve stimulator (article). Journal of ECT. 2009;25(3):195–7.
29. Bhat S, Lysenko L, Neiman ES, Rao GK, Chokroverty S. Increasing off-time improves sleep-disordered breathing induced by vagal nerve stimulation. Epileptic Disord. 2012;14(4):432–7.
30. Papacostas SS, Myrianthopoulou P, Dietis A, Papathanasiou ES. Induction of central-type sleep apnea by vagus nerve stimulation. Electromyogr Clin Neurophysiol. 2007;47(1):61–3.
31. De Herdt V, Boon P, Vonck K, Goossens L, Nieuwenhuis L, Paemeleire K, et al. Are psychotic symptoms related to vagus nerve stimulation in epilepsy patients? Acta Neurol Belg. 2003;103(3):170–5.
32. Duhaime AC, Melamed S, Clancy RR. Tonsillar pain mimicking glossopharyngeal neuralgia as a complication of vagus nerve stimulation: case report. Epilepsia. 2000;41(7):903–5.
33. Ackman C, Riviello JJ, Madsen JR, Bergin AM. Pharyngeal dysesthesia in refractory complex partial epilepsy: new seizure or adverse effect of vagal nerve stimulation? Epilepsia. 2003;44(6):855–8.
34. Carius A, Schulze-Bonhage A. Trigeminal pain under vagus nerve stimulation. Pain. 2005;118:271–3.
35. Shih JJ, Devier D, Behr A. Late onset laryngeal and facial pain in previously asymptomatic vagus nerve stimulation patients. Neurology. 2003;60:1214.
36. Burchiel KJ. A new classification for facial pain. Neurosurgery. 2003;53(5):1164–6.
37. Spitz MC, Winston KR, Maa EH, Ojemann SG. Insulation discontinuity in a vagus nerve stimulator lead: a treatable cause of intolerable stimulation-related symptoms. J Neurosurg. 2010;112:829–31.
38. Landy HJ, Ramsay RE, Slater J, Casiano RR, Morgan R. Vagus nerve stimulation for complex partial seizures: surgical technique, safety, and efficacy. J Neurosurg. 1993;78:26–31.
39. Kalkanis JG, Krishna P, Espinosa JA, Naritoku DK. Self-inflicted vocal cord paralysis in patients with vagus nerve stimulators. Report of two cases. J Neurosurg. 2002;96:949–51.
40. Rijkers K, Berfelo MW, Cornips EM, Majoie HJ. Hardware failure in vagus nerve stimulation therapy. Acta Neurochir. 2008;150:403–5.
41. Tran Y, Shah AK, Mittal S. Lead breakage and vocal cord paralysis following blunt neck trauma in a patient with vagal nerve stimulator. J Neurol Sci. 2011; 304(1-2):132–5.
42. Latremoliere A, Woolf CJ. Central sensitization: a generator of pain hypersensitivity by central neural plasticity. J Pain. 2009;10(9):895–926.
43. Ren K, Dubner R. The role of trigeminal interpolaris-caudalis transition zone in persistent orofacial pain. Int Rev Neurobiol. 2011;97:207–25.
44. Krahl SE. Vagus nerve stimulation for epilepsy: a review of the peripheral mechanisms. Surg Neurol Int. 2012;3(S1):47–52.
45. Bossut DF, Maixner W. Effect of cardiac vagal afferent electrostimulation on the responses of trigeminal and trigeminothelamic neurons to noxious orofacial stimulation. Pain. 1996;65:101–9.
46. Lyubashina OA, Sokolov AY, Panteleev SS. Vagal afferent modulation of spinal trigeminal responses to dural electrical stimulation in rats. Neuroscience. 2012;222:29–37.
47. Coimbra NC, Castro-Souza C, Segato EN, Nora JE, Herrero CF, Tedeschi-Filho W, et al. Post-ictal analgesia: involvement of opioid, serotoninergic and cholinergic mechanisms. Brain Res. 2001;888:314–20.
48. Krahl SE, Clark KB. Vagus nerve stimulation for epilepsy: a review of central mechanisms. Surg Neurol Int. 2012;3(4):255–9.
49. Felippotti TT, Ferreira CMR, Freitas RL, Oliveira RC, Paschoalin-Maurin T, Coimbra NC. Paradoxical effect of noradrenaline-mediated neurotransmission in the antinociceptive phenomenon that accompanies tonic–clonic seizures: role of locus coeruleus neurons and α2- and β-noradrenergic receptors. Epilepsy Behav. 2011;22:165–77.
50. Freitas RL, Ferreira CMR, Ribeiro SJ. Intrinsic neural circuits between dorsal midbrain neurons that control fear-induced response and seizure activity and nuclei of the pain inhibitory system elaborating postictal antinociceptive processes: a functional neuroanatomical and neuropharmacological study. Exp Neurol. 2005;191:225–42.

3

A systematic review and narrative synthesis of group self-management interventions for adults with epilepsy

Amelia Smith[1], Alison McKinlay[2], Gabriella Wojewodka[2] and Leone Ridsdale[2*]

Abstract

Background: Epilepsy is a serious and costly long-term condition that negatively affects quality of life, especially if seizures persist on medication. Studies show that people with epilepsy (PWE) want to learn more about the condition and some educational self-management courses have been trialled internationally. The objectives of this review were to evaluate research and summarise results on group self-management interventions for PWE.

Methods: We searched Medline and PsycINFO for results published in English between 1995 and 2015. Only studies evaluating face-to-face, group interventions for adults with epilepsy were included. Heterogeneity in study outcomes prevented the carrying out of a meta-analysis; however, a Cochrane style review was undertaken.

Results: We found eleven studies, nine of which were randomised controlled trials. There were variable standards of methodological reporting with some risk of bias. Seven of the studies used quality of life as an outcome, with four finding statistically significant improvements in mean total score. Two found an improvement in outcome subscales. One study included some additional semi-qualitative data.

Conclusions: We identified promising trends in the trials reviewed. In particular, there were significant improvements in quality of life scales and seizure frequency in many of the interventions. However, considerable heterogeneity of interventions and outcomes made comparison between the studies difficult. Courses that included psychological interventions and others that had a high number of sessions showed more effect than short educational courses. Furthermore, the evidence was predominantly from pilot studies with small sample sizes and short follow-up duration. Further research is needed to better evaluate the role of group self-management interventions in outpatient epilepsy management.

Keywords: Self-management education, Epilepsy, Patient-education, Quality of life

Background

Epilepsy is a long-term condition characterised by recurrent seizures, with a prevalence of around 1% in the general population [1, 2]. Common consequences of living with epilepsy include driving limitations, detrimental effects on education, unemployment, and diminished psychological wellbeing [3]. Stigma, frequency of seizures, and healthcare experiences also affect quality of life (QoL) in people with epilepsy (PWE) [4].

Epilepsy has significant financial and social costs. Direct costs are associated with a high rate of emergency admission that occurs with poorly-controlled epilepsy [5]. Emergency service use makes up the majority of admissions for epilepsy. Among all long-term conditions, epilepsy is the sixth most common cause of emergency admission in the United Kingdom [6, 7]. Reducing unnecessary emergency admissions is a key factor in helping to relieve financial pressure on healthcare services. Another major social issue is the indirect cost of epilepsy due to lost employment [8]. The health and social costs could be reduced and QoL improved via better outpatient management. However, around 40% of those diagnosed have poorly-controlled epilepsy and

* Correspondence: leone.ridsdale@kcl.ac.uk
[2]Institute of Psychiatry, Psychology & Neuroscience, Academic Neuroscience Centre, King's College London, PO Box 57, London SE5 8AF, UK
Full list of author information is available at the end of the article

continue to have two or more seizures per year, [3] despite using antiepileptic drugs (AEDs). These figures highlight missed opportunities for epilepsy self-management.

Management of long-term conditions requires self-efficacy and empowerment, enabling patients to live as independently as possible and reducing the need to go to hospital [9]. For other long-term conditions, strategies for enabling such behaviour have been attempted within self-management education courses. A diabetes group intervention used in the United Kingdom, called DESMOND, is a cost-effective intervention, shown to improve biopsychosocial outcomes [10–12]. The programme is structured and can be run over one to two days for six hours in total [12]. Content is based on social learning theory [13] and is integrated into standard outpatient care for diabetes.

Early research evidence from North America [14] and Germany [15] suggested that group self-management courses had the potential to have a positive effect on health outcomes in PWE. The interest in group self-management for PWE has grown; however, the evidence base for developing self-management groups as standard outpatient care for PWE is still small. The objectives of this review were to evaluate recent research and summarise results of group self-management interventions for PWE. This was undertaken in the context that our group was conducting a trial of group self-management education intervention in the UK [16].

Methods

Study eligibility criteria

Population

PWE, adults aged 16 or over, without learning disabilities (due to the markedly different approaches required for educational programs in these populations [17]).

Intervention

Group self-management interventions were the focus of this review, irrespective of the study objectives (i.e., education, behavioural therapy, or a combination were included). We were interested in the psychological and social elements of face-to-face, group self-management courses. Studies using telemedicine were therefore excluded, as they are not provided face-to-face in groups.

Comparison

Treatment as usual or waitlist control.

Outcomes of interest

There was particular interest in QoL as this is the outcome favoured by the National Institute for Health and Care Excellence (NICE) [18, 19]. However, as there is no fixed consensus on the best measure for evaluating group interventions, we also included studies assessing other outcomes such as seizure frequency, psychological state, self-efficacy, and knowledge of epilepsy.

Exclusion criteria

Studies reporting trial protocol without results, one-to-one interventions, web- or telephone-based interventions, and samples including people with learning disabilities, children or non-epileptic seizures.

We searched for papers published from 1990 to 2015. A randomised controlled trial is considered the "gold standard" research design for evaluating the efficacy of an intervention; [20] however, we extended search criteria to include other forms of clinical trial (i.e., controlled outcomes design).

Search strategy

We conducted electronic searches of the databases Medline and PsycINFO using the following keywords: epilepsy, seizures, self-care/self-efficacy, patient education/education programme, self-management, group intervention/complex intervention. A manual search of reference lists was performed to identify further relevant studies. For specific strategies for database searches refer to Appendix 1.

Quality appraisal

All studies were assessed for quality using the CONSORT guidelines for reporting clinical trials [21]. Studies were assigned a number between 0 (description absent) and 2 (satisfactory description) according to how fully they described the four sections: trial design (methodology), participants (study sample and characteristics), interventions and study outcomes. Appraisal was carried out by two independent assessors and studies were discussed as a group to resolve any disagreements. The Cochrane approach was used to categorise the studies into 'high', 'low' or 'unclear' risk of bias with regard to random sequence generation and allocation concealment [22]. As it is not possible to double-blind a group self-management intervention, this was not included in the quality assessment.

Results

Study selection

The first author conducted the initial literature search, which was repeated by the second author. The initial Medline search resulted in 42 papers being identified (Fig. 1). After examining the titles and abstracts, nine were unrelated and were excluded. Five studies on non-epileptic seizures (psychogenic seizures and febrile convulsions) were excluded also [23–27]. Five more were excluded as their participant population consisted of children (under 16) or patients with learning disabilities. Of the remaining papers, six were identified as involving a telephone or web-based intervention and were also excluded. Finally, some studies were excluded because no

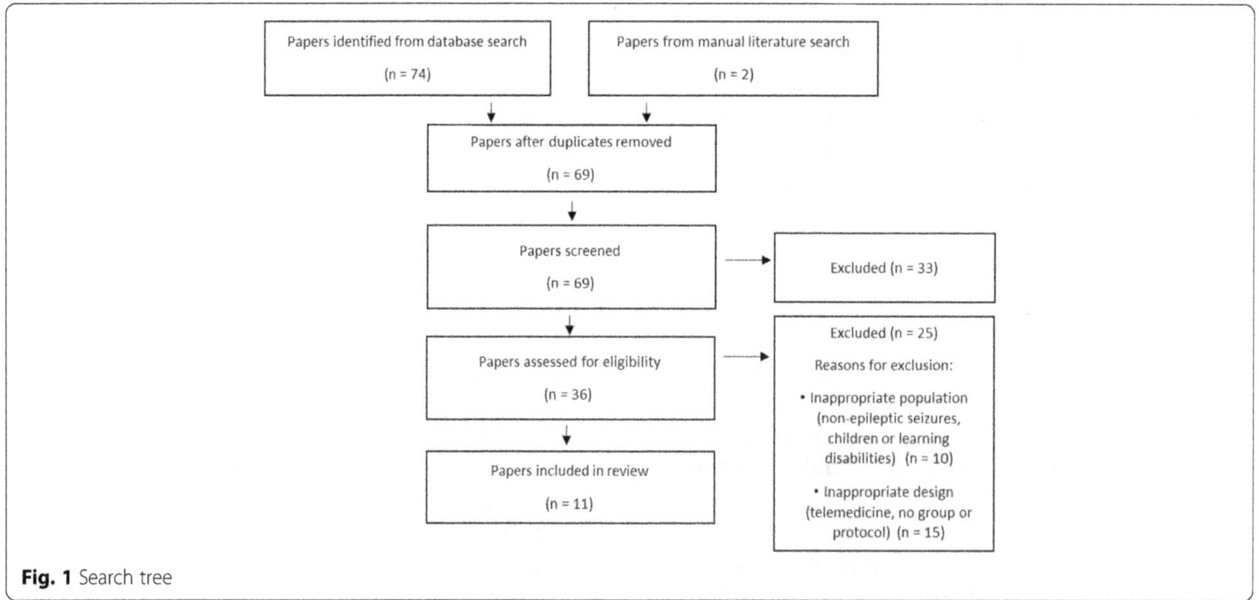

Fig. 1 Search tree

group intervention was administered. The papers described either individual care programmes or trial protocols with no results.

PsycINFO returned 32 results; three new papers were identified, but none were eligible for inclusion (two protocols, one telemedicine). Two studies were included from the manual literature search, resulting in 11 studies in total.

Search results

Of the 11 studies included with this review (Table 1), nine were described by their authors as randomised controlled trials [15, 28–30, 31, 32–35] and the remaining two as controlled outcome designs [36, 37]. The first study included a matching strategy for allocating participants to control or treatment group [37]. The second study used random assignment but did not provide more specific protocol information [36]. After synthesising review results, we established that due to outcome heterogeneity a meta-analysis would not be possible.

All studies focused on the effects of a group intervention in PWE, with one exclusively recruiting women [28] and another looking at older adults [32]. Most studies targeted poorly-controlled epilepsy; however, the definition of 'poorly-controlled' varied and four studies did not specify a minimum seizure frequency.

We assessed 11 studies for quality and risk of bias (Table 2). For most studies, the participants and outcome measures were well described. Trial design was the least well described throughout the 11 studies followed by the intervention description. Eight of the 11 studies had low risk of bias for the generation of the sequence allocating participants to treatment groups. In most study designs for self-management courses, the participants and facilitators will be un-blinded. Other research staff, such as those assessing participants and analysing data should have remained blinded to minimise bias. The concealment of group allocation was not described in the majority of studies.

Facilitators and treatment groups

Interventions were categorised as educational, [15, 28, 29, 33, 34] psychological (e.g. behavioural therapy) [30, 32, 37] and psychoeducational programmes (i.e. both) [31, 35]. Psychological and psychoeducational interventions were delivered by psychologists, whereas educational sessions were delivered by a range of practitioners. In two studies, [34, 36] instructors' qualifications were not clearly specified (e.g. 'researcher' or 'staff'). In one study, [15] facilitators were specified in a previous publication to be physicians, nurses, psychologists, social workers and occupational therapists.

The treatment of the control group varied across the studies. In six of the studies, [15, 28, 29, 31, 37, 33] controls received treatment as usual (TAU). Additional input was given to the controls alongside TAU in one study [33] in the form of two short telephone calls. In two, [30, 32] a control for attention was offered, for example, supportive therapy, involving equivalent attention from professionals, but without any active teaching or advice. Three studies [34–36] used a waitlist control design and offered intervention materials after follow-up.

Outcomes

The most frequently assessed outcome measure was QoL, used in seven studies included within this review [15, 28–30, 31, 35, 37]. The Quality of Life in Epilepsy questionnaire (QOLIE-31/QOLIE-89) [38, 39] was

Table 1 Summary of included papers

Author	Participants	Intervention (int.)	Facilitator	Control	Outcome measures	Main findings
Aliasgharpour et al. [33]	60 PWE randomised Aged 18–70 Diagnosed for ≥1 yr. Experienced seizures in the past year	1 month educational int. Four 2 hr sessions Face-to-face lectures with case histories, demonstrations and information leaflets to take away Group size: 4–6. Discrete intervention	Master's student in nursing	TAU	ESMS Pre-intervention and 1 month follow-up	Self-management score significantly improved in int. vs control
Au et al. [37]	17 adults with epilepsy (age range not specified) ≥ 2 seizures a month	8 week psychological CBT int. Eight 2 hr structured sessions Group size: 8 Discrete intervention	2 clinical psychologists trained in seizure management	TAU	QOLIE-31, ESES, seizure frequency 3 months pre-int. and 3 month follow-up	Significant improvement in QoL and self-efficacy scores in intervention group vs control No difference in seizure frequency
Fraser et al. [35]	83 PWE randomised Age ≥ 18 Diagnosed for ≥6 months	8 week psychoeducational int. Eight 75 min sessions Presentations, facilitated discussion and workbook Group size: 6–8. Discrete int.	Rehabilitation psychologist and trained peer mentor	WC	QOLIE-31, ESMS, ESES, PHQ-9, GAD-7 Pre-int., 8 week and 6 month follow-up	QoL, self-efficacy and PHQ-9 scores improved at 8 weeks in int. group but not significant at 6 months. Self-management significantly improved at 6 months
Helde et al. [29]	111 PWE aged 16–70 Diagnosed for ≥1 yr. ≥ 1 seizure in the past yr	1 day educational int. Information and discussion about epilepsy and psychosocial aspects Group size: 5–11 Additional input: telephone follow-up and 1–1 counselling from nurse	MDT (the study nurse, neurologist, social worker, and neurophysiologist)	TAU	QOLIE-89 and general patient satisfaction score Pre-randomisation and at 2 year follow-up	Significant improvement in QoL score in int. group at follow-up but no sig difference between int. and control Significant increase in satisfaction in int. vs control
Ibinda et al. [34]	738 PWE randomised 581 data analysed ≥ 1 seizure in the past yr	1 day educational int. Information about epilepsy provided using role play, discussion, narratives and brochure on the topics was given Group size: up to 20. Discrete int.	Non-specific 'researchers and field staff'	WC	AED adherence, seizure frequency, KEBAS (Kilifi epilepsy beliefs and Attitudes scores) Pre-int. and after 1 year follow-up	Significantly improved KEBAS scores in int. vs control at follow-up. No difference in adherence or seizure frequency between the groups (both improved significantly)
Losada-Comacho et al. [28]	182 women with epilepsy randomised Age ≥ 18 Diagnosed ≥1 yr. ≥ 1 seizure in the past 3 yrs	Educational int. part of pharmaceutical care programme Monthly lectures and information brochures Group size: not specified Additional input: 1–1 medication reviews. Given adherence aids and seizure journals	Pharmacist trained in epilepsy management	TAU and seizure Information brochure	QOLIE-31, seizure frequency, adverse events,CES-D (depression), Haynes-Sackett and Morinski-Green tests (medication adherence) Pre-int. and after 6 month follow-up	Highly significant improvement in QoL score between int. and control groups at follow-up. Other outcomes not reported in the paper
Lundgren et al. [30]	27 PWE randomised Aged 21–55 ≥ 4	Psychological ACT int. Two 3 hr sessions Group size: 6–8	2 clinical psychologists	Supportive therapy	WHOQOL-BREF, SWLS, seizure index	Significant improvement in seizure index at all time points post-int. in int. group vs control.

Table 1 Summary of included papers *(Continued)*

	seizures in the past 3 months	Additional input: Two individual 90 min sessions, individualised seizure control techniques			Pre-int, post-int, and at 6 month and 1 year follow-up	Significant improvement in QoL scores in int. group after 1 year
May and Pfafflin, [15]	383 PWE randomised Age ≥ 16 Any duration or severity of epilepsy	2 day educational int. Interactive course with 9 modules aiming to improve knowledge of epilepsy and psychosocial factors Group size: not specified. Discrete int.	Non-specific 'trainers'	TAU	SF-36, Depression Scale D-S', Rosenberg self-esteem, stigma, restrictions due to epilepsy, epilepsy-related fears and mobility and leisure scales, specifically developed epilepsy knowledge and coping with epilepsy scales. Seizure frequency Pre-int. and 6 month follow-up	Significant improvement in knowledge and coping scales (specifically developed) in int. group. Significant improvement in seizure frequency in int. group. No impact on QoL (SF-36 score)
McLaughlin and McFarland, [32]	37 older adults with epilepsy Age ≥ 60	6 week psychological CBT int. Six 2 h sessions Spector et al. protocol, modified for older adults with less content and diaries to aid memory Group size: 6–7. Discrete int.	Psychologist with epilepsy expertise	Relaxation training	GDS, CIDI-auto, WPSI, seizure frequency Pre-int, post-int. and after 3 month follow-up	Significant improvement in seizure frequency in int. group vs control. No significant difference between groups in other measures but depression and psychosocial functioning improved in both.
Olley et al. [36]	30 PWE allocated to groups Aged 21–65	2 day psychoeducational int. Educational sessions and group discussion on epilepsy, stigma & management Group size: not specified. Discrete int.	Non-specific 'researcher/therapist'	WC	CCEI, BDI (psychological symptoms), knowledge about epilepsy Pre-int, post-int and after 2 month follow-up	Significant improvement in int. group vs control in psychological scales and increased knowledge about epilepsy at follow-up
Pramuka et al. [31]	55 PWE randomised Age ≥ 18	6 week psychoeducational int. Six 2 hr sessions Presentations, activities and discussion on medical and self-management topics Written information provided Group size: 4–12. Discrete int.	2 psychologists and 1 research associate Guest lecture by nurse specialist	TAU	QOLIE-89, ESES, WPSI (psycho-social factors), locus of control scale, MCMI-III (depression) Pre-int. and 1 month follow-up	Trends in improved direction in all measures, but only one QoL subscale showed significant improvement in int. group vs control at follow-up.

PWE people with epilepsy; *yr.* year; *int* intervention; *hr.* hour; *TAU* treatment as usual; *ESMS* Epilepsy Self-Management Scale; *CBT* Cognitive Behaviour Therapy; *QOLIE* Quality of Life in Epilepsy; *ESES* Epilepsy Self-Efficacy Scale; *QoL* Quality of Life; *WC*waitlist control; *PHQ-9* Patient Health Questionnaire-9; *GAD-7* Generalised Anxiety Disorder-7; *MDT* multidisciplinary team; *ACT* Acceptance and Commitment Therapy; *WHOQOL-BREF* World Health Organisation quality of life – abbreviated version; *SWLS*: Satisfaction with Life Scale; *SF-36* 36-item short form survey; *GDS* Geriatric Depression Scale; *CIDI-auto* Composite International Diagnostic Interview; *WPSI* Washington Psychosocial Seizure Inventory; *CCEI* Crown-Crisp Experiential Index; *BDI* Beck Depression Inventory; *MCMI-III*: Millon Clinical Multiaxial Inventory -III

Table 2 Quality ratings and risk of bias

Study	Quality appraisal					Risk of bias appraisal			
	Trial design	Participants	Intervention	Outcomes	Total (max 8)	Sequence generation	Risk of bias	Allocation concealment	Risk of bias
Aliasgharpour et al. [33]	1	1.75	2	2	6.75	Random number table	Low	Not described	Unclear
Au et al. [37]	0.75	2	2	2	6.75	Matched design	Unclear	Not described	Unclear
Fraser et al. [35]	1.75	2	1.75	2	7.5	Random number generator	Low	Not described	Unclear
Helde et al. [29]	1.25	2	2	2	7.25	Computer-generated block randomisation	Low	Research assistant blinded	Low
Ibinda et al. [34]	1.25	1.25	0.5	1.5	4.5	Computer-generated randomisation	Low	Not described	Unclear
Losada-Camacho et al. [28]	2	2	1.75	2	7.75	Drawing of ballot papers	Low	Sequentially numbered, opaque, sealed envelopes	Low
Lundgren et al. [30]	1	2	2	2	7	Computer-generated randomisation	Low	Not described	Unclear
May and Pfafflin. [15]	1.25	2	0.75	1.5	5.5	Not described	Unclear	Not described	Unclear
McLaughlin and McFarland [32]	1	1.75	2	2	6.75	Computer-generated randomisation	Low	Not described	Unclear
Olley et al. [36]	1.5	2	1.25	1.75	6.5	Alternate clinic visit	High	Not described	Unclear
Pramuka et al. [31]	1.5	2	2	2	7.5	Random number table	Low	Consecutively numbered, sealed envelopes	Low

commonly chosen to assess it [28, 29, 31, 35, 37]. Six studies [15, 28, 30, 32, 34, 37] measured seizure frequency as a marker of control and three assessed self-efficacy, [31, 35, 37] using the Epilepsy Self-Efficacy Scale (ESES) [40]. Two studies [33, 35] used a specific self-management outcome measure called the Epilepsy Self-Management Scale (ESMS) [41]. Different measures were used to assess psychological symptoms, such as the Patient Health Questionnaire (PHQ-9) [42]. Comparison between the studies was complicated, due to the heterogeneity of outcome measures that were used.

Follow-up

The duration of follow-up ranged from one month [33] to two years [29] with a median follow-up period of six months. All studies recorded outcome measures at baseline before the intervention and at the end of follow-up. Four also took further measures immediately post-intervention or halfway through the follow-up period [30, 32, 35, 36].

Overview of findings

Quality of life

Of the seven studies using QoL outcome measures, three showed no significant difference in total QoL scores between the intervention and control groups [15, 29, 31]. Fraser et al. showed a significant improvement in QOLIE-31 scores eight weeks post-intervention, but no statistical significance between means after six months [35].

Two psychological interventions showed an improvement in QoL scores at follow-up. The cognitive behavioural therapy study demonstrated a significant QOLIE-31 score improvement in the intervention group compared with the control at the end of a three month follow-up [37]. Emotional Wellbeing was the only subscale that was significantly increased. In the trial by Lundgren et al [30]. there was a significant improvement in WHOQOL-BREF score (World Health Organisation Quality of Life Assessment abbreviated version) [43] in the acceptance and commitment therapy group, compared to supportive therapy at the final one year follow-up. The Satisfaction with Life Scale (SWLS) [44] score was improved at all three time points after the intervention.

One education-focused study showed an improvement in QoL score. The trial by Losada-Camacho et al. found significant improvement in QOLIE-31 after six months [28]. The intervention package was offered to women only, and focused on pharmaceutical aspects of epilepsy self-management. As one of the co-interventions, participants received advice and monitoring at set intervals from a pharmacist. At six-month follow-up, the total score increased in the intervention group by 12.45 points compared with a 2.61 increase in the controls.

Seizure frequency

Six studies measured seizure frequency. Three found that seizure frequency decreased significantly in the intervention group compared with controls [28, 30, 32]. However, two studies did not find a significant difference in seizure frequency post-intervention. Au et al. described a small improvement in the intervention group but this was not significant, [37] whereas, Ibinda et al. found a decrease in both groups but no difference between them [34]. One study did not report seizure frequency despite collecting this data [28]. The reason for this was unclear; however, it may be due to poor compliance with seizure diaries as only 37.5% of participants returned them.

Self-management and self-efficacy

Two studies using the ESMS showed promising findings after group intervention delivery. Aliasgharpour et al. found a significant difference between the groups post-intervention with an increase in self-management score in the intervention group but none in the control [33]. Likewise, Fraser et al. found a treatment effect favouring the intervention at eight weeks which, although small, remained significant at the six month follow-up [35].

Three studies used the ESES to measure self-efficacy [31, 35, 37]. Fraser et al. found a significant treatment effect in ESES score after eight weeks but this did not persist at six months. Au et al. found a significant improvement in score in the intervention group compared to control. Findings from Pramuka et al. showed a trend towards improvement in the intervention group but this was not significant.

Psychological symptoms

Two of the six studies which used symptom scales indicating psychological comorbidity showed statistically significant improvement [35, 36]. Fraser et al. found a statistical significant change in PHQ-9 [39] score with reductions in depressive symptom severity at eight weeks post-intervention; however, the difference between intervention and control was not statistically significant at six months. Olley et al. found an improvement in psychological state compared with controls but, with only two months follow-up, no long-term benefit was demonstrated [36]. The others found improvements which were not significant [28, 31, 32]. In the study by Losada-Camacho et al. the psychological outcome results were not reported, [28] nor were they published elsewhere.

Discussion

Quality assessment revealed gaps in the methodological reporting of many studies, especially regarding trial design. Risk of bias was assessed and most papers fell into the 'unclear' category due to insufficient description of treatment concealment. We paid particular attention to who delivered each intervention and how thoroughly this was described. Information about the role and training of facilitators is needed in order to replicate an intervention and apply it to other healthcare settings.

The usefulness of study findings is somewhat diminished in those that lacked thorough reporting of treatment fidelity. Most interventions were delivered multiple times, sometimes by different facilitators; however, only one study discussed means of ensuring treatment fidelity but the results were not presented [30]. Group interventions may not be delivered consistently and without reporting on measures to prevent deviation, it is uncertain whether interventions were delivered as planned.

All studies reported significant improvement in the intervention group compared with controls in at least one measure. More than half of the studies assessing QoL found some positive effect from the intervention but the duration of that effect is varied. Five studies repeated the QoL measures at least six months after the intervention and only two found a sustained significant improvement [28, 30]. These both consisted of sessions which were spread out over time, which may be a better intervention strategy than one-off courses. Fraser et al. also delivered their intervention over a period of 8 weeks but were unable to demonstrate a significant effect at 6 month follow-up [35]. They suggested the addition of a booster course to the programme. It is likely that other factors may also influence the duration of improvement.

It was difficult to identify mechanisms that make a group intervention for PWE effective. This is particularly true of co-interventions, where group effects cannot be separated out from additional support. Psychological interventions performed well on QoL and seizure frequency (Table 1) [36, 37, 32] although they had very small sample sizes (n = 17, 27 and 37). This suggests that including behavioural therapy in self-management interventions may be important to affect QoL.

Although some studies found positive trends for QoL improvements from baseline measurements, the scores were not necessarily statistically different between study groups. Many were pilot studies with small sample sizes and may not have had adequate power to detect important changes. One study that encountered this problem calculated a required sample size of 180 participants but recruitment difficulties resulted in a final sample of only 55 [31]. Larger-scale trials are needed to explore this further.

Another factor that may have contributed to the lack of significant effect is the use of unsuitable outcomes. Two studies found improvements only in measures developed specifically for the trial, despite including a variety of other outcomes [15, 34]. This suggests that the existing scales may not be optimal for evaluating effects of self-management interventions in this setting.

The diversity of outcome measures used across all studies made comparison difficult. There were five scales used to assess QoL, of which two were epilepsy-specific. Four studies did not use any QoL questionnaires although their chosen outcomes (e.g. seizure frequency) can be assumed to affect QoL. This highlights lack of consensus on the most appropriate measures for complex interventions in epilepsy.

Only one study used semi-qualitative data in their evaluation, collecting written comments from participants in an open-ended satisfaction survey [35]. They received positive comments about the intervention with 47% of respondents mentioning the value of meeting other PWE. However, response rates were uncertain and there were no interviews to explore participants' views. Guidelines from the Medical Research Council recommend the inclusion of qualitative methods as part of a process evaluation for complex interventions [45]. In light of this, it would be useful to collect further qualitative data on how and why group self-management interventions are beneficial.

The diversity of study settings also complicates interpretation. As trials were conducted across 13 countries with wide-ranging cultural and socioeconomic backgrounds, baseline standards of care and health literacy were likely different. Furthermore, participants in each setting may not be representative of the wider population. This was particularly relevant in the Seattle-based study which typically recruited highly educated participants, some of whom were volunteers, limiting the generalisability of their findings to other western countries in which health care is provided to all socio-economic groups [35].

There are several limitations associated with the present review. We were unable to perform a meta-analysis due to significant heterogeneity of outcome measures observed across the studies. Moreover, not all Cochrane review tools were utilised when evaluating the quality of studies included. Findings from the review may also be limited due to biases arising from initial search criteria (i.e., article language and publication date).

Suggestions for future research

Based on the evidence available to date, it seems that QoL is rarely affected long term by educational interventions. Thus to have a better chance of affecting QoL, self-management interventions should include psychological components. If group self-management education is to be offered as part of standard outpatient care for PWE, as DESMOND is for people with diabetes, then future research should examine the feasibility and cost-effectiveness of implementation. Although this review did not specifically search for published articles with health economics data, we found no discussion of the cost of implementing self-management education courses for PWE in the community. This would be valuable in the context of similar programmes being implemented in countries with public healthcare systems.

Conclusions

The studies evaluating group self-management interventions for PWE found encouraging results. There is some evidence that psychoeducational measures can be delivered to improve self-management, seizure control, and QoL in adults with poorly-controlled epilepsy. The MOSES programme has been offered in German-speaking countries for over a decade and other countries are investigating similar interventions [15]. Promising findings, along with demand from patients for more information about epilepsy, are indications for continued interest in group self-management interventions for PWE.

This review illustrates the need for clarity regarding outcome measures in this field of epilepsy research. Additionally, large-scale trials of group self-management interventions, combining quantitative, qualitative, and cost-effectiveness data, are required in the future.

Appendix 1

Search strategies

Medline (Ovid) search strategy

1. exp. Epilepsy/
2. epilep*
3. seizures
4. exp. Self Care/
5. exp. Self Efficacy/
6. exp. Patient Education as Topic/
7. educational program
8. self-management
9. group intervention
10. complex intervention
11. 1 or 2 or 3
12. Limit 11 to (English language and yr. = "1995 - Current")
13. 4 or 5 or 6 or 7 or 8 or 9 or 10
14. Limit 13 to (English language and yr. = "1995 - Current")
15. 12 and 14
16. Limit 15 to (clinical trial or controlled clinical trial or pragmatic clinical trial or randomized controlled trial)

PsycINFO search strategy

1. Exp Epilepsy/
2. epilep*
3. seizures
4. 1 or 2 or 3
5. self-management
6. exp. Self Efficacy/
7. group intervention
8. complex intervention
9. patient education
10. self care
11. educational program*
12. 5 or 6 or 7 or 8 or 9 or 10 or 11
13. 12 and 4
14. limit 13 to (English language and yr. = "1995- Current")

Abbreviations

DESMOND: Diabetes education and self-management for ongoing and newly diagnosed; ESES: Epilepsy self-efficacy scale; ESMS: Epilepsy self-management scale; MOSES: Modular service package epilepsy; PHQ-9: Patient health questionnaire 9; PWE: People with epilepsy; QoL: Quality of life; QOLIE: Quality of life in epilepsy; SWLS: Satisfaction with life scale; TAU: Treatment as usual; WHOQOL-BREF: World health organisation quality of life abbreviated version

Acknowledgements

The authors would like to acknowledge our clinical trial administrator, Carly Pearson.

Funding

This research was in part funded by the National Institute for Health Research (NIHR), under the Health Technology Assessment Programme (09/165/01), including salaries for AM and GW. There are no further funding sources to declare. The views and opinions expressed by authors in this publication are those of the authors and do not necessarily reflect those of the NHS, NIHR, MRC, CCF, NETSCC, HTA programme, or Department of Health.

Authors' contributions

AS was responsible for writing the first major draft of the manuscript, evaluating each article included with the review, and carrying out subsequent revisions of the manuscript. AM evaluated each of the articles included with the review and carried out moderate revisions of the manuscript in preparation for publication. GW evaluated each paper included with the review, contributed to the development of the manuscript and provided feedback throughout manuscript preparation. LR conceived of the study and its design and methods, and provided supervision and feedback throughout. All authors read and approved the final manuscript.

Competing interests

There are no further competing interests to declare.

Author details

[1]GKT School of Medicine, King's College London, London SE1 1UL, UK.
[2]Institute of Psychiatry, Psychology & Neuroscience, Academic Neuroscience Centre, King's College London, PO Box 57, London SE5 8AF, UK.

References

1. Longmore M, Wilkinson I, Baldwin A, Wallin E. Oxford handbook of clinical Medicine. 9th ed. Oxford: Oxford University Press; 2014.
2. Smithson WH, Walker MC, editors. ABC of epilepsy. 1st ed. Chichester: Wiley-Blackwell; 2012.
3. Moran NF, Poole K, Bell G, Solomon J, Kendall S, McCarthy M, et al. Epilepsy in the United Kingdom: seizure frequency and severity, anti-epileptic drug utilization and impact on life in 1652 people with epilepsy. Seizure. 2004; 13(6):425–33.
4. Jacoby A, Snape D, Baker GA. Determinants of quality of life in people with epilepsy. Neurol Clin. 2009;27(4):843–63.
5. Bruce M, Griffiths C, Brock A, Majeed A. Trends in mortality and hospital

admissions associated with epilepsy in England and Wales during the 1990s. Health Stat Q. 2004 Spring;21:23–9.

6. Noble AJ, Goldstein LH, Seed P, Glucksman E, Ridsdale L. Characteristics of people with epilepsy who attend emergency departments: prospective study of metropolitanhospital attendees. Epilepsia. 2012;53(10):1820–8.
7. Health and Social Care Information Centre (HSCIC), Clinical Indicators team. CCG Outcomes Indicator Set: Emergency Admissions. 2013; Available at: http://www.hscic.gov.uk/catalogue/PUB10584/ccg-ind-toi-mar-13-v4.pdf. Accessed October 28, 2015.
8. Cockerell OC, Hart YM, Sander JW, Shorvon SD. The cost of epilepsy in the United Kingdom: an estimation based on the results of two population-based studies. Epilepsy Res. 1994;18(3):249–60.
9. NHS England. Domain 2: Enhancing Quality Of Life For People With Long-Term Conditions. Available at: http://www.england.nhs.uk/resources/resources-for-ccgs/out-frwrk/dom-2/#help. Accessed 16 December 2015.
10. Carey ME, Mandalia PK, Daly H, Gray LJ, Hale R, Martin Stacey L, et al. Increasing capacity to deliver diabetes self-management education: results of the DESMOND lay educator non-randomized controlled equivalence trial. Diabetic Med. 2014;31(11):1431–8.
11. Gillett M, Dallosso HM, Dixon S, Brennan A, Carey ME, Campbell MJ. Delivering the diabetes education and self management for ongoing and newly diagnosed (DESMOND) programme for people with newly diagnosed type 2 diabetes: cost effectiveness analysis. BMJ. 2010;341
12. Davies MJ, Heller S, Skinner TC, Campbell MJ, Carey ME, Cradock S, et al. Effectiveness of the diabetes education and self management for ongoing and newly diagnosed (DESMOND) programme for people with newly diagnosed type 2 diabetes: cluster randomised controlled trial. BMJ. 2008; 336(7642):491–5.
13. Bandura A. Self-efficacy: toward a unifying theory of behavioral change. Psychol Rev. 1977;84(2):191–215.
14. Helgeson DC, Mittan R, Tan SY, Chayasirisobhon S. Sepulveda epilepsy education: the efficacy of a psychoeducational treatment program in treating medical and psychosocial aspects of epilepsy. Epilepsia. 1990;31(1):75–82.
15. May TW, Pfäfflin M. The efficacy of an educational treatment program for patients with epilepsy (MOSES): results of a controlled. Randomized Study Epilepsia. 2002;43(5):539–49.
16. Kralj-Hans I, Goldstein LH, Noble AJ, Landau S, Magill N, McCrone P. Self-management education for adults with poorly controlled epILEpsy (SMILE (UK)): a randomised controlled trial protocol. BMC Neurol. 2014;14
17. Durand M-A, Gates B, Parkes G, Zia A, Friedli K, Barton G, et al. Wordless intervention for epilepsy in learning disabilities (WIELD): study protocol for a randomized controlled feasibility trial. Trials. 2014;15(1):455.
18. National Institute for Health Care and Excellence. Guide to the methods of technology appraisal 2013. 2013; Available at: http://nice.org.uk/process/pmg9 accessed 4 March 2017.
19. Chidgey J, Leng G, Lacey T. Implementing NICE guidance. J R Soc Med. 2007;100(10):448–52.
20. Sibbald B, Roland M. Understanding controlled trials. Why are randomised controlled trials important?. BMJ: British Medical Journal. 1998;316(7126):201.
21. Schulz KF, Altman DG, Moher D, CONSORT Group. CONSORT 2010 Statement: updated guidelines for reporting parallel group randomised trials. BMJ. 2010;340:c332.
22. Higgins J, Altman D, Sterne J. Chapter 8: assessing risk of bias in included studies. 2011; Available at: http://handbook.cochrane.org/chapter_8/8_assessing_risk_of_bias_in_included_studies.htm. Accessed 13 December 2015.
23. Chen D, Maheshwari A, Franks R, Trolley G, Robinson J, Hrachovy R. Brief group psychoeducation for psychogenic nonepileptic seizures: a neurologist-initiated program in an epilepsy center. Epilepsia. 2014;55(1):156–66.
24. Paul F, Jones MC, Hendry C, Adair PM. The quality of written information for parents regarding the management of a febrile convulsion: a randomized controlled trial. J Clin Nurs. 2007;16(12):2308–22.
25. Huang MC, Liu CC, Huang CC. Effects of an educational program on parents with febrile convulsive children. Pediatr Neurol. 1998;18(2):150–5.
26. Riaz H, Comish S, Lawton L, Scheepers B. Non-epileptic attack disorder and clinical outcome: a pilot study. Seizure. 1998;7(5):365–8.
27. Thompson N, Connelly L, Peltzer J, Nowack WJ, Hamera E, Hunter EE. Psychogenic Nonepileptic seizures: a pilot study of a brief educational intervention. Perspectives in Psychiatric Care. 2013 Apr;49(2):78–83.
28. Losada-Camacho M, Guerrero-Pabon MF, Garcia-Delgado P, Martínez-Martinez F. Impact of a pharmaceutical care programme on health-related quality of life among women with epilepsy: a randomised controlled trial (IPHIWWE study). Health Qual Life Outcomes. 2014;12:162.
29. Helde G, Bovim G, Bråthen G, Brodtkorb E. A structured, nurse-led intervention program improves quality of life in patients with epilepsy: A randomized, controlled trial. Epilepsy & Behavior 2005 11;7(3):451–457.
30. Lundgren T, Dahl J, Melin L, Kies B. Evaluation of acceptance and commitment therapy for drug refractory epilepsy: a randomized controlled trial in South Africa - a pilot study. Epilepsia. 2006;47(12):2173–9.
31. Pramuka M, Hendrickson R, Zinski A, Van Cott AC. A psychosocial self-management program for epilepsy: a randomized pilot study in adults. Epilepsy Behav. 2007;11(4):533–45.
32. McLaughlin DP, McFarland K. A randomized trial of a group based cognitive behavior therapy program for older adults with epilepsy: the impact on seizure frequency, depression and psychosocial well-being. Journal of Behaviour Medicine. 2011;34(3):201–7.
33. Aliasgharpour M, Dehgahn Nayeri N, Yadegary MA, Haghani H. Effects of an educational program on self-management in patients with epilepsy. Seizure. 2013;22(1):48–52.
34. Ibinda F, Mbuba CK, Kariuki SM, Chengo E, Ngugi AK, Odhiambo R, et al. Evaluation of Kilifi epilepsy education Programme: a randomized controlled trial. Epilepsia. 2014;55(2):344–52.
35. Fraser R, Johnson E, Lashley S, Barber J, Chaytor N, Miller J, et al. PACES in epilepsy: results of a self-management randomized controlled trial. Epilepsia. 2015;56(8):1264–74.
36. Olley BO, Osinowo HO, Brieger WR. Psycho-educational therapy among Nigerian adult patients with epilepsy: a controlled outcome study. Patient Educ Couns. 2001;42(1):25–33.
37. Au A, Chan F, Li K, Leung P, Li P, Chan J. Cognitive-behavioral group treatment program for adults with epilepsy in Hong Kong. Epilepsy Behav. 2003;4(4):441–6.
38. Cramer JA, Perrine K, Devinsky O, Bryant-Comstock L, Meador K, Hermann B. Development and cross-cultural translations of a 31-item quality of life in epilepsy Inventory. Epilepsia. 1998;39(1):81–8.
39. Devinsky O, Vickrey BG, Cramer J, Perrine K, Hermann B, Meador K, et al. Development of the quality of life in epilepsy Inventory. Epilepsia. 1995; 36(11):1089–104.
40. Dilorio C, Faherty B, Manteuffel B. The development and testing of an instrument to measure self-efficacy in individuals with epilepsy. J Neurosci Nurs. 1992;24(1):9–13.
41. Dilorio C, Shafer PO, Letz R, Henry TR, Schomer DL, Yeager K. Behavioral, social, and affective factors associated with self-efficacy for self-management among people with epilepsy. Epilepsy Behav. 2006;9(1):158–63.
42. Kroenke K, Spitzer RL, Williams JB. The PHQ-9: validity of a brief depression severity measure. J Gen Intern Med. 2001;16(9):606–13.
43. WHOQOL Group. Development of the World Health Organization WHOQOL-BREF quality of life assessment. Psychol Med. 1998;28(03):551–8.
44. Diener E, Emmons RA, Larsen RJ, Griffin S. The satisfaction with life scale. J Pers Assess. 1985;49(1):71–5.
45. Craig P, Dieppe P, Macintyre S, Michie S, Nazareth I, Petticrew M. Developing and evaluating complex interventions: the new Medical Research Council guidance. Int J Nurs Stud. 2013;50(5):587–92.

Relationship between Azathioprine metabolites and therapeutic efficacy in Chinese patients with neuromyelitis optica spectrum disorders

Xindi Li[1,2], Shenghui Mei[3], Xiaoqing Gong[1,2], Heng Zhou[1,2], Li Yang[3], Anna Zhou[1,2], Yonghong Liu[1,2], Xingang Li[3], Zhigang Zhao[3*] and Xinghu Zhang[1,2*]

Abstract

Background: Neuromyelitis optica spectrum disorders (NMOSD) are demyelinating autoimmune diseases in the central nervous system (CNS) that are characterized by a high relapse rate and the presence of anti-aquaporin 4 antibodies (AQP4-IgG) in the serum. Azathioprine (AZA) is a first-line immunomodulatory drug that is widely used for the treatment of patients with NMOSD. However, the efficacy and safety of AZA vary in different individuals.

Method: Thirty-two patients with NMOSD who regularly took AZA were enrolled in the study at Beijing Tiantan Hospital, Capital Medical University. The efficacy of AZA was evaluated using the expanded disability status scale (EDSS) and the annual relapse rate (ARR). The erythrocyte concentrations of AZA metabolites were detected using an LC-MS/MS method.

Results: The erythrocyte concentrations of 6-thioguanine nucleotides (6-TGNs) and 6-methylmercaptopurine nucleotides (6-MMPNs) were 202.03 ± 63.35 pmol/8*10^8 RBC and 1618.90 ± 1607.06 pmol/8*10^8 RBC, respectively. After the patients had received AZA therapy for more than one year, the EDSS score decreased from 5.21 ± 0.24 to 2.57 ± 0.33 ($p < 0.0001$), and the ARR decreased from 1.41 ± 0.23 to 0.36 ± 0.09 ($p < 0.0001$). The 6-TGN and 6-MMPN levels were significantly different between the non-relapsed and relapsed groups ($p < 0.0001$, $p = 0.006$, respectively). A higher ARR was significantly correlated with higher erythrocyte concentrations of 6-TGNs ($p < 0.0001$) and 6-MMPNs ($p = 0.004$).

Conclusion: AZA can reduce the EDSS score and ARR in NMOSD patients. Additionally, the efficacy of AZA is significantly related to the erythrocyte concentrations of 6-TGNs and 6-MMPNs. Within the safe upper limits, a higher concentration of 6-TGNs is associated with better efficacy of AZA.

Keywords: Neuromyelitis optica spectrum disorders (NMOSD), Azathioprine (AZA), Thiopurine S-methyltransferase (TPMT), 6-thioguanine nucleotides (6-TGNs), 6-methylmercaptopurine nucleotides (6-MMPNs)

* Correspondence: ttyyzzg1022@126.com; xhzhtiantan@hotmail.com
[3]Department of Pharmacy, Beijing Tiantan Hospital, Capital Medical University, 6 TiantanXili, Dongcheng District, Beijing 100050, People's Republic of China
[1]Neuroinfection and Neuroimmunology Center, Department of Neurology, Beijing Tiantan Hospital, Capital Medical University, 6 TiantanXili, Dongcheng District, Beijing 100050, People's Republic of China
Full list of author information is available at the end of the article

Background

Neuromyelitis optica spectrum disorders (NMOSD) are demyelinating autoimmune diseases in the central nervous system (CNS) that are characterized by the presence of anti-aquaporin four antibodies (AQP4-IgG) in the serum [1]. The clinical disability progressively deteriorates, and the occurrence of relapses increases. Currently, azathioprine (AZA), which is a first-line immunomodulatory drug, is widely used for the prevention of relapse in NMOSD patients [2]. The efficacy of the AZA treatment in NMOSD patients has been mainly evaluated by expanded disability status scale (EDSS) values and the annual relapse rates (ARR). Elsone et al. reported that neurological function improved or remained stable in 78% of patients who received ASA therapy, with a mild reduction in the mean EDSS score from 5.5 to 4 in 103 NMOSD patients [3]. The ARR has been shown to decrease after treatment with AZA [4, 5]. In a Chinese retrospective study, 57.1% of NMOSD patients were in relapse-free status [6]. However, the efficacy and safety of AZA vary in different individuals. Severe adverse reactions to AZA, such as leukopenia and liver dysfunction, may limit its use [7]. Therefore, the identification of indicators to guide the safe and effective use of AZA is very important.

The immunosuppressive effects of AZA are mainly due to its metabolites. AZA rapidly transforms into 6-mercaptopurine (6-MP), which is further converted into thiopurine nucleotides (TPNs), including 6-thioguanine nucleotides (6-TGNs) and 6-methylmercaptopurine nucleotides (6-MMPNs), by a series of competitive enzymes [8]. 6-TGNs are produced by hypoxanthine-guanine phosphoribosyltransferase (HGPRT), and 6-MMPNs, which are the inactive by products of AZA, are formed by thiopurine-methyltransferase (TPMT) [9, 10]. The intracellular accumulation of 6-TGNs and 6-MMPNs can inhibit the biosynthesis of nucleic acids and prevent the proliferation of various lymphocytes [11]. The control of lymphocyte apoptosis is vital to the regulation of the immune system. Therefore, the immunosuppression effect of AZA was correlated with the accumulation of 6-TGNs and 6-MMPNs [12].

The AZA metabolites are mainly mediated by TPMT [13]. Allozymes encoded by certain *TPMT* mutant alleles displayed low TPMT activity that was undetectable after their expression in COS-1 cells [14]. *TPMT**2 (238G > C), *TPMT**3A (460G > A and719A > G), *TPMT**3B (460G > A) and *TPMT**3C (719A > G) account for 80–95% of patients with low TPMT activity [15, 16]. Pyrimidine and purine nucleosides, such as 6-TGNs and 6-MMPNs, are transported into the cells by the following two types of human nucleoside transporters: concentrative nucleoside transporters and equilibrative nucleoside transporters. These transporters are encoded by two gene families (i.e., *SLC28* and *SLC29*) [17, 18]. Badagnani et al. reported that CNT3 (i.e., *SLC28A3*) played an important role in the mediation of the cellular entry of a variety of physiological nucleosides and synthetic anticancer nucleoside analog drugs [19]. *SLC28A3* was also reported to have a significant influence on the transport of 6-MP [20]. The relationship between polymorphisms of *SLC28A3* and the erythrocyte concentrations of AZA metabolites in NMOSD has been demonstrated in our former study [21]. Based on the previous study, this study analyzed the relationship between the concentrations of AZA metabolites and the immunosuppressive efficacy of AZA to identify predictive biomarkers for efficacy evaluations of AZA in NMOSD patients.

Methods

Subjects

This study analyzed the clinical characteristics, AZA metabolites and genetic polymorphism of prospectively enrolled patients. The study was approved by the Ethics Committee of Beijing Tiantan Hospital Affiliated to Capital Medical University, Beijing, People's Republic of China (No. KY2015–031-02). Written informed consent was obtained from the patients or from their parents / legal guardians who were under 18 or from the close relatives whose participants had severe disability in the writing hand or the illiteracy. Forty-one patients with NMOSD were enrolled. All patients received steroids during the acute disease stage. The initial dosage of methylprednisolone was 1000 mg for 3 days, which was tapered as follows: 500 mg for 3 days, 250 mg for 3 days and 120 mg for 3 days. Then, oral prednisone (60 mg per day) was administered and slowly withdrawn within 12 weeks. AZA therapy was added at the beginning of the oral prednisone administration. The initial dosage of AZA was 50 mg per day for the first 5 days. If no severe adverse reactions appeared, the dosage of AZA was increased to 100 mg per day. Routine blood tests and hepatic and renal functions were monitored regularly (during the first month of the AZA intake, monitoring was performed once every week; during the 2nd month, monitoring was performed once every two weeks; during the 3rd month and thereafter, monitoring was performed once a month). The treatment was stopped if severe adverse reactions occurred. Nine patients withdrew from the study due to the appearance of severe adverse reactions. If relapse occurred, high-dose steroids were re-introduced and withdrawn as previously described.

The inclusion criteria in this study were as follows:

1. Met the International Consensus Diagnostic Criteria for Neuromyelitis Optica Spectrum Disorder 2015 [1].
2. Onset age: 12 to 80 years.
3. No previous exposure to any immunosuppressive agent.

4. Did not undergo blood transfusion three months before sampling.
5. Received more than 12 months of AZA treatment, and the dose has not been changed within the previous 4 weeks to ensure a stable AZA metabolite profile.

The exclusion criteria were as follows:

1. Intolerance to the AZA treatment due to any severe adverse reaction, such as the leukocyte counts less than 4×10^9/L, other severe cardiovascular disease or hepatopathy.
2. Planned or current pregnancy and/or breast feeding.
3. Other unsuitable characteristics as determined by the clinicians.

Methods

The disability was measured by the EDSS. The pretherapy EDSS was evaluated at the stable stage (more than one month after relapse), and the post-therapy EDSS was evaluated at the final visit (at least one year after the AZA treatment). The ARR was calculated according to the number of relapses per year. To remove the influence of the pretherapy ARR, we measure the ARR improvement as the pretherapy ARR minus the post-therapy ARR divided by the pretherapy ARR (the value of the ARR improvement was positive). A confirmed relapse was defined as the appearance of new neurological symptoms or worsening of preexisting symptoms that lasted for at least 24 h and was accompanied by an objective neurological change (worsening by 0.5 points on the EDSS or by ≥1.0 points on the pyramidal sign, cerebella, brainstem, or visual functional system scores) in patients who had been neurologically stable or improving in the previous 30 days [6]. The relapsed group included patients who had a confirmed relapse after taking AZA. The non-relapsed group included patients who did not experience any relapse event during the follow-up duration. The AZA efficacy was evaluated based on the changes in the EDSS score and the ARR after the therapy.

CSF and serum samples for the immunological tests, including CSF protein, CSF IgG and AQP4-IgG, were routinely collected during the acute phase before any therapy was administered. Cell-based assays were used for the serum AQP4-IgG detection [22]. Blood samples (5 mL) were collected in vacuum tubes (containing ethylenediaminetetraacetic acid) after 30 days of regular AZA therapy (during the remission phase). After centrifugation at 5000×*g* for 10 min, the plasma was removed, and the white blood cells were stored at −80 °C for genotyping. The erythrocytes were washed twice with 2 ml saline and centrifuged at 10000×*g* for 2 min to remove the supernatant, which was subsequently stored at −80 °C to detect the concentrations of erythrocyte 6-TGNs and 6-MMPNs using our previously reported method (high-performance liquid chromatographic tandem mass spectrometry) [21]. The measurements of TPNs were divided by the body mass index, total daily dose, and mean corpuscular volume to remove the influence of these variables.

Statistical analysis

SPSS (version 17, SPSS Inc., Chicago, IL, USA) was used for statistical analysis. The chi-square test was used to compare the ARR values (before and after the treatment) and the serum AQP4-IgG concentrations. Nonparametric independent-sample *k-s* test was used to analyze the differences in the EDSS scores. Independent-samples *t*-test was used to analyze the differences in the other related variables. The relationships between the concentrations of the AZA metabolites and ARR improvement were evaluated by 2-tailed *Spearman rank* correlation and *multiple linear-regression,* which was adjusted for onset age, disease duration, therapy duration, pretherapy and post-therapy EDSS scores, and laboratory tests. A two-tailed *p*-value <0.05 was considered statistically significant.

Results

Characteristics of NMOSD patients treated with AZA

All 32 NMOSD patients (30 females and 2 males) regularly received AZA therapy. The average onset age was 33.28 years (ranged from 18 to 62, SD = 12.77). The average duration of the disease was 85.56 months (ranged from 19 to 266, SD = 68.18), and the average duration of AZA therapy was 21.50 months (ranged from 12 to 40, SD = 6.19). In total, 21 (65.6%) patients presented with optic neuritis, and 29 (90.6%) patients presented with myelitis. The mean concentration of the CSF protein was 40.41 ± 32.67 mg/dl, and the mean CSF IgG index was 0.53 ± 0.10. Serum anti-AQP4 antibodies were positively detected in 14 (43.75%) patients. The concentrations of erythrocyte 6-TGNs were within the safe upper limits (6-TGN < 450 pmol/8 × 10^8 RBC), but a few patients had erythrocyte 6-MMPN concentrations above the safe upper limits (5700 pmol/8 × 10^8 RBC) [23]. The average 6-TGNs concentration was 202.03 pmol/8*10^8 RBC (ranged from 83.441 to 319.71, SD = 63.35), and the average 6-MMPN concentration was 1618.90 pmol/8*10^8 RBC (ranged from 235.04 to 7498.89, SD = 1607.06). The mean EDSS score decreased from 5.21 ± 0.24 to 2.57 ± 0.33 ($p < 0.0001$), and the mean ARR decreased from 1.41 ± 0.23 to 0.36 ± 0.09 ($p < 0.0001$). Detailed information is provided in Table 1. The individual relapse events within 10 years before AZA therapy and 2 years after AZA therapy are shown in Fig. 1, and two patients (No. 6 and No. 14) had worse ARRs after AZA therapy.

Table 1 The general characteristics of NMOSD patients

Variable	Patients (n = 32)
Mean Age of onset, year	33.28 (15–62)
Sex (n%)	
Female	30 (93.75%)
Male	2 (6.25%)
Mean BMI	24.17 (17.57–31.65)
Mean Disease duration, months	85.56 (19–266)
Mean Duration of AZA therapy, months	21.50 (12–40)
Clinical symptoms at onset (n%)	
Optic neuritis	21 (65.6%)
Bilateral Optic neuritis	17 (53.13%)
Myelitis	29 (90.6%)
Optic neuritis and Myelitis	19 (59.3%)
Mean Pre-therapy EDSS score	5.21 ± 0.24 (2.5–8)
Mean Post- therapy EDSS score	2.57 ± 0.33 (0–7)
Mean Concentration of CSF protein, mg/dl	40.41 ± 32.67 (12–184)
Mean Concentration of CSF IgG, mg/ml	0.04 ± 0.03 (0.01–0.19)
CSF IgG index (n%)	0.53 ± 0.10 (0.39–0.83)
Serum anti-AQP4 antibodies (n%)	14 (43.75%)
Mean Concentration of 6-TGNs, pmol/8 × 10^8 RBC	202.03
Mean Concentration of MMPNs, pmol/8 × 10^8 RBC	1618.90
Relapse, n%	12/32 (37.5%)
Pre- therapy ARR	1.42 ± 0.23 (0.2–3.5)
Post- therapy ARR	0.36 ± 0.09 (0–1.72)

NMOSD Neuromyelitisoptica spectrum disorders, *AZA* Azathioprine, *AQP4* anti-aquaporin 4, *BMI* Body mass index, *ARR* Annual relapse rate, *EDSS* Expanded disability status scale, *CSF* cerebrospinal fluid, *IgG* Immunoglobulin G

The differences in the related variables between the non-relapsed and relapsed groups

Except for the EDSS score, other variables were normally distributed with a homogeneity of variance. The mean values of the normalized 6-TGN levels (1.12 vs. 0.70, p < 0.0001) and 6-MMPN levels (10.60 vs. 3.62, p = 0.006) were significantly different between the non-relapsed and relapsed groups (See Table 2). No significant differences were observed in the other variables.

Relationships between the post-therapy ARR and the erythrocyte concentrations of 6-TGNs and 6-MMPNs

The normalized erythrocyte concentrations of 6-TGNs and 6-MMPNs followed a normal distribution. However, ARR improvement did not follow a normal distribution. Higher ARR improvements were significantly correlated with higher erythrocyte concentrations of both 6-TGNs (correlation coefficient (R) = 0.679, p < 0.0001) and 6-MMPNs (R = 0.493, p = 0.004) (See Table 3 and Fig. 2).

The ARR improvement (in log) was normally distributed. According to the multiple linear-regression, the ARR improvement (in log) was significantly influenced by the erythrocyte concentrations of 6-TGNs (adjusted R square = 0.206, constant = 0.417, standardized coefficients beta = −0.489, p = 0.013). The remaining variables, including the erythrocyte concentration of 6-MMPNs, onset age, disease duration, treatment duration, pretherapy and post-therapy EDSS scores, mean CSF protein, mean concentration of CSF IgG and the CSF IgG index, were excluded from the analysis due to underpowered statistical significance (p > 0.05) (See Table 4).

Discussion

The AZA treatment had a good efficacy in the NMOSD patients, and dramatic reductions in the EDSS scores (from 5.21 to 2.57, p < 0.0001) and ARR values (from 1.41 to 0.36, p < 0.0001) were observed. These results may be partially due to the concomitant use of corticosteroids, which was reported in the literature [6, 24]. The reduced ARR in our study was consistent with two large cohort studies in which the ARR decreased from 2.20 to 0.89 (p < 0.0001) and from 1.5 to 0 (p < 0.00005) [3, 5].

Elsone et al. posed an interesting question of whether the apparent reduction in relapses was simply a 'regression to the mean,' reflecting the natural course of the illness, or an immune-suppression effect of the AZA treatment [3]. In our study, no significant differences were observed in the pretherapy EDSS scores or onset of immunological status, including the CSF protein, CSF IgG index and serum AQP4-IgGs, between the relapsed and non-relapsed groups, and none of above parameters were correlated with the ARR improvement, which indicated homogeneity in individual disease activities. Therefore, we explored the relationships between the concentrations of the AZA metabolites and the post-therapy ARR. The mean normalized 6-TGNs levels (1.12 vs. 0.70, p < 0.0001) and mean normalized 6-MMPNs levels (10.60 vs. 3.62, p = 0.006) were significantly higher in the non-relapsed patients than in the relapsed patients. A greater ARR improvement was correlated with higher erythrocyte concentrations of 6-TGNs (R = 0.679, p < 0.0001) and 6-MMPNs (R = 0.493, p = 0.004). 6-TGNs are the main immunosuppressive compounds and have been proposed to induce the activation of non-specific apoptotic pathways in proliferating lymphocytes by distorting DNA and weakening its repair system, which leads to apoptosis [25]. 6-MMPNs, which are strong inhibitors of purine de novo synthesis (PDNS), can block the proliferation of various types of lymphocyte lines [26]. In addition, the AZA metabolites can also induce a very specific apoptosis pathway in the CD4+ subset of CD28 co-stimulated T lymphocytes [12]. NMOSD is a CNS immunological disease that can be

Before AZA										Patient	After AZA	
10y	9y	8y	7y	6y	5y	4y	3y	2y	1y	N	1y	2y
						/|	√		√	1		
					/|	√	√	√	√	2		
								/|	√ √	3	√	
√					√		√		√ √	4		
		/|	√	√	√	√		√	√ √	5		
√		√		√	√		√		√	6	√	√
				/|	√	√	√ √		√ √	7		
								/|	√	8		
								/|	√	9		
							/|	√	√ √	10	√	√
								/|	√	11		√
								/|	√	12		
							/|	√	√	13		√
			/|	√			√	√		14	√	√
								/|	√	15		
								/|	√	16		
							/|	√ √	√ √	17	√	√ √
√	√	√	√	√	√	√		√	√	18		√
							/|	√	√ √	19		
						/|	√		√	20		√
√	√	√	√	√						21		
								/|	√	22		
						/|	√ √	√ √	√	23		√
							/|	√	√ √	24		
						/|			√	25		
								/|	√	26		√
				/|	√	√	√	√ √		27		
√	√				√					28		
√	√	√		√			√			29		
								/|	√	30		
	/|	√		√		√				31		
							/|	√ √	√	32	√	

Fig. 1 The individual relapse times of each patient within 10 years before AZA therapy and 2 years after AZA therapy. "√" denotes the time of relapse. "I" denotes the beginning of AZA therapy. "/" indicates not available

Table 2 The difference of related variables between non-relapsed and relapsed groups

Variable	Non-relapsed (n = 20)	Relapsed (n = 12)	Mean Difference	Std. Error Difference	p-value
Age of onset, year	33.35	33.16	−0.183	4.740	0.969
Mean BMI	23.89	24.63	0.741	1.415	0.604
Disease duration, months	80.40	94.17	13.77	25.81	0.589
Duration of AZA therapy, months	22.10	20.50	−1.6	2.278	0.488
Mean CSF protein, mg/dl	39.82	41.43	1.613	13.275	0.904
Mean Concentration of CSF IgG, mg/ml	0.040	0.032	−0.008	0.014	0.577
CSF IgG index (n%)	0.546	0.494	−0.519	0.039	0.199
Serum anti-AQP4 antibodies (n%)	10 (50%)	4 (33.3%)	/	/	0.471
Pre-therapy EDSS score	5.17	5.29	/	/	0.687
Post- therapy EDSS score	2.43	2.83	/	/	0.893
Normalized concentration of 6-TGNs	1.12	0.70	−0.418	0.09	<0.0001*
Normalized concentration of 6-MMPNs	10.60	3.62	−6.983	2.32	0.006*

NMOSD, *AZA* Azathioprine, *BMI* Body mass index, *ARR* Annual relapse rate, *AQP4* anti-aquaporin 4, *EDSS* Expanded disability status scale, *6-TGN* 6-thioguanine nucleotides, *6-MMPN* 6-methylmercaptopurine nucleotides, *CSF* cerebrospinal fluid, *IgG* Immunoglobulin G. All two-tailed *P*-value <0.05 was considered statistically significant

Table 3 The correlation between ARR improvements and normalized erythrocyte concentrations of AZA metabolites

Variable	R	*P*-value
Normalized Concentration of 6-TGNs	0.679	<0.0001*
Normalized Concentration of MMPNs	0.493	0.004*

6-TGN 6-thioguanine nucleotides, *6-MMPN* 6-methylmercaptopurine nucleotides, *R* Spearman's correlation coefficient. All two-tailed *P*-value <0.05 was considered statistically significant

mediated by various lymphocytes, including Th17 lymphocytes, B lymphocytes and plasma-blasts [27]. After inhibiting the proliferation of lymphocytes by high levels of 6-TGNs and 6-MMPNs, the activation of immunoreactions decreased, and the mean ARR of the NMOSD patients subsequently declined.

The immunosuppressive effect of AZA was hypothesized to be achieved via a balanced contribution of pro-apoptotic (6-TGNs) and anti-metabolic (methylated ribonucleotides) pathways [8]. However, we found that the ARR improvement was only significantly influenced by the erythrocyte concentration of 6-TGNs (standardized coefficients beta = −0.489, p = 0.013), which could be due to the pro-apoptosis pathways in which lymphocytes are induced by 6-TGNs, causing widespread damage to lymphocytes in the short-term treatment, and the lethality of the anti-metabolic effect increased with the gradual accumulation of 6-TGNs levels in the long-term treatment [8]. Therefore, we believe that 6-TGNs may play a more important role in the immunosuppressive efficacy than previously thought, particularly during the early remission phase of NMOSD.

Furthermore, the internal variables that influence the erythrocyte concentrations of the AZA metabolites are unknown. The genetic polymorphisms of TPMT [28, 29] can affect TPMT activity, which directly regulates the formation of 6-MMPNs and subsequently influences the 6-TGNs concentration. However, in some recently published articles, no correlation among TPMT activity, 6-TGNs levels and 6-MMPNs levels was observed [30]. We found that rs10868138 (*SLC28A3*) was associated with a higher erythrocyte concentration of 6-TGNs, and rs12378361 (*SLC28A3*) was associated with a lower erythrocyte concentration of 6-TGNs in our former study [21]. The *SLC28A3* gene families correspond to human concentrative nucleoside transporters 3 (CNT3), which appears to be the best drug transporter because it can efficiently transport most of the pyrimidine and purine nucleoside analogs [31]. Our results indicated that the nucleoside transporter encoded by *SLC28A3* (rs10868138) may participate in the metabolism of AZA by transporting 6-TGNs out of the cells, and *SLC28A3* (rs12378361) may help transport 6-TGNs into the cells. In addition to its expression in the membranes of erythrocytes, CNT3 is also present in primary lymphocytes [32], monocytes, monocyte-derived macrophages, and monocyte-derived dendritic cell membranes [33]. Therefore, genetic polymorphisms of *SLC28A3* (encoding CNT3) may influence the activity of NMOSD by altering the concentration of intracellular 6-TGNs in various immune cells. However, considering that *SLC28A3* is not the only factor that influences the concentration of intracellular 6-TGNs, the direct correlation between the polymorphisms of *SLC28A3* and the outcomes of NMOSD must be investigation in further studies.

The disease activity in NMOSD is highly variable among individual patients, and some patients experience AZA efficacy after 6 months to 18 months in clinical practice. Some limitations were present in this study, including the use of patients from a single center, the small sample size and the short follow-up durations.

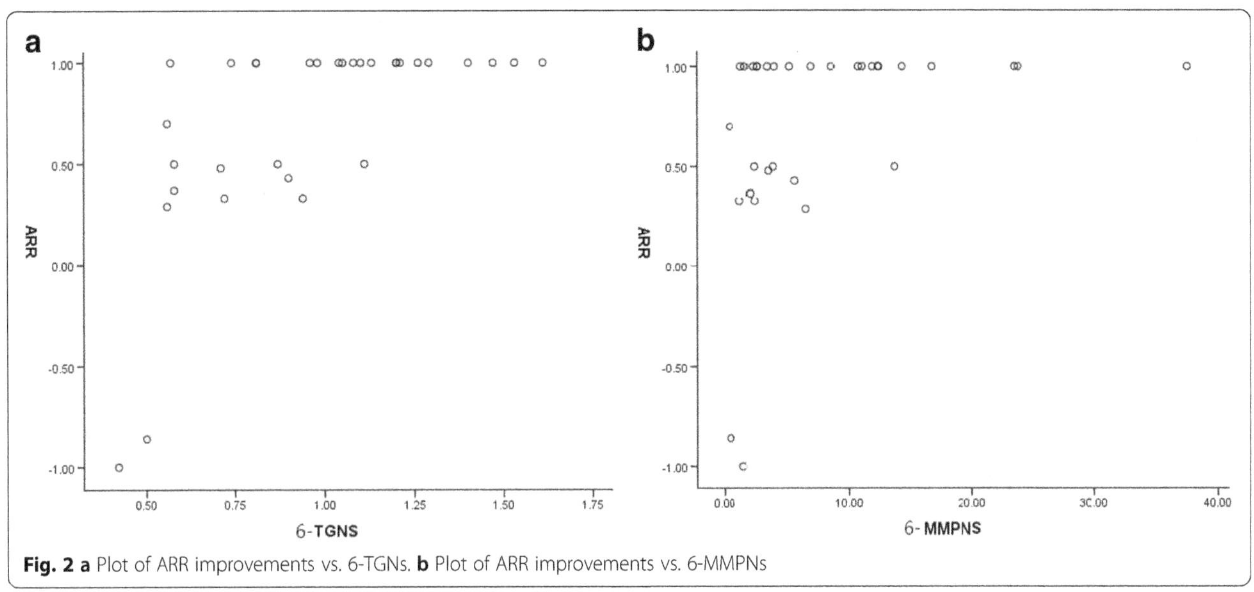

Fig. 2 a Plot of ARR improvements vs. 6-TGNs. **b** Plot of ARR improvements vs. 6-MMPNs

Table 4 The linear- regression between multiple variables and ARR improvements (in log)

Variable	Standardized coefficients- Beta	T	*P*-value
Constant (SE)	0.417 (0.116)	3.580	0.002
Normalized Concentration of 6-TGNs	−0.489	−2.689	0.013*
Excluded variables			
Age of onset, year	0.156	0.853	0.403
Disease duration, months	0.094	0.509	0.616
Treatment duration, months	−0.200	−1.106	0.281
Pre-therapy EDSS score	0.034	0.176	0.862
Post-therapy EDSS score	0.050	0.266	0.793
Mean CSF protein, mg/dl	−0.038	−0.198	0.845
Mean Concentration of CSF IgG, mg/ml	−0.158	−0.855	0.402
CSF IgG index (n%)	−0.287	−1.636	0.116
Normalized Concentration of MMPNs	−0.150	−0.751	0.461

NMOSD, AZA Azathioprine, *BMI* Body mass index, *ARR* Annual relapse rate, *EDSS* Expanded disability status scale, *6-TGN* 6-thioguanine nucleotides, *6-MMPN* 6-methylmercaptopurine nucleotides. All *P*-value <0.05 was considered statistically significant

Our preliminary conclusions must be verified in further large cohort studies with long follow-up durations.

Conclusion

AZA treatment in NMOSD patients can dramatically reduce post-therapy EDSS scores and ARRs, and this effect is significantly correlated with the erythrocyte concentrations of AZA metabolites, particularly 6-TGNs. A higher erythrocyte concentration of 6-TGNs is associated with better efficacy of AZA below the safe upper limits.

Abbreviations

6-MMPNs: 6-methylmercaptopurine nucleotides; 6-MP: 6-mercaptopurine; 6-TG: 6-thioguanine; 6-TGNs: 6-thioguanine nucleotides; ALL: Acute lymphoblastic leukemia; AQP4-IgG: Anti-aquaporin 4 antibodies; ARR: Annual relapse rates; AZA: Azathioprine; CNS: Central nervous system; EDSS: Expanded disability status scale; HGPRT: Hypoxanthine-guanine phosphoribosyltransferase; HWE: Hardy-Weinberg equilibrium; MAF: Minor allele frequency; NMOSD: Neuromyelitis optica spectrum disorders; PDNS: Purine de novo synthesis; SD: Standard deviation; SLC28A: Solute carrier family 28; SLC29A: Solute carrier family 29; SNPs: Single nucleotide polymorphisms; TPMT: Thiopurine S-methyltransferase; TPNs: Thiopurine nucleotides

Acknowledgements

Not applicable.

Funding

The design of the study and collection, analysis, and interpretation of data and in writing the manuscript were all supported by the Beijing Municipal Science & Technology Commission (No. Z141107002514124).

Authors' contributions

XDL: study design, data analysis, manuscript writing and revising. SM: study design, azathioprine metabolites concentration detection and analysis. XG: study design, serum and CSF sample collection. HZ: patient's clinical information collection and follow-up. LY: azathioprine metabolites concentration detection. AZ: patient's clinical information collection and follow-up. YL: patient's clinical information collection and follow-up. XGL: Genetic variants and azathioprine metabolites concentration detection and analysis. ZZ: study design and manuscript revising. XZ: study design and manuscript revising. All authors read and approved the final manuscript.

Competing interests

The authors declare that they have no competing interests.

Author details

[1]Neuroinfection and Neuroimmunology Center, Department of Neurology, Beijing Tiantan Hospital, Capital Medical University, 6 TiantanXili, Dongcheng District, Beijing 100050, People's Republic of China. [2]China National Clinical Research Center for Neurological Diseases, Beijing Tiantan Hospital, Capital Medical University, 6 TiantanXili, Dongcheng District, Beijing 100050, People's Republic of China. [3]Department of Pharmacy, Beijing Tiantan Hospital, Capital Medical University, 6 TiantanXili, Dongcheng District, Beijing 100050, People's Republic of China.

References

1. Wingerchuk DM, Banwell B, Bennett JL, Cabre P, Carroll W, Chitnis T, et al. International consensus diagnostic criteria for neuromyelitis optica spectrum disorders. Neurology. 2015;85:177 –89.
2. Sellner J, Boggild M, Clanet M, Hintzen RQ, Illes Z, Montalban X, et al. EFNS guidelines on diagnosis and management of neuromyelitis optica. Eur J Neurol. 2010;17:1019–32.
3. Elsone L, Kitley J, Luppe S, Lythgoe D, Mutch K, Jacob S, et al. Long-term efficacy, tolerability and retention rate of azathioprine in 103 aquaporin-4 antibody-positive neuromyelitis optica spectrum disorder patients: a multicentre retrospective observational study from the UK. Mult Scler. 2014;20:1533–40.
4. Mandler RN, Ahmed W, Dencoff JE. Devic's neuromyelitis optica: a prospective study of seven patients treated with prednisone and azathioprine. Neurology. 1998;51:1219–20.
5. Costanzi C, Matiello M, Lucchinetti CF, Weinshenker BG, Pittock SJ, Mandrekar J, et al. Azathioprine: tolerability, efficacy, and predictors of benefit in neuromyelitis optica. Neurology. 2011;77:659–66.
6. Qiu W, Kermode AG, Li R, Dai Y, Wang Y, Wang J, et al. Azathioprine plus corticosteroid treatment in Chinese patients with neuromyelitis optica. J Clin Neurosci. 2015;22:1178–82.
7. Amin J, Huang B, Yoon J, Shih DQ. Update 2014: advances to optimize 6-mercaptopurine and azathioprine to reduce toxicity and improve efficacy in the management of IBD. Inflamm Bowel Dis. 2015;21:445–52.
8. Cara CJ, Pena AS, Sans M, Rodrigo L, Guerrero-Esteo M, Hinojosa J, et al. Reviewing the mechanism of action of thiopurine drugs: towards a new paradigm in clinical practice. Med Sci Monit. 2004;10:Ra247–54.
9. Sahasranaman S, Howard D, Roy S. Clinical pharmacology and pharmacogenetics of thiopurines. Eur J Clin Pharmacol. 2008;64:753–67.
10. Fung C, Vaughn DJ, Mitra N, Ciosek SL, Vardhanabhuti S, Nathanson KL, et al. Chemotherapy refractory testicular germ cell tumor is associated with a variant in armadillo repeat gene deleted in Velco-cardio-facial syndrome (ARVCF). Front Endocrinol (Lausanne). 2012;3:163.

11. Fairchild CR, Maybaum J, Kennedy KA. Concurrent unilateral chromatid damage and DNA strand breakage in response to 6-thioguanine treatment. Biochem Pharmacol. 1986;35:3533–41.
12. Tiede I, Fritz G, Strand S, Poppe D, Dvorsky R, Strand D, et al. CD28-dependent Rac1 activation is the molecular target of azathioprine in primary human CD4+ T lymphocytes. J Clin Invest. 2003;111:1133–45.
13. Burnett HF, Tanoshima R, Chandranipapongse W, Madadi P, Ito S, Ungar WJ. Testing for thiopurine methyltransferase status for safe and effective thiopurine administration: a systematic review of clinical guidance documents. Pharmacogenomics J. 2014;14:493–502.
14. Salavaggione OE, Wang L, Wiepert M, Yee VC, Weinshilboum RM. Thiopurine S-methyltransferase pharmacogenetics: variant allele functional and comparative genomics. Pharmacogenet Genomics. 2005;15:801–15.
15. Collie-Duguid ES, Pritchard SC, Powrie RH, Sludden J, Collier DA, Li T, et al. The frequency and distribution of thiopurine methyltransferase alleles in Caucasian and Asian populations. Pharmacogenetics. 1999;9:37–42.
16. Umamaheswaran G, Kumar DK, Adithan C. Distribution of genetic polymorphisms of genes encoding drug metabolizing enzymes & drug transporters - a review with Indian perspective. Indian J Med Res. 2014;139:27–65.
17. Gray JH, Owen RP, Giacomini KM. The concentrative nucleoside transporter family, SLC28. Pflugers Arch. 2004;447:728–34.
18. Errasti-Murugarren E, Molina-Arcas M, Casado FJ, Pastor-Anglada M. A splice variant of the SLC28A3 gene encodes a novel human concentrative nucleoside transporter-3 (hCNT3) protein localized in the endoplasmic reticulum. FASEB J. 2009;23:172–82.
19. Badagnani I, Chan W, Castro RA, Brett CM, Huang CC, Stryke D, et al. Functional analysis of genetic variants in the human concentrative nucleoside transporter 3 (CNT3; SLC28A3). Pharmacogenomics J. 2005;5:157–65.
20. Fotoohi AK, Lindqvist M, Peterson C, Albertioni F. Involvement of the concentrative nucleoside transporter 3 and equilibrative nucleoside transporter 2 in the resistance of T-lymphoblastic cell lines to thiopurines. Biochem Biophys Res Commun. 2006;343:208–15.
21. Mei S, Li X, Gong X, Li X, Yang L, Zhou H, Liu Y, Zhou A, Zhu L, Zhang X et al. LC-MS/MS analysis of erythrocyte thiopurine nucleotides and their association with genetic variants in patients with neuromyelitis optica spectrum disorders taking azathioprine. Ther Drug Monit 2016; doi: 10.1097/FTD.0000000000000362.
22. Ketelslegers IA, Modderman PW, Vennegoor A, Killestein J, Hamann D, Hintzen RQ. Antibodies against aquaporin-4 in neuromyelitis optica: distinction between recurrent and monophasic patients. Mult Scler. 2011;17:1527–30.
23. Rae W, Burke G, Pinto A. A study of the utility of azathioprine metabolite testing in myasthenia gravis. J Neuroimmunol. 2016;293:82–5.
24. Watanabe S, Misu T, Miyazawa I, Nakashima I, Shiga Y, Fujihara K, et al. Low-dose corticosteroids reduce relapses in neuromyelitis optica: a retrospective analysis. Mult Scler. 2007;13:968–74.
25. Swann PF, Waters TR, Moulton DC, Xu YZ, Zheng Q, Edwards M, et al. Role of postreplicative DNA mismatch repair in the cytotoxic action of thioguanine. Science (New York, NY). 1996;273:1109–11.
26. Elion GB. The purine path to chemotherapy. Science (New York, NY). 1989;244:41–7.
27. Jasiak-Zatonska M, Kalinowska-Lyszczarz A, Michalak S, Kozubski W. The immunology of Neuromyelitis Optica-current knowledge, clinical implications, controversies and future perspectives. Int J Mol Sci. 2016;17:273.
28. Lu HF, Shih MC, Chang YS, Chang JY, Ko YC, Chang SJ, et al. Molecular analysis of thiopurine S-methyltransferase alleles in Taiwan aborigines and Taiwanese. J Clin Pharm Ther. 2006;31:93–8.
29. Umamaheswaran G, Krishna Kumar D, Kayathiri D, Rajan S, Shewade DG, Dkhar SA, et al. Inter and intra-ethnic differences in the distribution of the molecular variants of TPMT, UGT1A1 and MDR1 genes in the south Indian population. Mol Biol Rep. 2012;39:6343–51.
30. Lowry PW, Franklin CL, Weaver AL, Pike MG, Mays DC, Tremaine WJ, et al. Measurement of thiopurine methyltransferase activity and azathioprine metabolites in patients with inflammatory bowel disease. Gut. 2001;49:665–70.
31. Fernandez-Calotti PX, Colomer D, Pastor-Anglada M. Translocation of nucleoside analogs across the plasma membrane in hematologic malignancies. Nucleosides Nucleotides Nucleic Acids. 2011;30:1324–40.
32. Molina-Arcas M, Marce S, Villamor N, Huber-Ruano I, Casado FJ, Bellosillo B, et al. Equilibrative nucleoside transporter-2 (hENT2) protein expression correlates with ex vivo sensitivity to fludarabine in chronic lymphocytic leukemia (CLL) cells. Leukemia. 2005;19:64–8.
33. Minuesa G, Purcet S, Erkizia I, Molina-Arcas M, Bofill M, Izquierdo-Useros N, et al. Expression and functionality of anti-human immunodeficiency virus and anticancer drug uptake transporters in immune cells. J Pharmacol Exp Ther. 2008;324:558–67.

Nasal administration of the neuroprotective candidate NeuroEPO to healthy volunteers

Orestes Santos-Morales[1], Alina Díaz-Machado[2], Daise Jiménez-Rodríguez[3], Yaisel Pomares-Iturralde[1], Tatiana Festary-Casanovas[3], Carlos A. González-Delgado[2], Sonia Pérez-Rodríguez[2], Eulalia Alfonso-Muñoz[2], Carmen Viada-González[1], Patricia Piedra-Sierra[1], Idrian García-García[3*], Daniel Amaro-González[1] and for the NeuroEPO Study Group

Abstract

Background: Delivery of therapeutic agents as erythropoietin (EPO) into Central Nervous System through intranasal route could benefit patients with neurological disorders. A new nasal formulation containing a non-hematopoietic recombinant EPO (NeuroEPO) has shown neuroprotective actions in preclinical models. In the current study, the safety of NeuroEPO was evaluated for the first time in humans.

Methods: A phase I, randomized, parallel, open-label study was carried out in healthy volunteers. They received, intranasally, 1 mg of NeuroEPO every 8 h during 4 days (Group A) or 0.5 mg of NeuroEPO (Group B) with the same schedule. The working hypothesis was that intranasal NeuroEPO produce <10% of severe adverse reactions in the evaluated groups. Therefore, a rigorous assessment of possible adverse events was carried out, which included tolerance of the nasal mucosa and the effect on hematopoietic activity. Clinical safety evaluation was daily during treatment and laboratory tests were done before and on days 5 and 14 after starting treatment.

Results: Twenty-five volunteers, 56% women, with a mean age of 27 yrs. were included. Twelve of them received the highest NeuroEPO dose. Twenty types of adverse events occurred, with headache (20%) and increase of hepatic enzymes (20%) as the most reported ones. Nasopharyngeal itching was the most common local event but only observed in four patients (16%), all of them from the lowest dose group. About half of the events were very probably or probably caused by the studied product. Most of the events were mild (95.5%), did not require treatment (88.6%) and were completely resolved (81.8%). No severe adverse events were reported. During the study the hematopoietic variables were kept within reference values.

Conclusions: NeuroEPO was a safe product, well tolerated at the nasal mucosa level and did not stimulate erythropoiesis in healthy volunteers.

Keywords: Non-hematopoietic recombinant erythropoietin, NeuroEPO, Stroke, Neurodegenerative diseases, Healthy volunteers, Safety, Hematopoietic activity

* Correspondence: idrian.garcia@cidem.cu
[3]Clinical Trials Group, Research Direction, Center for Drug Research and Development (CIDEM), Ave. 26 and Puentes Grandes, No. 1605, Nuevo Vedado, Havana, Cuba
Full list of author information is available at the end of the article

Background

The search of neuroprotective agents in stroke has been intended for more than 25 years to interfere with the molecular events taking place into nerve cells during or after exposure to ischemia. Nevertheless, none of them have met efficacy and safety criteria in controlled clinical trials [1, 2]. Neuroprotective actions of recombinant human erythropoietin (rHu-EPO) have been evaluated both in vitro and in vivo, demonstrating antiapoptotic, antioxidative, antiinflammatory, neurotrophic and angiogenic properties [3, 4]. However, rHu-EPO's action on erythropoiesis could be inconvenient by triggering an increase in cardiovascular and thromboembolic events [5].

The use of EPO, similar to that produced in the brain during hypoxia, without erythropoietic but with neuroprotective activity, could be preferable [6]. Such molecule might be administered by delivery to the upper third of nasal cavity to contact both the olfactory [7] and trigeminal [8] neural pathways. This method has been reported to effectively bypass the blood-brain barrier (BBB) providing a direct connection of therapeutic proteins including EPO with the Central Nervous System (CNS) to treat neurodegenerative disorders such as Alzheimer's and stroke while reducing systemic exposure [9, 10]. By these pathways, intranasal EPO is able to rapidly reaches many brain regions [11, 12] to effectively protect against focal cerebral ischemia [13].

Center for Drug Research and Development (CIDEM, in Spanish) developed a nasal formulation containing EPO with non-hematopoietic activity produced by the Center of Molecular Immunology (CIM, in Spanish). This formulation named NeuroEPO incorporates bioadhesive polymers and other ingredients which increase the residence time in the nasal cavity to enhance its therapeutic effect [14–16].

Mongolian gerbils treated with 30 μg of rHu-EPO by intranasal route daily during 4 days showed a lower expression of clinical signs of ischemia and edema and a better functional integrity compared with vehicle-treated animals. The molecule was detected either in the olfactory bulbs or in the cerebellum 5 min after administration [17]. Mortality of NeuroEPO-treated gerbils decreased after surgery, and the sensory and motor function was significantly improved. Histopathological mapping showed that NeuroEPO significantly reduced the delayed neuronal death in the brain [18]. NeuroEPO had a better neuroprotective effect than systemic rHu-EPO, evidenced by the significant improvement of neurological, cognitive, and histological status [19, 20]. Additionally, NeuroEPO also improved significantly neurologic behavior in rats that which underwent transitory focal ischemia, decreasing infarction area [21].

This product did not stimulate the erythropoiesis when it was administered through intranasal route in several rodent models [22, 23]. In the *Macaca fascicularis* model a 0.15% of NeuroEPO dose was determined in the cerebrospinal fluid after 15 min of intranasal administration. In this specie treatment related-changes in blood parameters were neither observed [24].

These results suggested that nasal route may be a successful, non-invasive and a safe mode to brain access for non-hematopoietic EPO, which can be used as neuroprotective agent in patients with neurological diseases. Nevertheless, is necessary to obtain primary evidences of the tolerability of NeuroEPO in humans, which will allow subsequent clinical trials to evaluate its efficacy. The present clinical investigation aims to evaluate the safety of NeuroEPO in healthy volunteers using two dosing schedules by nasal route.

Methods

A phase I, randomized, uncontrolled, parallel, open-label safety study was carried out at the National Center for Toxicology, in Havana, a certified reference unit for this type of studies.

Subjects

Cuban citizens of both genders, aged between 18 and 40 years, without organic or psychological diseases in the questioning and non-symptoms or signs at physical examination and laboratory tests were included in the trial. The absence of HIV and hepatitis B and C virus infection markers in serum was required. Exclusion criteria were: women who are pregnant or breastfeeding, hypersensitivity to EPO or to any other of the ingredients of the formulation, rhinitis, nasal septum deviation, mental disorders, history of alcoholism, record of chronic diseases, treatment with any drug in the previous 15 days, surgical intervention in the previous 6 months, blood donations in the previous 3 months and participation in a clinical trial during the prior 6 months. No more than 14 days between pre-screening and the beginning of the trial were allowed. Subjects could withdraw from the trial voluntarily, due to occurrence of severe adverse events, or by the appearance of any exclusion criteria.

Hypothesis and treatment

In this study was expected that after intranasal administration of NeuroEPO the frequency of severe adverse events certainly caused by the product was less than 10%.

NeuroEPO [CIMAB S.A, Havana, Cuba] was a stabilized liquid formulation, multidose vials, containing 6 mg (1 mg/mL) of non-hematopoietic rHu-EPO, produced in Chinese hamster ovary (CHO) cells. Each vial also contains buffer salts, polysorbate 80, sodium EDTA, NaCl, benzalkonium chloride, HPMC F4 M, and water for injection to complete 6 mL. A placebo formulation containing the same ingredients (except EPO) was also used.

Before administration, vials were kept at rest room temperature during 50 min. After this time, vials were gently shaken in form of eight, to guarantee homogenization before volume extraction. A graduated type-insulin syringe was used to administer the prefixed doses.

The Maximum Safe Starting Dose (MSSD) in healthy humans was calculated according to established guidelines [25]. This dose, estimated from the whole preclinical data, was 3.3 mg for 60 kg average bodyweight. Due to practical reasons MSSD was 3 mg daily for this clinical trial. A second dose of daily 1.5 mg was also evaluated. Taking into account that intranasal drug administration capacity is limited by the maximum volume that can be used [26, 27], it was decided to divide doses into three administrations (every 8 h). These treatments were extended for 4 days considering the data from ischemia models, acute and sub-acute toxicology and previous clinical trials with rHu-EPO [17–23, 28, 29].

Subjects were distributed according to a computer-generated simple random number list to two groups of treatment with 15 individuals each one. Subjects from Group A received 1 mg of NeuroEPO every 8 h during 4 days by nasal route. Subjects included in Group B received 0.5 mg of NeuroEPO with the same schedule, by the same route of administration. Each multidose NeuroEPO vial could be used in five subjects from Group A and ten subjects from Group B.

For each group, doses were given in two moments with the same volumes. For Group A, firstly, a volume of 250 μL (0.25 mg) of NeuroEPO into each nostril was applied and 15 min later the same application was repeated to obtain a final volume of 500 μL (0.5 mg) in each nostril. For Group B, firstly, a volume of 250 μL (0.25 mg) of NeuroEPO into each nostril was applied and 15 min later 250 μL of placebo were administered into each nostril to obtain a final volume of 250 μL (0.25 mg) in each nostril. These procedures were carried out daily at 8:00 am, 4:00 pm and 12:00 am in all the individuals.

The products were administered slowly into one of the nostrils, drop by drop, to assure a full instillation into the nasal mucous. The subjects were lying in *decubitus supine* position, with the head dorsally bowed 45 degrees from the axis of the body, to guarantee the product bypass the BBB and reach their site of action. At the same time a pressure in the opposite nostril was exerted. After this, the volunteers rested 1 min and the method was applied in the other nostril. They were requested to sustain a normal breathing during the process.

Other concomitant treatments could be administered to mitigate adverse events, after medical consent. None of these treatments could affect the results by interactions or direct effects on the tested safety variables.

Volunteers were regularly checked for vital signs and adverse manifestations during the study. They were hospitalized during the 4 days of treatment and were given discharge the following day, after evaluation. Two weeks after beginning the treatment, final evaluation was done under outpatient conditions.

Safety evaluation

Tolerability was monitored during the whole study by means of adverse events control. Data related to adverse events were obtained through questioning or were spontaneously referred by the subject. When the event was presented, the medical investigator acted according to their nature and severity taking the required actions (pharmacological or not) for their reduction and elimination.

Events were considered severe if produce subject's death, threatens subject's life, requires or prolongs hospitalization or produce a significant or persistent disability. Additionally, those events that required medical or surgical intervention to prevent the occurrence of bronchial allergic spasm at home, blood dyscrasias and seizures that do not provoke hospitalization were considered as severe.

The medical terminology for adverse events and their intensity classification (grades 1–5) was applied according to the Common Terminology Criteria for Adverse Events [30]. The causal relationship was classified as very probable/certain, probable (likely), possible, unlikely, not related or unassessable/unclassifiable, according to WHO criteria for causality [31].

Blood samples were taken for hematological and biochemical determinations before (day 0) and after treatment (day 5, day 14). Hematological counts (reticulocytes, hemoglobin, hematocrit, leukocytes), coagulation parameters (platelet count, partial thromboplastin and prothrombin times) and blood chemistry (glycemia, creatinine, urea, liver enzymes) were done according to usual clinical laboratory procedures at the Clinical Laboratory of the Center for Medical-Surgical Research, Havana, Cuba, a laboratory certified by the Cuban Regulatory Agency. Advanced automated analyzers (Mindray, Shenzhen, China; Cobas, Roche Diagnostics, Basel, Switzerland) were used for these purposes. After treatment, those values outside reference limits established by this laboratory were considered as adverse events excepting transient and very close variations without clinical relevance. Laboratory evaluations were done blindly regarding the subject' group allocation.

Before and after each administration and in each evaluation time, vital signs taking and physical examination were carried out. The presence of toxicity signs in the nasal mucous, such as: redness, swelling and nasal congestion was evaluated by means of thorough medical examination of the nasal cavity by the same Otorhinolaryngology Specialist.

Statistical analysis

Sample size was determined in correspondence with the aim of the study, the international trend in this type of study, the predominant descriptive nature of the analysis of the variables and the need to minimize the number of subjects exposed to the investigational medicinal product [32, 33]. A sample size of 30 subjects (15 per group) was chosen. The possibility of compensating withdrawals was not foreseen.

Data were double entered and validated and then imported into SPSS for Windows (version 15.0, IBM Analytics 2006, Armonk, North Castle, NY, USA) and Epidat (version 3.1, Directorate General of Public Health (Xunta de Galicia) 2006, Santiago de Compostela, Spain) for further analysis. Continuous variables were expressed as mean ± standard deviation (SD) or median ± interquartile range (QR) and categorical variables (e.g. adverse events) were given as frequencies and percentages. For laboratory measurements and vital signs normality analysis (Kolmogorov-Smirnov's test or Shapiro Wilk's test) and homogeneity of variance (Levene's test) were carried out. These variables were analyzed through paired analysis (non-parametrical Wilcoxon's test) comparing initial values with those obtained on 5th and 14th day for each group. Additionally, groups were compared at each time using the Mann-Whitney's U test. Significance level was 0.05.

Results

After medical check-up, 30 apparently healthy volunteers were selected among a universe of 93 subjects who expressed their consent to participate in the study (Fig. 1). The causes of no inclusion were: abnormal clinical laboratory values (27 subjects), presence of organic or psychic disease (13), presence of rhinitis (10), blood donation in the previous 3 months (3), nasal septum deviation (7) and voluntary abandonment before inclusion (3).

Included volunteers were randomly assigned to one of the two treatment groups (15 per group). However, five withdrawals, three of them from Group A, occurred prior to first dose, four were voluntary abandonment and the other case was the appearance of an exclusion criterion (rhinitis). Consequently, 25 subjects, 12 from Group A and 13 from Group B received NeuroEPO treatment. This final sample was big enough to study the hypothesis. During the study, there were no losses in the follow-up and evaluation and analysis included all subjects (Fig. 1).

Groups of treatment were homogenous according to demographic and baseline characteristics as shown in Table 1. Women slightly prevailed (56%) and white and non-white skin color proportions were similar. The subjects weighed around 65 Kg and were 167 cm tall; the mean age was 27 years.

Eighty percent of treated subjects reported at least one clinical manifestation (local or systemic) or laboratory alteration (Table 2). Individuals with adverse events were two thirds in Group A and 92.3%. in Group B. Sixteen types of adverse events occurred during the trial, 13 recorded during clinical examinations and three identified during the monitoring of hematological and biochemical parameters. There were seven types of events in Group A and 12 in Group B. Upper respiratory tract events (related with nasal administration) prevailed in Group B as observed. The groups had in common three types of events: nasal mucous ardor, headache and increase of liver enzymes.

The most frequent adverse events were headache and increase of liver enzymes, but both were reported in only two subjects from Group A and three subjects from Group B. Nasopharyngeal itching was the most common local event, only detected in four volunteers from Group B. Other events, such as: nasal mucous ardor, sneezing, fever and anemia occurred in two or three subjects in general. The rest of events, mostly systemic, were recorded in a single subject of one or the other group (Table 2).

The number of adverse events was also superior in the Group B since 61.4% of the 44 reports arose in this group (Table 3). One subject from Group B had the maximum number of reports with seven. Non-severe adverse events were recorded, thus no subject withdrew from the trial due to adverse reactions. Regarding intensity, events were mostly (95.5%) classified as grade 1 (mild). Only two events (headache and epicondylitis), both in patients from Group A, were classified as grade 2 (moderate).

The number of events with certain or probable causal relationship rounded 50%. In the Group A 47% of the events had a probable relation, none certain, whereas in Group B 41% of the events were certainly caused by the product. These last ones were those produced at the site of administration. Only some systemic events or laboratory alterations (mostly in Group B) were unlikely or not related to NeuroEPO treatment. Just one increase of hepatic enzymes was unclassifiable (Table 3).

Most of the events did not require treatment (88.6%) and were well solved (81.8%). It was necessary

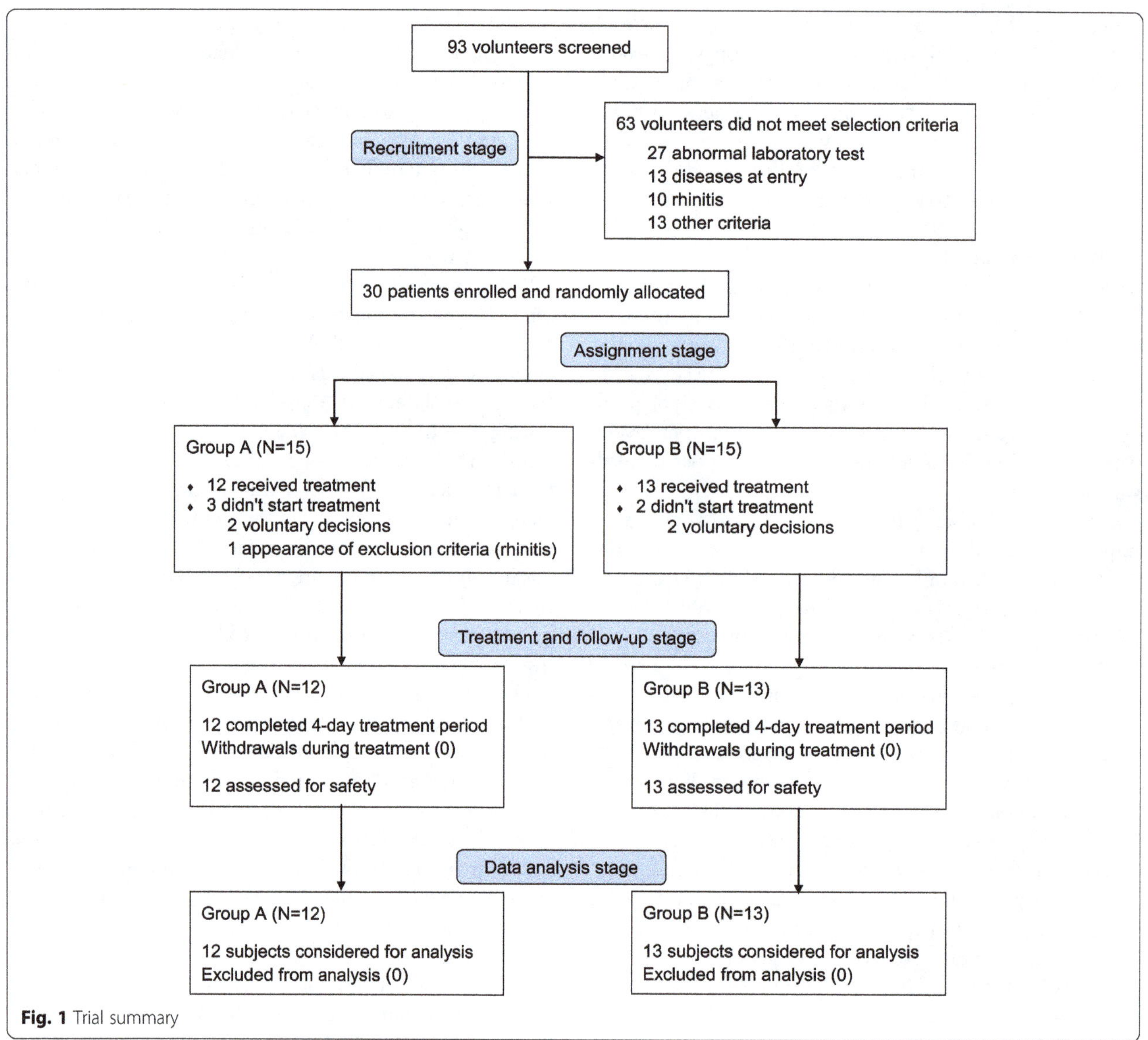

Fig. 1 Trial summary

to administer dipyrone to treat headache and fever. Ibuprofen was used to treat epicondylitis. Only seven events, five of them in the Group B, persisted at the end of the study, but these were mostly alterations in laboratory parameters which returned spontaneously to normal values, few weeks later.

Vital signs did not change significantly during the study in both groups (data non-shown). Otorhinolaryngological study proved normality in most of the subjects throughout the study, except for some individuals with the above-mentioned local events. Physical examination was also normal after the 4 days of treatment (day 5) as well as on the final evaluation (day 14).

Concerning hematological toxicity, values in both evaluation times were kept within normal ranges (Fig. 2, see legend). Some changes detected in reticulocytes count (Fig. 2a) and hematocrit Fig. 2c) had non-clinical significance. For hemoglobin, there were no significant changes throughout the study (Fig. 2b). A mild anemia was recorded in two subjects from Group B, whose values descended to 115 and 97 g/L, respectively, on day 14. Differences between groups of treatment were no significant at each time. Other clinical laboratory measurements were not markedly affected (data non-shown).

Discussion

The findings support the hypothesis that the frequency of severe adverse events following intranasal administration of NeuroEPO would be less than 10% since no severe events occurred. This is in accordance with the literature since the use of rHu-EPO in healthy subjects apparently does not affect

Table 1 Demographic and baseline characteristics of the subjects who received 1 mg (Group A) or 0.5 mg (Group B) of NeuroEPO every 8 h, during 4 days, by nasal route

Characteristic	Group A *N* = 12	Group B *N* = 13	Total *N* = 25
Female gender	7 (58.3%)	7 (53.8%)	14 (56.0%)
Skin color			
White	7 (58.3%)	6 (46.2%)	13 (52.0%)
Non-white	5 (41.7%)	7 (53.8%)	12 (48.0%)
Age (years)	28 ± 6	26 ± 4	27 ± 5
Weight (Kg)	67 ± 13	63 ± 10	65 ± 11
Height (cm)	164 ± 9	169 ± 11	167 ± 10

Data are reported as number of subjects (%) or mean ± standard deviation

physiological indexes and its use is safe for experimental purposes [34].

The current first NeuroEPO-in-human trial demonstrated the absence of hematopoietic activity according to the safety profile. This result is expected due to this EPO possesses a low content of sialic acid, a component that plays a key role in the preservation of EPO structure thereby avoiding its destruction by the liver. Low sialic acid content rHu-EPO molecules are rapidly metabolized by the liver and therefore eliminated without being able to exert their hematopoietic action [3]. This is the main expected safety benefit of NeuroEPO and has already been demonstrated in laboratory animals since the product did not modify hematopoietic activity even when used at high doses [23].

Table 2 Frequency of adverse events during the study

Adverse event	Group A *N* = 12	Group B *N* = 13	Total *N* = 25
Any adverse event	8 (66.7%)	12 (92.3%)	20 (80.0%)
Site of administration (local events)			
Nasopharyngeal itching	–	4 (30.8%)	4 (16.0%)
Nasal mucous ardor	1 (8.3%)	2 (15.4%)	3 (12.0%)
Sneezing	–	2 (15.4%)	2 (8.0%)
Reddened nasal mucous	–	1 (7.7%)	1 (4.0%)
Systemic events			
Headache	2 (16.7%)	3 (23.1%)	5 (20.0%)
Fever	2 (16.7%)	–	2 (8.0%)
Arterial hypertension	1 (8.3%)	–	1 (4.0%)
Diarrheas	–	1 (7.7%)	1 (4.0%)
Pruritus	–	1 (7.7%)	1 (4.0%)
Colics	–	1 (7.7%)	1 (4.0%)
Epicondylitis	1 (8.3%)	–	1 (4.0%)
Insomnia	–	1 (7.7%)	1 (4.0%)
Cough	–	1 (7.7%)	1 (4.0%)
Laboratory alterations			
Hepatic enzymes increased[a]	2 (16.7%)	3 (23.1%)	5 (20.0%)
Anemia[b]	–	2 (15.4%)	2 (8.0%)
Platelet count decreased[c]	1 (8.3%)	–	1 (4.0%)

Data are presented as number of individuals with each adverse reaction (%)
[a]ALT > 41 U/L (men) or >33 U/L (women); AST > 40 U/L (men) or >32 U/L (women); GGT > 60 U/L (men) or >40 U/L (women)
[b]Hgb: < 130 g/L (men) or <120 g/L (women)
[c] < 150 × 10^9 cells/L

Table 3 Characterization of the adverse events registered

Characteristic	Classification	Group A	Group B	Total
Number of events		17 (38.6%)	27 (61.4%)	44 (100%)
Severity	Non-severe	17 (100%)	27(100%)	44 (100%)
Intensity	Grade 1	15 (88.2%)	27 (100%)	42 (95.5%)
	Grade 2	2 (11.8%)	–	2 (4.5%)
Causality	Certain	–	11 (40.7%)	11 (25.0%)
	Probable	8 (47.1%)	2 (7.4%)	10 (22.7%)
	Possible	7 (41.1%)	5 (18.5%)	12 (27.3%)
	Unlikely	–	4 (14.8%)	4 (9.1%)
	Not related	2 (11.8%)	4 (14.8%)	6 (13.6%)
	Unclassifiable	–	1 (3.7%)	1 (2.3%)
Conduct	Pharmacotherapy	3 (17.7%)	1 (3.7%)	4 (9.1%)
	Other intervention	–	1 (3.7%)	1 (2.3%)
	Observational	14 (82.3%)	25 (92.6%)	39 (88.6%)
Result	Resolved	14 (82.3%)	22 (81.5%)	36 (81.8%)
	Improved	1 (5.9%)	–	1 (2.3%)
	Persisted	2 (11.8%)	5 (18.5%)	7 (15.9%)

Data are reported as number of events (%)

A good local tolerance was evidenced. The mild local adverse events described correspond to those observed in the preclinical studies both with NeuroEPO and controls in the nasal irritation test [23] and could also be considered common when this route of administration is used. The recorded events support the role of trigeminal pathway in the entrance of NeuroEPO to CNS. Sensory nerves of the afferent trigeminal system including myelinated Aδ-fibres and thin, non-myelinated C-fibres of the nasal mucosa transmit signals generating sensations, including itching and motor reflexes, such as sneezing [35]. The trigeminal nerve is also the primary nerve involved in headache [36].

Although rHu-EPO increases blood pressure in patients with chronic renal failure and cancer [37, 38], the mild event observed in one subject could be considered an isolated event within the framework of the study, considering that the rest of subjects preserved normal values.

A mild rise of the liver enzymes values was founded in some individuals. There is no history of increase of these enzymes in acute toxicological studies with NeuroEPO.

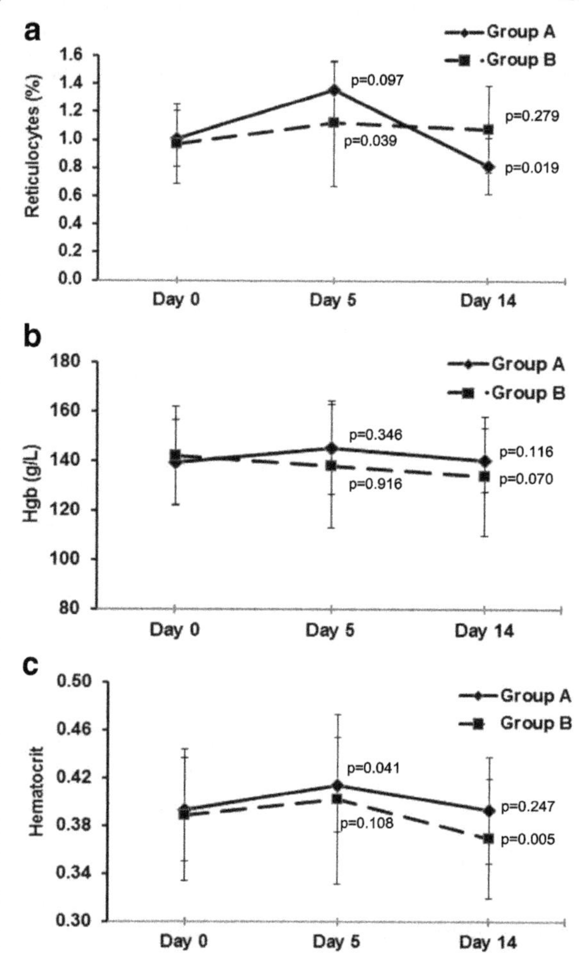

Fig. 2 Hematological parameters before and after treatment with NeuroEPO. Data correspond to the healthy subjects who received 1 mg of NeuroEPO (Group A, $N = 12$) or 0.5 mg of NeuroEPO (Group B, $N = 13$) every 8 h, during 4 days, by nasal route. Points correspond to median and deviations for each measure before treatment (day 0) and after it (day 5, day 14). **a** Reticulocytes count (0.5–1.5%). **b** Hemoglobin (M: 130–175 g/L; W: 120–165 g/L). **c** Hematocrit (M: 0.41–0.54; W: 0.37–0.47). Post-treatment vs. initial analysis (Wilcoxon's test) is showed for the three variables. Differences between groups of treatment were no significant at each time ($p > 0.05$, Mann-Whitney's U test)

However, considering temporal relationship between NeuroEPO administration and the appearance of the event, this aspect should continue being studied as part of the clinical development of the product.

Considering that Group B received the lowest NeuroEPO dose, a direct relationship between dose and the frequency of adverse events was not evidenced. Later studies will confirm or not if patients treated with smaller doses have a higher frequency of local events. The contribution of formulation components to these adverse events should be also considered.

Erythropoietin has been proposed for neuroprotection [39]. It has shown to have more than one mechanism of action, and continues to be a promising choice in the future, concerning the data review of brain ischemia models [40]. This molecule is able to reach CNS minimally between 9 and 24 h after intravenous administration [41]. The first clinical evidence of the utility of rHu-EPO in the treatment of stroke was obtained in the early 2000s [28]. A further attempt to replicate this outcome failed because of safety concerns that the authors associated with errors in the execution of the trial [29].

Nasal administration provides a promissory route of administration for EPO [42]. Intranasal rHu-EPO was able to recover spontaneous motor activity, without induction of peripheral erythropoiesis in a focal brain hypoxia model [43]. The information now obtained indicates us a dose frame to which rHu-EPO can be safely administered through nasal route. The NeuroEPO dosing scheme was previously validated in a cerebral ischemia model improving neurological status and increasing viability and spontaneous exploratory activity, also showed a therapeutic window up to 12 h [20]. Moreover, this product confirmed their high neuroprotective activity since it relieved memory alterations, oxidative stress, neuroinflammation, apoptosis induction and amyloid load in a reference transgenic mouse model of Alzheimer's disease [44].

The results in healthy volunteers justified the approval of further clinical trials with NeuroEPO formulation in stroke [45] and spinocerebellar ataxia [46]. These trials are ongoing and preliminary results in ataxia are encouraging.

Conclusions

Intranasal administration of NeuroEPO in healthy volunteers was well tolerated without undesired hematopoietic effects. These results strongly validate the continuity of clinical development of this product in patients with stroke and neurodegenerative diseases.

Abbreviations

ALT: Alanine aminotransferase; AST: Aspartate aminotransferase; BBB: Blood-brain barrier; CHO: Chinese hamster ovary; CNS: Central Nervous System; EDTA: Ethylenediaminetetraacetic acid; GGT: Gamma-glutamyltransferase; Hgb: Hemoglobin; HPMC: Hydroxypropyl methylcellulose; MSSD: Maximum safe starting dose; NaCL: Sodium chloride; rHu-EPO: Recombinant human erythropoietin; WHO: World Health Organization

Acknowledgments

The authors wish to thank Adriana Muñoz, Anay Cordero, Alina González, Otman Fernández and Alejandro Pando for protocol review and suggestions, Ernesto Pérez, Moisés González, Niurka Verdecia, Noelia Jiménez, Lissette Barrero, Odelay Ramírez, Marbelis Campo, Alina Mazorra and Yordanka González for their participation as laboratory technicians, Mabel Álvarez and Aliuska Frías for their assistance in the data management, Teresita Rodríguez, Carmen Valenzuela and Alexey García for manuscript review, and especially the 25 young people who served as volunteers.

Funding
The study was financed by CIMAB S.A, Havana, Cuba, from its design and execution until collection, analysis, and interpretation of data. The authors received NeuroEPO formulation free from CIMAB S.A. The Ministry of Public Health of Cuba also supported the clinical trial (hospital facilities and general medical care of the volunteers as in-patients).

Authors' contributions
OSM participated in the design and coordination of the study, analysis of the results as well as manuscript writing. ADM was the main investigator and analyzed the results. DJR, YPI and TFC coordinated the study and analyzed the results; DJR also participated in the manuscript writing. CAGD, SPR and EAM were involved in subject recruitment, management, clinical examinations and follow-up. CVG contributed as data processor and statistician. PPS took part in the study design. IGG analyzed the results and wrote the manuscript draft. DAG conceived the study and revised the manuscript. All authors read and approved the final manuscript.

Competing interests
Authors OSM, YPI, CMG, PPS and DAG are employees of the Center of Molecular Immunology (CIM), Havana, Cuba, where NeuroEPO intranasal formulation is produced. Authors DJR, TFC and IGG are employees of the Center for Drug Research and Development (CIDEM), Havana, Cuba, where this formulation was developed and partly preclinically developed. Drs. García-Rodríguez and Sosa-Teste are co-inventors of the patent of rHu-EPO nasal formulations (see ref. [14]). The rest of the authors have no competing interests concerning this paper.

Author details
[1]NeuroEPO Research and Development Group, Center of Molecular Immunology, Havana, Cuba. [2]National Center for Toxicology, "Carlos J. Finlay" University Hospital, Havana, Cuba. [3]Clinical Trials Group, Research Direction, Center for Drug Research and Development (CIDEM), Ave. 26 and Puentes Grandes, No. 1605, Nuevo Vedado, Havana, Cuba.

References

1. Ginsberg MD. Neuroprotection for ischemic stroke: past, present and future. Neuropharmacology. 2008;55:363–89.
2. Wang YL, Liang H, Song SL. The intervention treatment of neuroprotection for ischemic stroke. Sheng Li Ke Xue Jin Zhan. 2012;43:279–82.
3. García-Rodríguez JC, Sosa-Teste I. The nasal route as a potential pathway for delivery of erythropoietin in the treatment of acute ischemic stroke in humans. Sci World J. 2009;9:970–81.
4. Parra AL, Rodriguez JC. Nasal Neuro EPO could be a reliable choice for neuroprotective stroke treatment. Cent Nerv Syst Agents Med Chem. 2012;12:60–8.
5. Chateauvieux S, Grigorakaki C, Morceau F, Dicato M, Diederich M. Erythropoietin, erythropoiesis and beyond. Biochem Pharmacol. 2011;82:1291–303.
6. Erbayraktar S, Grasso G, Sfacteria A, Xie QW, Coleman T, Kreilgaard M, Torup L, Sager T, Erbayraktar Z, Gokmen N, Yilmaz O, Ghezzi P, Villa P, Fratelli M, Casagrande S, Leist M, Helboe L, Gerwein J, Christensen S, Geist MA, Pedersen LO, Cerami-Hand C, Wuerth JP, Cerami A, Brines M. Asialoerythropoietin is a nonerythropoietic cytokine with broad neuroprotective activity in vivo. Proc Natl Acad Sci U S A. 2003;100:6741–6.
7. Frey WH II, Liu J, Chen X, Thorne RG, Fawcett JR, Ala TA, Rahman YE. Delivery of ^{125}I-NGF to the brain via the olfactory route. Drug Delivery. 1997;4:87–92.
8. Thorne RG, Pronk GJ, Padmanabhan V, Frey WH 2nd Delivery of insulin-like growth factor-I to the rat brain and spinal cord along olfactory and trigeminal pathways following intranasal administration. Neuroscience 2004;127:481–496.
9. Hanson LR, Frey WH 2nd. Intranasal delivery bypasses the blood-brain barrier to target therapeutic agents to the central nervous system and treat neurodegenerative disease. BMC Neurosci. 2008;9 Suppl 3:S5.
10. Williams GS. Intranasal drug delivery bypasses the blood-brain barrier. Neurol Rev. 2016;24:1,4041.
11. Alcalá-Barraza SR, Lee MS, Hanson LR, McDonald AA, Frey WH 2nd, McLoon LK. Intranasal delivery of neurotrophic factors BDNF, CNTF, EPO, and NT-4 to the CNS. J Drug Target. 2010;18:179–90.
12. Lochhead JJ, Wolak DJ, Pizzo ME, Thorne RG. Rapid transport within cerebral perivascular spaces underlies widespread tracer distribution in the brain after intranasal administration. J Cereb Blood Flow Metab. 2015;35(3):371–81.
13. Yu YP, Xu QQ, Zhang Q, Zhang WP, Zhang LH, Wei EQ. Intranasal recombinant human erythropoietin protects rats against focal cerebral ischemia. Neurosci Lett. 2005;387:5–10.
14. Muñoz-Cernada A, García-Rodríguez JC, Núñez-FigueredoY, Pardo-Ruiz Z, García-Salman JD, Sosa-Testé I, Curbelo-Rodríguez D, Cruz-Rodríguez J, Subirós-Martínez, N. rh-EPO nasal formulations with low sialic acid concentration for the treatment of diseases of the central nervous system. 2005; PCT/CU2006/000007 [WO/2007/009404].
15. Muñoz-Cernada A, Pardo-Ruiz Z, Montero-Alejo V, Fernández-Cervera M, Sosa-Testé I, García-Rodríguez JC. Effect of nonionic surfactants and HPMC F4M on the development of formulations of Neuro-EPO as a neuroprotective agent. JAPST. 2014;1:22–35.
16. Muñoz-Cernada A, Cardentey-Fernández J, Pardo-Ruiz Z, Díaz-Sánchez D, Montero-Alejo V, Sosa-Testé I, Fernández-Cervera M, García-Rodríguez JC, Amaro-González D. Physicochemical and biological evaluation of bioadhesive polymers for the development of intranasal low sialic acid erythropoietin formulations. Bioprocess J. 2014;13:23.
17. Sosa I, García JC, García JD, Santana J, Subirós N, González C, Rodríguez Y, Cruz J. Intranasal administration of recombinant human erythropoietin exerts neuroprotective effects on post-ischemic brain injury in Mongolian gerbils. Pharmacol Online. 2006;1:100–12.
18. Gao Y, Mengana Y, Cruz YR, Muñoz A, Testé IS, García JD, Wu Y, Rodríguez JC, Zhang C. Different expression patterns of Ngb and EPOR in the cerebral cortex and hippocampus revealed distinctive therapeutic effects of intranasal delivery of Neuro-EPO for ischemic insults to the gerbil brain. J Histochem Cytochem. 2011;59:214–27.
19. Rodríguez Cruz Y, Mengana Támos Y, Muñoz Cernuda A, Subirós Martines N, González-Quevedo A, Sosa Testé I, García Rodríguez JC. Treatment with nasal Neuro-EPO improves the neurological, cognitive, and histological state in a gerbil model of focal ischemia. Sci World J. 2010;10:2288–300.
20. Teste IS, Tamos YM, Cruz YR, Cernada AM, Rodríguez JC, Martínez NS, Antich RM, González-Quevedo A, Rodríguez JC. Dose effect evaluation and therapeutic window of the Neuro-EPO nasal application for the treatment of the focal ischemia model in the Mongolian gerbil. Sci World J. 2012;2012:607498.
21. Núñez-Figueredo Y, Bueno V, Carrillo C, Jiménez N, Valdés O, Muñoz-Cernada A, Alonso E. Neuroprotective effect of a nasal formulation of erythropoietin with low sialic acid content. Rev Cuba Farm. 2009;43:1–13.
22. Sosa I., Mengana TY, Portillo A, Ruiz E, Cruz J, Muñoz A, García-Salman JD, García Rodríguez JC. Ensayo de seguridad de la aplicación nasal de la molécula de rHu-EPO con bajo contenido de ácido siálico en el modelo de ratón B6D2F1. CD VI Congreso Internacional de Ciencias Veterinarias 2007. ISBN: 978–959–282-047-3 Animales de laboratorio:164–71.
23. Lagarto A, Bueno V, Guerra I, Valdés O, Couret M, López R, Vega Y. Absence of hematological side effects in acute and subacute nasal dosing of erythropoietin with a low content of sialic acid. Exp Toxicol Pathol. 2011;63:563–7.
24. Sosa I, Cruz J, Santana J, Mengana Y, García-Salman JD, Muñoz A, Ozuna TG, García JC. Recombinant human erythropoietin with low sialic acid pathway to the central nervous system by intranasal route in *Meriones unguiculatus* and no human primate *Macaca Fascicularis* models. Rev Salud Anim. 2008;30:39–44.
25. U.S. Department of Health and Human Services, Food and Drug Administration, Center for Drug Evaluation and Research (CDER): Guidance for industry: estimating the maximum safe starting dose in initial clinical trials for therapeutics in adult healthy volunteers. 2005.
26. Dhuria SV, Hanson LR, Frey WH 2nd. Intranasal delivery to the central nervous system: mechanisms and experimental considerations. J Pharm Sci 2010;99:1654–1673.
27. Muñoz-Cernada A, Fernández-Cervera M, García-Rodríguez JC. Factors involved in the design of nasal delivery systems for peptides and proteins. Biotecnol Apl. 2013;30:88–96.
28. Ehrenreich H, Hasselblatt M, Dembowski C, Cepek L, Lewczuk P, Stiefel M, Rustenbeck HH, Breiter N, Jacob S, Knerlich F, Bohn M, Poser W, Rüther E, Kochen M, Gefeller O, Gleiter C, Wessel TC, De Ryck M, Itri L, Prange H,

Cerami A, Brines M, Sirén AL. Erythropoietin therapy for acute stroke is both safe and beneficial. Mol Med. 2002;8:495–505.

29. Ehrenreich H, Weissenborn K, Prange H, Schneider D, Weimar C, Wartenberg K, Schellinger PD, Bohn M, Becker H, Wegrzyn M, Jähnig P, Herrmann M, Knauth M, Bähr M, Heide W, Wagner A, Schwab S, Reichmann H, Schwendemann G, Dengler R, Kastrup A, Bartels C, EPO Stroke Trial Group. Recombinant human erythropoietin in the treatment of acute ischemic stroke. Stroke. 2009;40:e647–56.
30. Common Terminology Criteria for Adverse Events (CTCAE), Version 4.0, Published: May 28, 2009 (v4.03: June 14, 2010), DCTD, NCI, NIH, DHHS, https://ctep.cancer.gov/. Last accessed 4 Jan 2017.
31. The use of the WHO-UMC system for standardized case causality assessment. Available from: http://www.who.int/medicines/areas/quality_safety/safety_efficacy/WHOcausality_assessment.pdf. Last accessed 4 Jan 2017.
32. Buoen C, Bjerrum OJ, Thomsen MS. How first-time-in-human studies are being performed: a survey of phase I dose-escalation trials in healthy volunteers published between 1995 and 2004. J Clin Pharmacol. 2005;45:1123–36.
33. European Medicines Agency. Committee for Medicinal Products for Human Use (CHMP). Guideline on strategies to identify and mitigate risks for first-in -human and early clinical trials with investigational medicinal products. Draft. 2016.
34. Lundby C, Olsen NV. Effects of recombinant human erythropoietin in normal humans. J Physiol. 2011;589:1265–71.
35. Pfaar O, Raap U, Holz M, Hörmann K, Klimek L. Pathophysiology of itching and sneezing in allergic rhinitis. Swiss Med Wkly. 2009;139:35–40.
36. Costa A, Antonaci F, Ramusino MC, Nappi G. The Neuropharmacology of cluster headache and other trigeminal autonomic Cephalalgias. Curr Neuropharmacol. 2015;13:304–23.
37. Tonia T, Mettler A, Robert N, Schwarzer G, Seidenfeld J, Weingart O, Hyde C, Engert A, Bohlius J. Erythropoietin or darbepoetin for patients with cancer. Cochrane Database Syst Rev. 2012;12:CD003407.
38. Żebrowski P, Mieczkowski M. Erythropoietin stimulating agents in chronic kidney disease: indications and contraindications. Wiad Lek. 2016;69:753–5.
39. Chatagner A, Hüppi PS, Ha-Vinh Leuchter R, Sizonenko S. Erythropoietin and neuroprotection. Arch Pediatr. 2010;17:S78–84.
40. Minnerup J, Heidrich J, Rogalewski A, Schäbitz WR, Wellmann J. The efficacy of erythropoietin and its analogues in animal stroke models: a meta-analysis. Stroke. 2009;40:3113–20.
41. Xenocostas A, Cheung WK, Farrell F, Zakszewski C, Kelley M, Lutynski A, Crump M, Lipton JH, Kiss TL, Lau CY, Messner HA. The pharmacokinetics of erythropoietin in the cerebrospinal fluid after intravenous administration of recombinant human erythropoietin. Eur J Clin Pharmacol. 2005;61:189–95.
42. Genc S, Zadeoglulari Z, Oner MG, Genc K, Digicaylioglu M. Intranasal erythropoietin therapy in nervous system disorders. Expert Opin Drug Deliv. 2011;8:19–32.
43. Merelli A, Caltana L, Girimonti P, Ramos AJ, Lazarowski A, Brusco A. Recovery of motor spontaneous activity after intranasal delivery of human recombinant erythropoietin in a focal brain hypoxia model induced by $CoCl_2$ in rats. Neurotox Res. 2011;20:182–92.
44. Rodríguez Cruz Y, Strehaiano M, Rodríguez Obaya T, García Rodríguez JC, Maurice T. An intranasal formulation of erythropoietin (Neuro-EPO) prevents memory deficits and Amyloid toxicity in the APPSwe transgenic mouse model of Alzheimer's disease. J Alzheimers Dis. 2017;55:231–48.
45. Cuban Public Registry of Clinical Trials. Safety and efficacy of NeuroEPO in patients with stroke. Phase I-II. http://registroclinico.sld.cu/ensayos/RPCEC00000185-Sp. Last accessed 4 Jan 2017.
46. Cuban Public Registry of Clinical Trials. Evaluation of the safety and effect of treatment with intranasal NeuroEPO in patients with type 2 spinocerebellar ataxia. http://registroclinico.sld.cu/ensayos/RPCEC00000187-Sp. Last accessed 4 Jan 2017.

6

Injury of ascending reticular activating system associated with delayed post-hypoxic leukoencephalopathy

Sung Ho Jang[1] and Hyeok Gyu Kwon[2*]

Abstract

Background: Delayed post-hypoxic leukoencephalopathy (DPHL) is a demyelinating syndrome characterized by neurological relapse after an initial recovery from hypoxic brain injury. We describe a patient with impaired consciousness following DPHL, concurrent with injury of the ascending reticular activating system (ARAS) shown using diffusion tensor tractography (DTT).

Case presentation: A 50-year-old male patient was in a drowsy mental state after exposure to carbon monoxide (CO) for about ten hours. About a day after the CO exposure, his mental state recovered to an alert condition. However, his consciousness deteriorated to drowsy 24 days after the exposure and worsened to a semi-coma state at 26 days after onset. When he started rehabilitation six weeks after the CO exposure, he had impaired consciousness, with a Glasgow Coma Scale score of 8 and a Coma Recovery Scale-Revised score of 8. On 6-week DTT, decreased neural connectivity of the upper ARAS between the intralaminar thalamic nucleus and the cerebral cortex was observed in both frontal cortices, basal forebrains, basal ganglia and thalami. The lower dorsal ARAS was not reconstructed on the right side, and was thin on the left side. The lower ventral ARAS was not reconstructed on either side.

Conclusions: Using DTT, we demonstrated injury of the ARAS in a patient with impaired consciousness following DPHL. Our result suggests that injury of the ARAS is a plausible pathogenetic mechanism of impaired consciousness in patients with DPHL.

Keywords: Delayed post-hypoxic leukoencephalopathy, Hypoxic brain injury, Ascending reticular activating system, Consciousness, Diffusion tensor tractography

Background

Delayed post-hypoxic leukoencephalopathy (DPHL), a rare clinical condition, is a demyelinating syndrome characterized by neurological relapse after an initial recovery from hypoxic brain injury caused by carbon monoxide (CO) poisoning, overdose of drug, and myocardial infarction [1–3]. The majority of DPHL cases are associated with CO poisoning [4]. Lee and Marsden divided DPHL into two general clinical categories: parkinsonism (masked face, rigidity, tremor, dystonic posturing, agitation) and akinetic mutism (apathetic and developed functional bowel and minimal primitive responses to pain) [5–13]. However, very little is known about impaired consciousness following DPHL.

Hypoxic brain injury predominantly involves the gray matter. MRI is recognized as the most sensitive and common imaging tool for hypoxic brain injury [14]. In contrast, DPHL predominantly involves the white matter. Many studies have reported abnormality of the white matter including basal ganglia following DPHL using neuroimaging tools such as conventional MRI, diffusion weight imaging, and MR spectroscopy [5–13].

* Correspondence: khg0715@hanmail.net
[2]Department of Physical Therapy, College of Health Sciences, Catholic University of Pusan, 57 Oryundae-ro, Geumjeong-gu, Pusan 46252, Republic of Korea
Full list of author information is available at the end of the article

Recently developed diffusion tensor tractography (DTT), derived from diffusion tensor imaging (DTI), has the unique capability to estimate the neural tract in the white matter and is able to find the subtle or invisible neural injury by detection of characteristics of water diffusion [15]. Injury of the ascending reticular activating system (ARAS), which is responsible for consciousness, has been reported in patients with hypoxic brain injury [16, 17]. However, no study of injury of the ARAS in patients with DPHL has been reported.

In this study, using DTT, we report on a patient with impaired consciousness concurrent with injury of the ARAS following DPHL.

Case presentation

A 50-year-old male patient showed drowsy mental state after exposure to carbon monoxide released from a coal briquette stove for about ten hours while he was sleeping. He underwent conservative management at a local hospital and his drowsy mental state recovered to an alert state approximately one day later without any neurological sequelae. However, he was transferred to the nephrology department of a university hospital for management of an acute kidney injury due to rhabdomyolysis ten days later. At that time, his Glasgow Coma Scale (GCS) and mini-mental state examination were full scores (15 and 30 scores, respectively) and results of blood test were as follows: creatine phosphokinase - 3273 IU/L (57 ~ 374), blood urea nitrogen - 133 mg/dL (8 ~ 23), creatinine - 5.67 mg/dL (0.6 ~ 1.5), aspartate aminotransferase - 53 IU/L (10 ~ 35), and alanine aminotransferase - 2 IU/L (0 ~ 40). Deep second degree contact burn wound was observed on his left buttock and he was diagnosed as a rhabdomyolysis which was caused by the contact burn. We assumed that the contact burn was occurred by the contact with the briquette stove during sleeping because there was no observer. At 16 days after the CO exposure, he began to show mild dysarthria and myoclonus on the right fingers. He developed clumsy movement 22 days after onset. His consciousness deteriorated to a drowsy state 24 days after onset and worsened to a semi-coma state at 26 days after onset. Brain MR images at three weeks after onset showed lesions in both basal ganglia (Fig. 1a). Six weeks after the CO poisoning, he was transferred to the rehabilitation department of the same university hospital. The patient showed impaired consciousness, with a Glasgow Coma Scale score of 8 (eye opening: 4, best verbal response: 1, and best motor response: 3) and a Coma Recovery Scale-Revised score of 8 (auditory function: 0, visual function: 3, motor function: 2, verbal function: 1, communication: 0, and arousal: 2) [18, 19]. The patient's wife provided signed, informed consent, and the study protocol was approved by our Institutional Review Board.

Magnetic resonance imaging and diffusion tensor imaging

Imaging parameters for T2-weighted MRI were as follows: acquisition matrix = 265 × 224, field of view = 210 × 210 mm^2, repetition time = 4224.1 ms, echo time = 100 ms, number of excitations = 2, and a slice thickness of 5 mm with a gap of 2.2 mm. DTI data were acquired at six weeks after onset using a six-channel head coil on a 1.5 T Philips Gyroscan Intera with single-shot echo-planar imaging. Imaging parameters were as follows: acquisition matrix = 96 × 96; reconstructed to matrix = 192 × 192; field of view = 240 × 240 mm^2; repetition time = 10,398 ms; echo time = 72 ms; echo-planar imaging factor = 59; b = 1000s/mm^2; and a slice thickness = 2.5 mm. Affine multi-scale two-dimensional registration at the Oxford Centre for Functional Magnetic Resonance Imaging of Brain (FMRIB) Software Library was used to correct head motion effect and image distortion. Fiber tracking used FMRIB Diffusion (5000 streamline samples, 0.5 mm step lengths, curvature thresholds = 0.2), a probabilistic tractography method [20]. Three portions of the ARAS were reconstructed by selection of fibers passing through region of interest (ROI) as follows [21–23]: the upper ARAS, in which the neural connectivity of the intralaminar thalamic nucleus (ILN, ROI 1) to the cerebral cortex was analyzed, the dorsal lower ARAS, between the pontine reticular formation (RF, ROI 1) and the ILN (ROI 2), and the ventral lower ARAS, between the pontine RF (ROI 1) and the hypothalamus (ROI 2). Out of 5000 samples generated from the seed voxel, results for fiber tracking were applied at a threshold of two streamlines for the dorsal and ventral lower ARAS and 10 streamlines for the upper ARAS.

On 6-week DTT, decreased neural connectivity of the upper ARAS between the ILN and the cerebral cortex was observed in both frontal cortices, basal forebrains, basal ganglia and thalami (Fig. 1). The dorsal lower ARAS between the pontine RF and the ILN was not reconstructed on the right side and thin on the left side. The ventral lower ARAS between the pontine RF and the hypothalamus was not reconstructed on either side.

Discussion and conclusions

In the current study, three portions of the ARAS (the dorsal lower ARAS, ventral lower ARAS and upper ARAS) in a patient with impaired consciousness following DPHL caused by CO poisoning were evaluated using DTT. We found that these three portions of the ARAS were injured in both hemispheres: the upper ARAS – decreased neural connectivity to both frontal cortexes, basal forebrains, basal ganglia and thalami, the dorsal

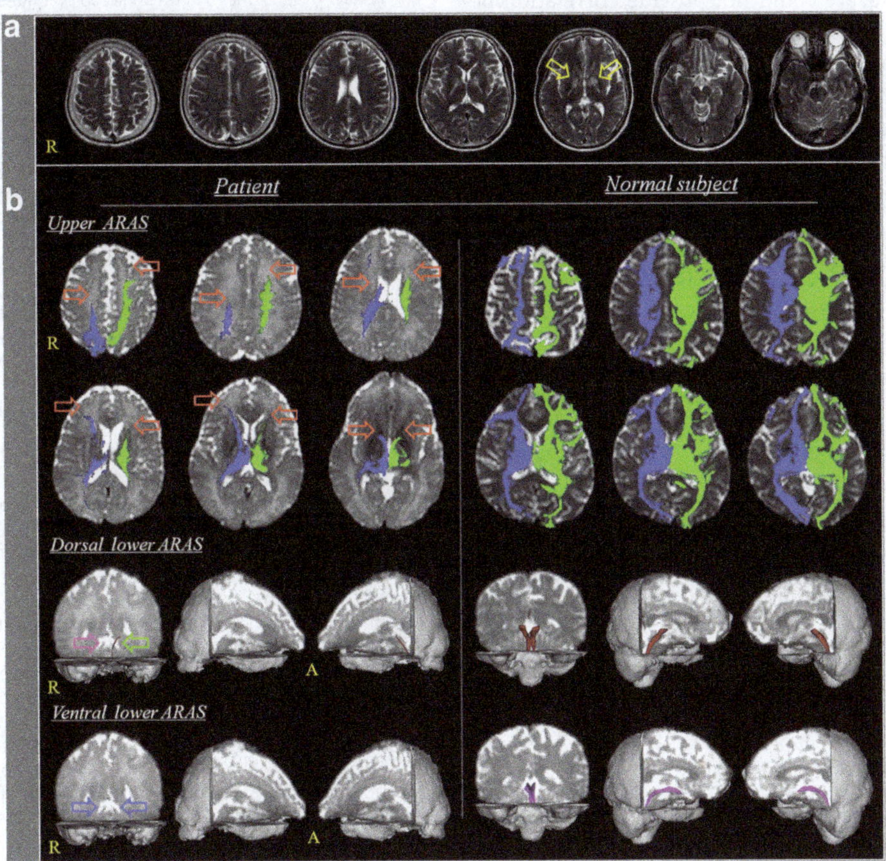

Fig. 1 **a** Brain MR images at three weeks after onset show lesions in both basal ganglia (*yellow arrows*). **b** Results of diffusion tensor tractography (DTT) for the ascending reticular activation system (ARAS). On 6-week DTT, decreased neural connectivity of the upper ARAS between the intralaminar thalamic nucleus and the cerebral cortex is observed in both frontal cortices, basal forebrains, basal ganglia and thalami (*red arrows*). The dorsal lower ARAS between the pontine reticular formation and the intralaminar thalamic nucleus is not reconstructed on the right side (*purple arrow*) and thinning on the left side (*green arrow*). The ventral lower ARAS between the pontine reticular formation and the hypothalamus is not reconstructed on both sides (*blue arrows*). Results of DTT for the ARAS in a normal subject (53 year-old male). ARAS: ascending reticular activation system

lower ARAS – non-reconstruction in the right side and narrowing in the left side and the ventral lower ARAS – non-reconstruction in both sides. We believe that the impaired consciousness in this patient was ascribed to the injury of the three portions of the ARAS.

Many studies have reported abnormality of the white matter including basal ganglia (caudate nucleus, putamen, and globus pallidus) in patients with DPHL using various neuroimaging tools including conventional MRI [5–13]. Neurological manifestations were observed as follows: 1) cognitive impairments - confusion, disorientation, executive dysfunction, attention deficit, and akinetic mutism 2) motor symptoms - spasticity, hyper-reflexia, bradykinesia, rigidity, tremor, gait disturbance, dystonia 3) hallucinations, and 4) dysautonomia [5–13]. Regarding DTI, as far as we are aware, only one study was reported on patients with DPHL [24]. In 2008, Kenshi et al. demonstrated extensive white matter injury using DTI parameters (fractional anisotropy and mean diffusivity) in two patients with carbon monoxide intoxication (patient 1: frontal and parietal regions, globus pallidus, and corpus callosum and patient 2: globus pallidus) and showed neurological manifestations as follows: 1) patient 1 - akinetic mutism, disorientation, gait disturbance and 2) patient 2 - akinetic mutism [24]. To the best of our knowledge, this is the first DTT study to demonstrate injury of the ARAS in a patient with DPHL.

In conclusion, using DTT, we demonstrated injury of the ARAS in a patient with impaired consciousness following DPHL. Our result suggests injury of the ARAS is a plausible pathogenetic mechanism of impaired consciousness in patients with DPHL. However, because it is a single case report, this study is limited. In addition, several limitations of this study should be considered. First, use of DTT could lead to both false positive and negative results due to multiple fiber orientations in a voxel [25]. Second, we could not provide correlation between cognitive function and DTI anatomical site. Third, based on the blood test, we could not completely ruled out whether it affected neurogical status of the patient. Therefore, we suggest that further studies including large numbers of patients and overcoming limitations of this study should be encouraged.

Acknowledgements
None.

Funding
Analysis and interpretation of data in writing the manuscript was supported by the Medical Research Center Program (2015R1A5A2009124) through the National Research Foundation of Korea (NRF) funded by the Ministry of Science, ICT and Future Planning.

Authors' contributions
SHJ participated the design of this study and collected the clinical raw data, writing the manuscript. HGJ carried out analysis of data, writing the manuscript. Both authors read and approved the final manuscript.

Competing interests
The authors declare that they have no competing interests.

Author details
[1]Department of Physical Medicine and Rehabilitation, College of Medicine, Yeungnam University, Gyeongsan, South Korea. [2]Department of Physical Therapy, College of Health Sciences, Catholic University of Pusan, 57 Oryundae-ro, Geumjeong-gu, Pusan 46252, Republic of Korea.

References
1. Plum F, Posner JB, Hain RF. Delayed neurological deterioration after anoxia. Arch Intern Med. 1962;110:18–25.
2. Shprecher D, Mehta L. The syndrome of delayed post-hypoxic leukoencephalopathy. NeuroRehabilitation. 2010;26(1):65–72.
3. Zamora CA, Nauen D, Hynecek R, Ilica AT, Izbudak I, Sair HI, Gujar SK, Pillai JJ. Delayed posthypoxic leukoencephalopathy: a case series and review of the literature. Brain Behav. 2015; 5(8):e00364. doi:10.1002/brb3.364.
4. Choi IS. Delayed neurologic sequelae in carbon monoxide intoxication. Arch Neurol. 1983;40(7):433–5.
5. Lee MS, Marsden CD. Neurological sequelae following carbon monoxide poisoning clinical course and outcome according to the clinical types and brain computed tomography scan findings. Mov Disord. 1994;9(5):550–8. doi:10.1002/mds.870090508.
6. Barnett MH, Miller LA, Reddel SW, Davies L. Reversible delayed leukoencephalopathy following intravenous heroin overdose. J Clin Neurosci. 2001;8(2):165–7. doi:10.1054/jocn.2000.0769.
7. Lam SP, Fong SY, Kwok A, Wong T, Wing YK. Delayed neuropsychiatric impairment after carbon monoxide poisoning from burning charcoal. Hong Kong Med J. 2004;10(6):428–31.
8. Hsiao CL, Kuo HC, Huang CC. Delayed encephalopathy after carbon monoxide intoxication–long-term prognosis and correlation of clinical manifestations and neuroimages. Acta Neurol Taiwanica. 2004;13(2):64–70.
9. Shprecher DR, Flanigan KM, Smith AG, Smith SM, Schenkenberg T, Steffens J. Clinical and diagnostic features of delayed hypoxic leukoencephalopathy. J Neuropsychiatry Clin Neurosci. 2008;20(4):473–7. doi:10.1176/appi.neuropsych.20.4.473. 10.1176/jnp.2008.20.4.473.
10. Rozen TD. Rapid resolution of akinetic mutism in delayed post-hypoxic leukoencephalopathy with intravenous magnesium sulfate. NeuroRehabilitation. 2012;30(4):329–32. doi:10.3233/NRE-2012-0763.
11. Meyer MA. Delayed post-hypoxic leukoencephalopathy: case report with a review of disease pathophysiology. Neurol Int. 2013;5(3):e13. doi:10.4081/ni.2013.e13.
12. Huisa BN, Gasparovic C, Taheri S, Prestopnik JL, Rosenberg GA. Imaging of subacute blood-brain barrier disruption after methadone overdose. J Neuroimaging. 2013;23(3):441–4. doi:10.1111/j.1552-6569.2011.00669.x.
13. Geraldo AF, Silva C, Neutel D, Neto LL, Albuquerque L. Delayed leukoencephalopathy after acute carbon monoxide intoxication. J Radiol Case Rep. 2014;8(5):1–8. doi:10.3941/jrcr.v8i5.1721.
14. Huang BY, Castillo M. Hypoxic-ischemic brain injury: imaging findings from birth to adulthood. Radiographics. 2008; 28(2):417–439; quiz 617. doi:10.1148/rg.282075066.
15. Behrens TE, Berg HJ, Jbabdi S, Rushworth MF, Woolrich MW. Probabilistic diffusion tractography with multiple fibre orientations: What can we gain? Neuroimage. 2007;34(1):144–55. doi:10.1016/j.neuroimage.2006.09.018.
16. Jang SH, Kim SH, Lim HW, Yeo SS. Injury of the lower ascending reticular activating system in patients with hypoxic-ischemic brain injury: diffusion tensor imaging study. Neuroradiology. 2014;56(11):965–70. doi:10.1007/s00234-014-1419-y.
17. Jang SH, Hyun YJ, Lee HD. Recovery of consciousness and an injured ascending reticular activating system in a patient who survived cardiac arrest: A case report. Medicine (Baltimore). 2016;95(26):e4041. doi:10.1097/MD.0000000000004041.
18. Teasdale G, Jennett B. Assessment of coma and impaired consciousness. A practical scale. Lancet. 1974;2(7872):81–4.
19. Giacino JT, Kalmar K, Whyte J. The JFK coma recovery scale-revised: measurement characteristics and diagnostic utility. Arch Phys Med Rehabil. 2004;85(12):2020–9.
20. Smith SM, Jenkinson M, Woolrich MW, Beckmann CF, Behrens TE, Johansen-Berg H, Bannister PR, De Luca M, Drobnjak I, Flitney DE, et al. Advances in functional and structural MR image analysis and implementation as FSL. Neuroimage. 2004;23(Suppl 1):S208–19. doi:10.1016/j.neuroimage.2004.07.051.
21. Yeo SS, Chang PH, Jang SH. The ascending reticular activating system from pontine reticular formation to the thalamus in the human brain. Front Hum Neurosci. 2013; 7:416. doi:10.3389/fnhum.2013.00416.
22. Jang SH, Lim HW, Yeo SS. The neural connectivity of the intralaminar thalamic nuclei in the human brain: a diffusion tensor tractography study. Neurosci Lett. 2014;579:140–4. doi:10.1016/j.neulet.2014.07.024.
23. Jang SH, Kwon HG. The ascending reticular activating system from pontine reticular formation to the hypothalamus in the human brain: a diffusion tensor imaging study. Neurosci Lett. 2015;590:58–61. doi:10.1016/j.neulet.2015.01.071.
24. Terajima K, Igarashi H, Hirose M, Matsuzawa H, Nishizawa M, Nakada T. Serial assessments of delayed encephalopathy after carbon monoxide poisoning using magnetic resonance spectroscopy and diffusion tensor imaging on 3.0T system. Eur Neurol. 2008;59(1–2):55–61. doi:10.1159/000109262.
25. Yamada K. Diffusion tensor tractography should be used with caution. Proc Natl Acad Sci U S A. 2009; 106(7):E14; author reply E5. doi:10.1073/pnas.0812352106.

7

Serum melatonin levels in survivor and non-survivor patients with traumatic brain injury

Leonardo Lorente[1*], María M. Martín[2], Pedro Abreu-González[3], Antonia Pérez-Cejas[4], Luis Ramos[5], Mónica Argueso[6], Jordi Solé-Violán[7], Juan J. Cáceres[8], Alejandro Jiménez[9] and Victor García-Marín[10]

Abstract

Background: Circulating levels of melatonin in patients with traumatic brain injury (TBI) have been determined in a little number of studies with small sample size (highest sample size of 37 patients) and only were reported the comparison of serum melatonin levels between TBI patients and healthy controls. As to we know, the possible association between circulating levels of melatonin levels and mortality of patients with TBI have not been explored; thus, the objective of our current study was to determine whether this association actually exists.

Methods: This multicenter study included 118 severe TBI (Glasgow Coma Scale <9) patients. We measured serum levels of melatonin, malondialdehyde (to assess lipid peroxidation) and total antioxidant capacity (TAC) at day 1 of severe TBI. We used mortality at 30 days as endpoint.

Results: We found that non-survivor (n = 33) compared to survivor (n = 85) TBI patients showed higher circulating levels of melatonin (p < 0.001), TAC (p < 0.001) and MDA (p < 0.001). We found that serum melatonin levels predicted 30-day mortality (Odds ratio = 1.334; 95% confidence interval = 1.094–1.627; p = 0.004), after to control for GCS, CT findings and age. We found a correlation between serum levels of melatonin levels and serum levels of TAC (rho = 0.37; p < 0.001) and serum levels of MDA (rho = 0.24; p = 0.008).

Conclusions: As to we know, our study is the largest series providing circulating melatonin levels in patients with severe TBI. The main findings were that non-survivors had higher serum melatonin levels than survivors, and the association between serum levels of melatonin levels and mortality, peroxidation state and antioxidant state.

Keywords: Melatonin, Brain trauma, Patients, Mortality, Injury

Background

Severe traumatic brain injury (TBI) leads to resources consumption, disabilities, and deaths [1]. TBI causes primary and secondary brain injuries. Primary brain injury is produced due to physical forces at the moment of impact. Secondary brain injury, during following hours or days to TBI, leads to neuroinflammation and brain oxidative damage [2–6].

There has been suggested that the administration of melatonin on TBI could have different beneficial effects, such as antioxidant effects, anti-inflammatory effects, anti-apoptotic effects, a reduction in brain edema [2–6].

Circulating levels of melatonin in patients with traumatic brain injury (TBI) have been determined in a little number of studies with small sample size [7–11] (the highest sample size was of 37 patients [11]). Some studies found lower melatonin levels in salive [7] or serum [8–10] in TBI patients compared to healthy controls; however, one study found higher levels of melatonin in cerebrospinal fluid in TBI patients compared to healthy controls [11]. As to we know, circulating melatonin levels in survivor and non-survivor patients with TBI, the possible association between serum levels of melatonin levels and mortality and peroxidation state in patients with TBI, and the possible prognostic value of

* Correspondence: lorentemartin@msn.com
[1]Intensive Care Unit, Hospital Universitario de Canarias, Ofra s/n. La Laguna, 38320 Santa Cruz de Tenerife, Spain
Full list of author information is available at the end of the article

serum levels of melatonin in patients with TBI have not been explored; thus, the objectives of our current study were to determine whether those acts actually exists. For those reasons, we determined in our study serum levels of melatonin, malondialdehyde (to assess lipid peroxidation) and total antioxidant capacity (to assess antioxidant state). The clinical interest of this study lies in that if we find these associations, then the determination of serum melatonin levels in clinical practice to estimate the prognosis of the patients could be proposed, and new lines of research in the treatment of these patients could be opened.

Methods

Design and subjects

This was a prospective and observational study in 6 spanish Intensive Care Units, and was approved by the Ethic Review Board of all participating hospitals: H. U. de Canarias (La Laguna), H. U. Nuestra Señora de Candelaria (Santa Cruz de Tenerife), H. General de La Palma (La Palma), H. U. de Valencia (Valencia), H. U. Insular (Las Palmas de Gran Canaria), H. U. Dr. Negrín (Las Palmas de Gran Canaria). Legal guardians of patients written the informed consent. The study adheres to the ethical conduct of research involving human subjects by World Medical Association Declaration of Helsinki.

We included 118 severe TBI patients. We classified TBI severity by Glasgow Coma Scale (GCS) [12]. We defined severe TBI as GCS < 9 points.

We excluded patients with Injury Severity Score (ISS) in non-cranial aspects > 9 points [13], inflammatory or malignant disease, age < 18 years, and pregnancy.

Previously, we used the same patient cohort with severe TBI with lower number of patients (n = 100) to analyse serum concentrations of malondialdehyde (MDA) [14] and total antioxidant capacity (TAC) [15]. The aims of our current research were to analyse serum concentrations of melatonin in 118 patients with severe TBI, and the association between serum concentrations of melatonin, MDA and TAC in patients with a severe TBI.

Variables recorded

In each patient were recorded the following variables: temperature, sex, sodium, glycemia (basal determination previously to start nutrition), leukocytes, bilirrubin, creatinine, hemoglobin, lactic acid, ISS, platelets, GCS, international normalized ratio (INR), activated partial thromboplastin time (aPTT), fibrinogen, Acute Physiology and Chronic Health Evaluation II (APACHE II) score [16], age, and brain lesion according to the Marshall computed tomography (CT) classification [17]. Serum samples and clinical variables were recorded approximately at the same moment.

CT lesion according Marshall classification [17] is as follows: Class I (not visible pathology), Class II (cisterns are present and midline shift < 5 mm and there is not lesion > 25 cm^3), Class III (cisterns are compressed and midline shift < 5 mm and there is not lesion > 25 cm^3), Class IV (midline shift > 5 mm and there is not lesion > 25 cm^3), Class V (evacuated lesion) or Class VI (lesion > 25 cm^3 not surgically evacuated).

End-point

We used mortality at 30 days as endpoint.

Blood sample collection

We collected blood samples on day 1 of TBI (within 4 h after TBI) in tubes with separator gel. After 10 min at room temperature, serum was obtained by centrifugation during 15 min at 1000 g, and frozen at –80 °C on each hospital until serum concentration determinations. Afterwards, the samples were transported between different locations in refrigerated boxes with dry ice.

Determination of serum levels of melatonin, total antioxidant capacity (TAC) and malondialdehyde (MDA)

All serum concentrations were determined at the same moment (to avoid the possible dispersion of results), when recruitment process was finished, and were determined by personnel without access to clinical data.

The determination of total antioxidant capacity (TAC) give more information about patient antioxidant status than determining concentrations of each antioxidant compounds [18]. It is due to that antioxidant compounds establish complex interactions with other antioxidant compounds and do not work alone [19].

Malondialdehyde (MDA) appears during the lipid peroxidation from cellular membrane phospholipids degradation, afterwards is released into extracellular space, and finally appears in the blood [20, 21].

In the Physiology Department at Faculty of Medicine of University of La Laguna (Tenerife, Spain) was performed the determination of serum concentrations of melatonin using a kit from Immuno Biological Laboratories (IBL Hamburg GmbH, Hamburg, Germany) based in ELISA method, which has a detection limit of 0.13 pg/ml, an intra-assay coefficient of variation (CV) of 6.4% and an inter-assay CV of 11.1%.

In the Laboratory Department at Hospital Universitario de Canarias (La Laguna, Tenerife, Spain) was performed the determination of serum concentrations of TAC using a kit from Cayman Chemical Corporation (Ann Arbor, USA) based in the ability of the sample to inhibit the oxidation of 2,2′-azino-di-[3-ethylbenzthiazoline sulphonate] (ABTS) by metmyoglobin, which has a detection limit of 0.04 mmol/L, an intra-assay CV of 3.4% and an inter-assay CV of 3.0%.

In the Physiology Department at Faculty of Medicine of University of La Laguna (Tenerife, Spain) was performed the determination of serum concentrations MDA using a thiobarbituric acid-reactive substance (TBARS) assay according to Kikugawa et al. [22], which has a detection limit of 0.079 nmol/mL, an intra-assay CV of 1.82% and an inter-assay CV of 4.01%.

Statistical methods

Medians and interquartile ranges were used to report continuous variables, and frequencies and percentages to report categorical variables. Wilcoxon-Mann-Whitney test was used to compare continuous variables between groups, and chi-square test to compare categorical variables.

We used logistic regression analysis to determine the association with 30-day mortality. We carried out two logistic regression models with four variables because 33 patients died. We included in logistic regression analysis the statistically significant variables in the bivariate analysis. We included serum melatonin levels, GCS, CT classification, and age in the first model. We included serum melatonin levels, APACHE-II score, CT classification, and sex in the second model. We recoded the CT classification variable previously to include it in the logistic regression analysis. We found the following mortality rates according CT classification: 5/29 (12.5%) in patients with class 2, 6/20 (30.0%) with class 3, 9/21 (42.9%) with class 4, 5/35 (14.3%) with class 5 and 8/13 (61.5%) with class 6. Then we recoded the CT classification variable as low risk of death (CT class 2 or 5) and high risk of death (CT class 3, 4 or 6). The group of patients with CT with low risk of death (CT class 2 or 5) had a mortality rate of 10/64 (15.6%); and the group of patients with CT with high risk of death (CT class 3, 4 or 6) had a mortality rate of 23/54 (42.6%). We calculate Odds Ratio and 95% confidence intervals to measure the association of variables with mortality.

Receiver operator characteristic (ROC) curve was constructed with serum levels of melatonin as prognostic variable and 30-day survival as classification variable. To select cut-off prognostic value of serum melatonin level (3.53 pg/mL), Youden J index was used. Kaplan-Meier analysis was constructed with survival at 30 days and with cut-off serum melatonin levels (> or <3.53 pg/mL), and both curves were compared using log-rank test.

Correlation between continuous variables was analysed using coefficient of Spearman. We considered p-values < 0.05 as statistically significant. NCSS 2000 (Kaysville, Utah), SPSS 17.0 (SPSS Inc., Chicago, IL, USA), and LogXact 4.1, (Cytel Co., Cambridge, MA) were used to carry out statistical analyses.

Results

Biochemical and clinical characteristics of survivor (n = 85) and non-survivor (n = 33) TBI patients are showed in Table 1. Non-survivor TBI patients compared to survivor had higher serum levels of melatonin (p < 0.001), TAC (p < 0.001), and MDA (p < 0.001). In addition, non-survivor TBI patients compared to survivor patients had higher APACHE-II score, female rate and age, and lower GCS than survivors. Besides, non-survivor and survivor TBI patients had differences in CT classification.

Logistic regression analyses are showed in Table 2. Serum melatonin levels are associated with 30-day mortality (OR = 1.334; 95% CI = 1.094–1.627; p = 0.004) after to control for age, GCS and CT lesions. Besides, serum melatonin levels are associated with 30-day mortality (OR = 1.364; 95% CI = 1.108–1.678; p = 0.003) after to control for sex, APACHE-II and CT lesions.

Area under the curve (AUC) to predict 30-day mortality for serum melatonin levels was of 0.84 (95% CI = 0.76–0.90; p < 0.001) (Fig. 1). We have not found differences in AUC for GCS (0.77; 95% CI = 0.68–0.84) and serum melatonin levels (p = 0.19).

Kaplan-Meier analysis showed a higher mortality at 30 days in patients with serum melatonin levels > 3.53 pg/mL (Hazard ratio = 10.5; 95% CI = 4.99–22.13; p < 0.001) (Fig. 2).

We found a positive correlation of serum melatonin levels with serum TAC levels (rho = 0.37; p < 0.001), and with serum MDA levels (rho = 0.24; p = 0.008).

Discussion

As we know, this study is the series of higher sample size providing serum levels of melatonin levels in patients with TBI. The new findings were that non-survivor compared to survivor patients had higher serum melatonin levels, that an association between serum melatonin levels, peroxidation state, antioxidant state, and mortality exists, and that serum melatonin levels could be used as biomarker for mortality prediction in patients with TBI.

Previously, circulating levels of melatonin in patients with TBI have been determined in a little number of studies [7–11], and was reported only the comparison of serum melatonin levels between TBI patients and healthy controls. Thus, our study is the first providing serum melatonin levels in survivor and non-survivor patients with TBI, and higher levels in non-survivors compared to survivors. Besides, to our knowledge, our study (including 118 TBI patients) is the study with largest sample size reporting serum melatonin levels in patients with TBI.

In the Seifman et al. study [11] was found a weak positive correlation of serum levels of melatonin and 6-month Glasgow outcome score extended (GOSE) in 39 severe TBI patients (r = 0.189; p = 0.004), and higher

Table 1 Clinical and biochemical characteristics of survivor and non-survivor patients

	Non-survivors (n = 33)	Survivors (n = 85)	*P value*
Gender female – n (%)	13 (39.4)	15 (17.6)	0.02
Age (years) - median (p 25–75)	66 (55–75)	46 (28–62)	<0.001
Temperature (°C) - median (p 25–75)	36.0 (35.0–37.0)	37.0 (36.0–37.3)	0.12
Sodium (mEq/L)- median (p 25–75)	142 (138–148)	140 (138–143)	0.19
Glycemia (g/dL) - median (p 25–75)	160 (134–189)	139 (122-167)	0.08
Leukocytes-median*10^3/mm^3 (p 25–75)	16.3 (9.8–22.7)	14.5 (10.3–19.0)	0.46
PaO2 (mmHg) - median (p 25–75)	133 (98–180)	148 (110–203)	0.34
PaO2/FIO_2 ratio - median (p 25–75)	274 (173–393)	336 (240–400)	0.11
Bilirubin (mg/dl) - median (p 25–75)	0.70 (0.58–0.95)	0.50 (0.40–0.80)	0.045
Creatinine (mg/dl) - median (p 25–75)	0.80 (0.70–1.10)	0.80 (0.63–1.00)	0.44
Hemoglobin (g/dL) - median (p 25–75)	11.9 (9.8–13.1)	11.4 (10.2–13.0)	0.87
GCS score - median (p 25–75)	3 (3–6)	7 (5–8)	<0.001
Lactic acid (mmol/L)-median (p 25–75)	2.40 (1.30–4.60)	1.70 (1.10–2.50)	0.06
Platelets - median*10^3/mm^3 (p 25–75)	180 (125–237)	184 (134–244)	0.52
INR - median (p 25–75)	1.12 (1.03–1.40)	1.11 (1.00–1.21)	0.29
aPTT (seconds) - median (p 25–75)	29 (25–36)	28 (25–31)	0.31
Fibrinogen (mg/dl) - median (p 25–75)	361 (269–520)	366 (283–448)	0.99
APACHE-II score - median (p 25–75)	25 (23–28)	18 (14–22)	<0.001
ISS - median (ppe 25–75)	25 (25–25)	25 (25–29)	0.43
ICP (mmHg) - median (p 25–75)	25 (13–34)	15 (14–20)	0.28
CPP (mmHg) - median (p 25–75)	61 (54–69)	68 (57–70)	0.48
CT classification - n (%)			0.006
Type 1	0	0	
Type 2	5 (15.2)	24 (28.2)	
Type 3	6 (18.2)	14 (16.5)	
Type 4	9 (27.3)	12 (14.1)	
Type 5	5 (15.2)	30 (35.3)	
Type 6	8 (24.2)	5 (5.9)	
CT with high risk of death (types 3,4,6)- n (%)	23 (69.7)	31 (36.5)	0.002
Melatonin (pg/mL) - median (p 25–75)	6.74 (3.78–7.34)	2.49 (2.13–3.24)	<0.001
TAC (mmol/mL) - median (p 25–75)	5.09 (2.45–9.63)	2.36 (1.82–2.94)	<0.001
MDA (nmol/mL) - median (p 25–75)	2.01 (1.35–4.24)	1.36 (1.05–1.79)	<0.001

P 25–75 percentile 25th - 75th, *PaO_2* pressure of arterial oxygen/fraction inspired oxygen, *FIO_2* pressure of arterial oxygen/fraction inspired oxygen, *GCS* Glasgow Coma Scale, *ISS* Injury Severity Score, *INR* international normalized ratio, *aPTT* activated partial thromboplastin time, *APACHE II* Acute Physiology and Chronic Health Evaluation, *ICP* intracranial pressure, *CPP* cerebral perfusion pressure, *CT* computer tomography, *TAC* total antioxidant capacity, *MDA* Malondialdehyde

serum melatonin levels may indicate a better outcome. Our findings are in contrast with those of Seifman et al. Posibles explanations for those different findings could be the outcome chosen (mortality in our study, and GOSE in the study of Seifman et al.), the moment to assess the outcome (30 days in our study, and 6 months in the work by Seifman et al.), and the sample size (118 patients in our study, and 39 patients in the research of Seifman et al.). We chosen mortality at 30 days as outcome due to that in previous studies by us and by other researchers was used this outcome.

In addition, we found that an association of serum levels of melatonin with mortality exists in patients with TBI for the first time. Besides, to our knowledge, our study is the first suggested that serum melatonin levels could be used as biomarker for mortality prediction in patients with TBI. Also, as to we know, the association of serum levels of melatonin, TAC and MDA found in our study has been reported for the first time. We found, as previously were described, higher serum levels of MDA [14, 23] and TAC [15, 24] in non-survivor compared to survivors.

Table 2 Multiple binomial logistic regression analysis to predict 30-day mortality

Variable	Odds Ratio	95% Confidence Interval	*P*
First Model			
Serum melatonin levels (pg/mL)	1.334	1.094–1.627	0.004
GCS score (points)	0.574	0.426–0.773	<0.001
Age (years)	1.047	1.014–1.082	0.006
Computer tomography classification (reference category: low risk of death)	4.526	1.375–14.895	0.013
Second Model			
Serum melatonin levels (pg/mL)	1.364	1.108–1.678	0.003
APACHE-II score (points)	1.315	1.148–1.505	<0.001
Sex (reference category: female)	0.477	0.125–1.823	0.280
Computer tomography classification (reference category: low risk of death)	4.360	1.246–15.253	0.021

GCS Glasgow Coma Scale, *APACHE II* Acute Physiology and Chronic Health Evaluation

In the Seifman et al. study were found higher levels of melatonin and isoprostane (to assess oxidative stress) in cerebrospinal fluid in TBI patients compared to healthy controls, and a positive association of cerebrospinal fluid levels of melatonin with isoprostane [11]. However, in the study by Seifman et al. were not found differences in serum levels of melatonin in TBI patients compared to healthy controls, and they found a negative association of serum levels of melatonin with isoprostane. These authors believed that the increase of melatonin levels in CSF after TBI likely represents a response to oxidative stress. Besides, they believed that that negative correlation of serum levels of melatonin with isoprostane that they found could represent that patients with higher oxidative stress may have higher melatonin consumption and antioxidant activity.

We think that non-survivor compared to survivor TBI patients have higher ROS production, which leads to a higher oxidant state (assessed by increased serum levels of MDA); and that increased serum levels of TAC and melatonin are an attempt to maintain the balance between oxidant and antioxidant state due to the high production of oxidant products. However, in non-survivors those increase of serum levels of TAC and melatonin are not enough for the compensation of high production of oxidants species and then they present higher peroxidation of proteins, lipids, carbohydrates and nucleic acids, contributing to cellular dysfunction, vasogenic edema [2–6].

The administration of melatonin could be suggested for the treatment of patients with severe TBI according to animal model results [25–33]. The administration of melatonin has been associated with antioxidant effects [25–31], anti-inflammatory effects [28, 33], a reduction in brain edema [29, 30, 32], and anti-apoptotic effects [31]. We think that the melatonin administration could help to compensate the increased oxidant products production in patients with higher oxidant state and higher risk of death. In addition, we think that the melatonin administration could contribute to reduce cellular dysfunction and vasogenic edema, and finally reduce the risk of death.

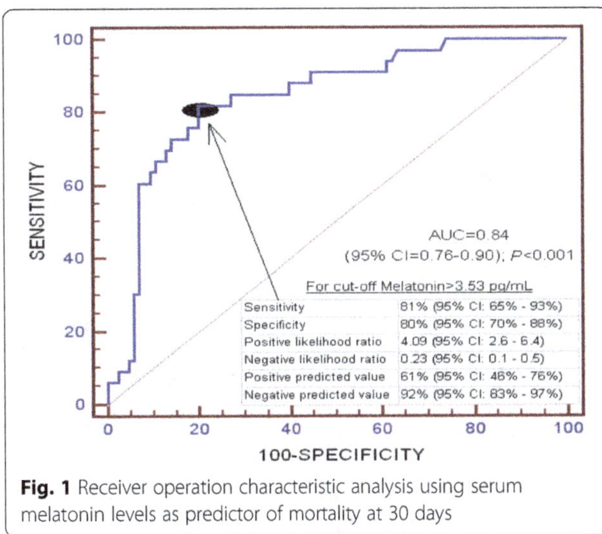

Fig. 1 Receiver operation characteristic analysis using serum melatonin levels as predictor of mortality at 30 days

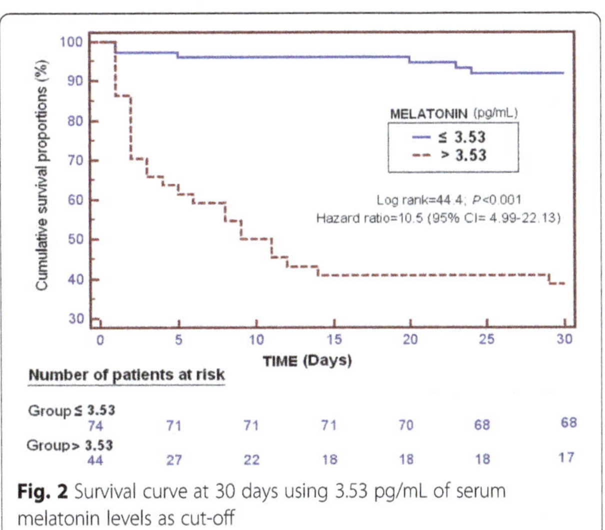

Fig. 2 Survival curve at 30 days using 3.53 pg/mL of serum melatonin levels as cut-off

Our study presents several limitations. First, serum melatonin levels in non-surviving and surviving during follow-up were not described. Second, the determination of other compounds of oxidant and antioxidant states would have been interesting. Third, we did not analyse concentrations of melatonin in cerebrospinal fluid; however, we proposed a low invasiveness protocol and this was the motive to determine melatonin levels in serum. Fourth, due to that the objective of the study was recollect blood samples early after TBI (within 4 h after TBI) then the moment of day to obtain blood samples was not the same for all patients, and the melatonin circadian rhythm is known. Fifth, serum melatonin concentations in control subjects were not analysed; however, our objective study was to analyse whether there is an association of serum melatonin levels with 30-day mortality, and not to determine whether severe TBI modify serum melatonin levels. However, as circulating melatonin levels could be differents according to laboratory kits and moment of day, then the determinations in control subjects could have been interesting. Finally, we think that our study could open the perspective for an interventional trial in patients with TBI.

Conclusions

As to we know, our study is the largest series providing circulating melatonin levels in patients with severe TBI. The main findings were that non-survivors had higher serum melatonin levels than survivors, and the association between serum levels of melatonin levels and mortality, peroxidation state and antioxidant state.

Abbreviations

APACHE: Acute physiology and chronic health evaluation; APTT: Activated partial thromboplastin time; CPP: Cerebral perfusion pressure; CT: Computed tomography; FIO_2: Fraction inspired of oxygen; GCS: Glasgow coma scale; ICP: Intracranial pressure; ICU: Intensive care unit; INR: International normalized ratio; ISS: Injury severity score; MDA: Malondialdehyde; PaO_2: Pressure of arterial oxygen; SOFA: Sepsis-related organ failure assessment score; TAC: Total antioxidant capacity; TBI: Trauma brain injury

Acknowledgments

None.

Funding

This study was supported by a grant from Grupo de Expertos Neurológicos de Canarias (GEN-Canarias. Santa Cruz de Tenerife. Spain), and by a grant from Instituto de Salud Carlos III (INT16/00165) (Madrid, Spain) and co-financed with Fondo Europeo de Desarrollo Regional (FEDER). Fundings influenced no in the study design, the collection, analysis, and interpretation of data, the manuscript writing, and the decision to submit it for publication.

Authors' contributions

LL conceived and designed the protocol study. LL, MMM, LR, MA, JSV, JJC and VGM acquired clinical data and blood samples. PAG determined serum concentrations of melatonin and malondialdehyde. APC determined serum concentrations of total antioxidant capacity. LL and AJ analyzed the data. LL wrote the paper. All authors revised critically the manuscript and approved the final version.

Competing interests

The authors declare that they have no competing interests.

Author details

[1]Intensive Care Unit, Hospital Universitario de Canarias, Ofra s/n. La Laguna, 38320 Santa Cruz de Tenerife, Spain. [2]Intensive Care Unit, Hospital Universitario Nuestra Señora de Candelaria, Crta del Rosario s/n, 38010 Santa Cruz de Tenerife, Spain. [3]Deparment of Physiology. Faculty of Medicine, University of the La Laguna, Ofra s/n. La Laguna, 38320 Santa Cruz de Tenerife, Spain. [4]Laboratory Deparment, Hospital Universitario de Canarias, Ofra, s/n. La Laguna, 38320 Tenerife, Spain. [5]Intensive Care Unit, Hospital General La Palma, Buenavista de Arriba s/n, 38713 Breña Alta, La Palma, Spain. [6]Intensive Care Unit, Hospital Clínico Universitario de Valencia, Avda. Blasco Ibáñez n°17-19, 46004 Valencia, Spain. [7]Intensive Care Unit, Hospital Universitario Dr. Negrín. CIBERES, Barranco de la Ballena s/n, 35010 Las Palmas de Gran Canaria, Spain. [8]Intensive Care Unit, Hospital Insular, Plaza Dr. Pasteur s/n, 35016 Las Palmas de Gran Canaria, Spain. [9]Research Unit, Hospital Universitario de Canarias, Ofra s/n. La Laguna, 38320 Santa Cruz de Tenerife, Spain. [10]Deparment of Neurosurgery, Hospital Universitario de Canarias, Ofra, s/n. La Laguna, 38320 Santa Cruz de Tenerife, Spain.

References

1. Brain Trauma Foundation; American Association of Neurological Surgeons; Congress of Neurological Surgeons. Guidelines for the management of severe traumatic brain injury. J Neurotrauma. 2007;24:S1–106.
2. Esposito E, Cuzzocrea S. Antiinflammatory activity of melatonin in central nervous system. Curr Neuropharmacol. 2010;8:228–42.
3. Samantaray S, Das A, Thakore NP, Matzelle DD, Reiter RJ, Ray SK, Banik NL. Therapeutic potential of melatonin in traumatic central nervous system injury. J Pineal Res. 2009;47:134–42.
4. Maldonado MD, Murillo-Cabezas F, Terron MP, Flores LJ, Tan DX, Manchester LC, Reiter RJ. The potential of melatonin in reducing morbidity-mortality after craniocerebral trauma. J Pineal Res. 2007;42:1–11.
5. Naseem M, Parvez S. Role of melatonin in traumatic brain injury and spinal cord injury. Sci World J. 2014;2014:586270.
6. Fernández-Gajar do R, Matamala JM, Carrasco R, Gutiérrez R, Melo R, Rodrigo R. Novel therapeutic strategies for traumatic brain injury: acute antioxidant reinforcement. CNS Drugs. 2014;28:229–48.
7. Shekleton JA, Parcell DL, Redman JR, Phipps-Nelson J, Ponsford JL, Rajaratnam SM. Sleep disturbance and melatonin levels following traumatic brain injury. Neurology. 2010;74:1732–8.
8. Seifman MA, Gomes K, Nguyen PN, Bailey M, Rosenfeld JV, Cooper DJ, Morganti-Kossmann MC. Measurement of serum melatonin in intensive care unit patients: changes in traumatic brain injury, trauma, and medical conditions. Front Neurol. 2014;5:237.
9. Paul T, Lemmer B. Disturbance of circadian rhythms in analgosedated intensive care unit patients with and without craniocerebral injury. Chronobiol Int. 2007;24:45–61.
10. Paparrigopoulos T, Melissaki A, Tsekou H, Efthymiou A, Kribeni G, Baziotis N, Geronikola X. Melatonin secretion after head injury: a pilot study. Brain Inj. 2006;20:873–8.
11. Seifman MA, Adamides AA, Nguyen PN, Vallance SA, Cooper DJ, Kossmann T, Rosenfeld JV, Morganti-Kossmann MC. Endogenous melatonin increases in cerebrospinal fluid of patients after severe traumatic brain injury and correlates with oxidative stress and metabolic disarray. J Cereb Blood Flow Metab. 2008;28:684–96.
12. Teasdale G, Jennett B. Assessement of coma and impaired conciousness. A practical scale. Lancet. 1974;2:81–4.
13. Baker SP, O'Neill B, Haddon W, Jr Long WB. The injury severity score: a method for describing patients with multiple injuries and evaluating emergency care. J Trauma. 1974;14:187–96.
14. Lorente L, Martín MM, Abreu-González P, Ramos L, Argueso M, Cáceres JJ, Solé-Violán J, Lorenzo JM, Molina I, Jiménez A. Association between serum malondialdehyde levels and mortality in patients with severe brain trauma injury. J Neurotrauma. 2015;32:1–6.
15. Lorente L, Martín MM, Almeida T, Abreu-González P, Ramos L, Argueso M, Riaño-Ruiz M, Solé-Violán J, Jiménez A. Total antioxidant capacity is associated with mortality of patients with severe traumatic brain injury. BMC Neurol. 2015;15:115.
16. Knaus WA, Draper EA, Wagner DP, Zimmerman JE. APACHE II: a severity of disease classification system. Crit Care Med. 1985;13:818–29.
17. Marshall LF, Marshall SB, Klauber MR, Van Berkum CM, Eisenberg H, Jane JA,

Luerssen TG, Marmarou A, Foulkes MA. The diagnosis of head injury requires a classification based on computed axial tomography. J Neurotrauma. 1992;9(Suppl 1):S287–92.
18. Ghiselli A, Serafini M, Natella F, Scaccini C. Total antioxidant capacity as a tool to assess redox status: critical view and experimental data. Free Radic Biol Med. 2000;29:1106–14.
19. Young IS, Woodside JV. Antioxidants in health and disease. J Clin Pathol. 2001;54:176–86.
20. Draper HH, Hadley M. Malondialdehyde determination as index of lipid peroxidation. Methods Enzymol. 1990;186:421–31.
21. Dalle-Donne I, Rossi R, Colombo R, Giustarini D, Milzani A. Biomarkers of oxidative damage in human disease. Clin Chem. 2006;52:601–23.
22. Kikugawa K, Kojima T, Yamaki S, Kosugi H. Interpretation of the thiobarbituric acid reactivity of rat liver and brain homogenates in the presence of ferric ion and ethylediaminotetraacetic acid. Anal Biochem. 1992;202:249–55.
23. Paolin A, Nardin L, Gaetani P, Rodriguez Y, Baena R, Pansarasa O, Marzatico F. Oxidative damage after severe head injury and its relationship to neurological outcome. Neurosurgery. 2002;51:949–54.
24. Kavakli HS, Erel O, Karakayali O, Neselioglu S, Tanriverdi F, Coskun F, Kahraman AF. Oxidative stress in isolated blunt traumatic brain injury. Sci Res Essays. 2010;5:2832–6.
25. Messenge C, Margail I, Verrechia C, Allix M. Protective effect of melatonin in a model of traumatic brain injury in mice. J Pineal Res. 1998;25:41–6.
26. Horakova L, Onrejickova O, Barchrrata K, Vajdova M. Preventive effect of several antioxidants after oxidative stress on rat brain homogenates. Gen Physiol Biophys. 2000;19:195–205.
27. Kerman M, Cirak B, Ozguner MF, Dagtekin A, Sutcu R, Altuntas I, Delibas N. Does melatonin protect or treat brain damage from traumatic oxidative stress? Exp Brain Res. 2005;163:406–10.
28. Tsai MC, Chen WJ, Tsai MS, Ching CH, Chuang JI. Melatonin attenuates brain contusion-induced oxidative insult, inactivation of signal transducers and activators of transcription 1, and upregulation of suppressor of cytokine signaling-3 in rats. J Pineal Res. 2011;51:233–45.
29. Dehghan F, Khaksari Hadad M, Asadikram G, Najafipour H, Shahrokhi N. Effect of melatonin on intracranial pressure and brain edema following traumatic brain injury: role of oxidative stresses. Arch Med Res. 2013;44:251–8.
30. Ding K, Wang H, Xu J, Li T, Zhang L, Ding Y, Zhu L, He J, Zhou M. Melatonin stimulates antioxidant enzymes and reduces oxidative stress in experimental traumatic brain injury: the Nrf2-ARE signaling pathway as a potential mechanism. Free Radic Biol Med. 2014;73:1–11.
31. Yürüker V, Nazıroğlu M, Şenol N. Reduction in traumatic brain injury-induced oxidative stress, apoptosis, and calcium entry in rat hippocampus by melatonin: possible involvement of TRPM2 channels. Metab Brain Dis. 2015;30:223–31.
32. Kabadi SV, Maher TJ. Posttreatment with uridine and melatonin following traumatic brain injury reduces edema in various brain regions in rats. Ann N Y Acad Sci. 2010;1199:105–13.
33. Ding K, Wang H, Xu J, Lu X, Zhang L, Zhu L. Melatonin reduced microglial activation and alleviated neuroinflammation induced neuron degeneration in experimental traumatic brain injury: possible involvement of mTOR pathway. Neurochem Int. 2014;76:23–31.

A novel frameshift *GRN* mutation results in frontotemporal lobar degeneration with a distinct clinical phenotype in two siblings

Takashi Hosaka[1†], Kazuhiro Ishii[1*†], Takeshi Miura[2,3], Naomi Mezaki[2,3], Kensaku Kasuga[2], Takeshi Ikeuchi[2] and Akira Tamaoka[1]

Abstract

Background: Progranulin gene (*GRN*) mutations are major causes of frontotemporal lobar degeneration. To date, 68 pathogenic *GRN* mutations have been identified. However, very few of these mutations have been reported in Asians. Moreover, some *GRN* mutations manifest with familial phenotypic heterogeneity. Here, we present a novel *GRN* mutation resulting in frontotemporal lobar degeneration with a distinct clinical phenotype, and we review reports of *GRN* mutations associated with familial phenotypic heterogeneity.

Case presentation: We describe the case of a 74-year-old woman with left frontotemporal lobe atrophy who presented with progressive anarthria and non-fluent aphasia. Her brother had been diagnosed with corticobasal syndrome (CBS) with right-hand limb-kinetic apraxia, aphasia, and a similar pattern of brain atrophy. Laboratory blood examinations did not reveal abnormalities that could have caused cognitive dysfunction. In the cerebrospinal fluid, cell counts and protein concentrations were within normal ranges, and concentrations of tau protein and phosphorylated tau protein were also normal. Since similar familial cases due to mutation of *GRN* and microtubule-associated protein tau gene (*MAPT*) were reported, we performed genetic analysis. No pathological mutations of MAPT were identified, but we identified a novel *GRN* frameshift mutation (c.1118_1119delCCinsG: p.Pro373ArgX37) that resulted in progranulin haploinsufficiency.

Conclusion: This is the first report of a *GRN* mutation associated with familial phenotypic heterogeneity in Japan. Literature review of *GRN* mutations associated with familial phenotypic heterogeneity revealed no tendency of mutation sites. The role of progranulin has been reported in this and other neurodegenerative diseases, and the analysis of *GRN* mutations may lead to the discovery of a new therapeutic target.

Keywords: Progranulin, Primary progressive aphasia, Corticobasal syndrome, Frontotemporal lobar degeneration, Phenotypic heterogeneity, Case report

Background

Frontotemporal lobar degeneration (FTLD) is characterized by degeneration of the frontal and temporal lobes, and presents as a clinically heterogeneous disease. The pathological classification of FTLD is based on the molecular features of the disease-associated inclusion-forming proteins: FTLD-tau, FTLD-TDP, FTLD-FUS, and FTLD-UPS. Clinically, FTLD is classified into two subsets: behavioral variant FTLD (bvFTLD) and primary progressive aphasia (PPA), the latter of which includes semantic dementia and progressive non-fluent aphasia. In addition, FTLD can be concomitant with corticobasal degeneration (CBD), progressive supranuclear palsy (PSP), and motor neuron disease (MND) [1].

Progranulin is widely expressed in the central nervous system and is involved in immunomodulation as well as cell growth and proliferation. Since the first demonstration of

* Correspondence: kazishii@md.tsukuba.ac.jp
†Equal contributors
[1]Department of the Neurology, Division of Clinical Medicine, Faculty of Medicine, University of Tsukuba, 1-1-1 Ten'noudai, Tsukuba, Ibaraki 305-8575, Japan
Full list of author information is available at the end of the article

FTLD-associated progranulin gene (*GRN*) mutation in 2006 [2, 3], more than 150 *GRN* mutations have been identified, including 68 pathogenic mutations. FTLD due to a *GRN* mutation is histopathologically characterized by ubiquitin-positive and TDP-43-positive inclusion bodies. While the most frequent clinical phenotype is bvFTLD, PPA and corticobasal syndrome (CBS) have also been reported [4–6]. There are also reports of clinical heterogeneity within a family [7, 8]. In addition, FTLD due to a *GRN* mutation is rare in Asian individuals, with an incidence of < 1% in Asians compared to an incidence of 5–10% in Europeans [9, 10].

In this report, we present the case of a 74-year-old Japanese woman with left-side atrophy in the frontal and temporal lobes and symptoms of progressive anarthria and non-fluent aphasia. We identified the cause to be a novel frameshift mutation in *GRN* that caused progranulin haploinsufficiency.

Case presentation

A 74-year-old woman was referred to our hospital and admitted for progressive speech and language difficulties. The patient was unable to recall the names of things or persons and was unable to communicate with others for about 1 year prior to admission, though she was able to shop and do housework without difficulty. She had no significant medical history; however, regarding her family history, her elder brother had developed word-finding difficulty with verbal paraphasia and right-hand limb-kinetic apraxia at the age of 62 years of age, and was diagnosed with CBS at 69 years of age. He had frontal lobe signs such as forced grasping, total aphasia, and right-limb kinetic apraxia; moreover, brain magnetic resonance imaging (MRI) demonstrated frontal and temporal lobar atrophy dominantly affecting the left side (Fig. 1a). The patient's brother and parents had passed away; therefore, we could not obtain their detailed clinical information.

Neurological findings indicated that our patient was lucid, but showed thought laziness. The cranial nerves, including those related to eye movement, were normal. The patient had normal muscle tonus and did not show muscle weakness or involuntary movement, but all extremity tendon reflexes were slightly increased. There was no evidence of sensory impairment or cerebellar ataxia. It was noted that speech required significant effort, was slow and non-fluent, and showed anarthria and aphasia. The patient's Mini-Mental Scale Examination score was 4/30.

Language function was assessed using the Western Aphasia Battery (WAB) Japanese edition once and SLTA (standard language test of aphasia) two times within 2 months. The scores of WAB subtests were as follows: spontaneous speech, 13 points; auditory verbal comprehension, 5.5 points; repetition, 0 points; naming, 0 points; reading, 4.3 points; writing, 2.2 points; praxis, 6.8 points; and construction, drawing, block design & calculation, 6.6 points. Raven's score was 25/37 (average ± standard deviation: 26.9 ± 5.4). Aphasia quotient was 36.8. The results of SLTA were similar to those of

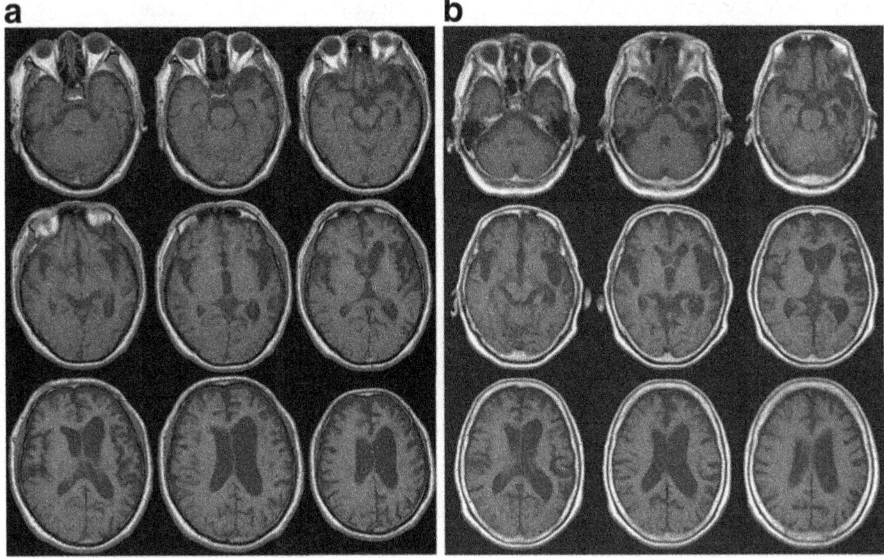

Fig. 1 Brain MRI (axial T1-weighted images) of the patient's brother (**a**) and the patient (**b**). **a** T1-weighted brain images of the patient's brother at 4 years after disease onset. Atrophy was predominantly observed in the left hemisphere affecting the frontotemporal lobes. **b** T1-weighted brain images of the patient at 1 year after disease onset. Similar to her brother, atrophy was predominantly observed in the left hemisphere affecting the frontal and temporal lobes

WAB. Naming, writing, and repetition were impaired. However, auditory verbal comprehension and reading concerning words and short sentences were relatively preserved. Spatial perception and visual perception were also normal. Verbal comprehension via visual perception was approximately normal. Therefore, it is likely that auditory verbal comprehension was complemented by visual perception. Constructional dysfunction, limb-kinetic apraxia, ideational apraxia, and motor apraxia were not observed. Laboratory blood examinations did not reveal any particular abnormalities that could have caused cognitive dysfunction. Cell counts and protein concentrations in the patient's cerebrospinal fluid were within normal ranges, and concentrations of tau protein (282 pg/mL) and phosphorylated tau protein (31.3 pg/mL or lower) were also normal. Brain MRI demonstrated cerebral atrophy dominantly affecting the left frontotemporal lobes (Fig. 1b).

Clinically, the main patient symptoms were difficulty in verbal expression and non-fluent aphasia in the absence of visual memory impairment or behavioral abnormalities. On this premise, the patient was diagnosed with PPA according to Mesulam's criteria [11]. Furthermore, the aphasia was classified as non-fluent progressive aphasia because, while speech itself required effort, the patient retained knowledge about objects and the ability to understand words. Brain MRI demonstrated cerebral cortical atrophy dominantly affecting the left frontal and temporal lobes, consistent with previous reports of non-fluent aphasia [4, 12]. Thus, FTLD was diagnosed according to the patient's clinical symptoms. Since the patient's elder brother had been diagnosed with CBS, and similar familial cases of FTLD due to *GRN* and microtubule-associated protein tau gene (*MAPT*) mutations had been reported [13], we performed genetic analyses on the patient.

Genomic deoxyribonucleic acid (DNA) was extracted from peripheral leukocytes isolated from the patient. The exon/intron boundary of *GRN* was amplified by polymerase chain reaction (PCR) according to a previously reported method [2] and the PCR products were sequenced in both directions. Briefly, blood was collected into a PAXgene® RNA tube, total ribonucleic acid (RNA) was extracted from the sample, and cDNA was prepared from total RNA by a reverse transcriptase reaction. cDNA was then amplified by reverse transcriptase–polymerase chain reaction (RT-PCR) (forward primer: 5′-ACCCAGGCTGT GTGCTG-3′; reverse primer: 5′-GACAGCCTCTGGG ATTGGAC-3′) and the gene expression of *GRN* was analyzed. Then, the amplified PCR product was extracted and its sequence was analyzed.

The genetic examination identified a novel mutation (c.1118_1119delCCinsG) in exon10 of *GRN,* which was thought to cause a frameshift mutation (p.Pro373ArgX38). No pathological mutations of *MAPT* were identified. The *GRN* mRNA sequence was analyzed by RT-PCR; however, a mutant allele product was not detected, suggesting degradation of the mutant allele by the nonsense-mediated RNA decay system. Accordingly, haploinsufficiency due to reduced expression of progranulin was considered to be a possible pathogenic mechanism of FTLD in these cases (Fig. 2).

Discussion and conclusions

Various types of mutations including aberrant splicing, gene deletion, frameshift, and nonsense mutations of *GRN* have been reported. These mutations are known to cause familial FTLD via progranulin haploinsufficiency [2, 3]. In the present case, our patient displayed PPA as a main symptom of progranulin haploinsufficiency due to a novel frameshift mutation of *GRN*. PPA, progressive difficulties with word recall and usage, and language comprehension impairments were apparent, whereas behavioral disinhibition, executive function, and memory impairments were not impaired in the early stages of disease (within 1 year after diagnosis). Other diseases known to cause PPA include FTLD, Alzheimer's disease (AD), CBS, and Creutzfeldt–Jakob disease (CJD) [11]; however, a large number of studies reporting a link between *GRN* mutations and PPA suggest that *GRN* mutations should always be considered in the differential diagnosis of PPA. Similar symptoms, neuropsychological profile, and neuroimaging findings have been reported in a monozygotic twin pair with a *GRN* mutation [14]. In contrast, in our case, the patient's brother presented distinct phenotypic characteristics (i.e., FTLD with PPA and CBS in the early stage). However, because the patient's brother had already passed away, we could not obtain sufficient information to perform a genetic

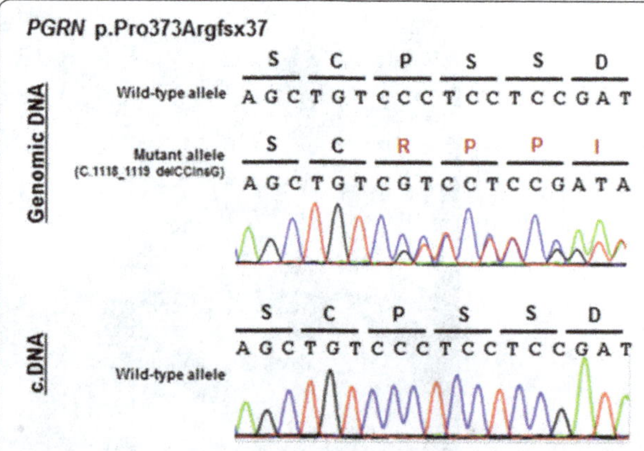

Fig. 2 Genomic DNA and mRNA analyses. A sequential analysis of genomic DNA obtained from the patient revealed a novel mutation in *GRN* (c.1118_1119delCCinsG; p.Pro373ArgX38). RT-PCR analysis using cDNA prepared from the patient's peripheral lymphocytes revealed no expression of the mutant allele, suggesting haploinsufficiency due to nonsense-mediated mRNA decay

Table 1 Familial cases presenting with distinct clinical phenotypes

Case	Age onset; number of patients	First symptom	Phenotype	Brain atrophy	Ethnic origin	*GRN* mutation
Rovelet-Lecrux et al., 2008 [15]	67,77; 2 patients	Language dysfunction	PPA	left > right	French	g.95_4390del
		Resting tremor	PD			
Spina et al., 2007 [13]	45,73; 2 patients	Involuntary arm movement	CBS	right > left	N/A	g.26C >A
		Cognitive decline	AD			
Beck et al., 2008 [4]	54–67; 10 patients	Language dysfunction	PPA	left > right (*n* = 2)	United Kingdom	g.90_91insCTGC
		Limb apraxia	CBS	right > left (*n* = 1)		
Skoglund et al., 2009 [12]	46–59; 10 patients	Language dysfunction	PPA	N/A	Swedish	g.102delC
		Limb apraxia	CBS			
Rademakers et al., 2007 [16]	62,66; 2 patients	N/A	FTLD, CBS	N/A	American	g.3240C > T
Masellis et al., 2006 [17]	57,62; 2 patients	Behavioral changes	FTLD	right > left	Canadian family of Chinese origin	g.1637G > A
		Axial and extremity rigidity	CBS			
Leverenz et al., 2007 [18]	35–69; 9 patients	Language dysfunction	FTLD	left > right (*n* = 3) right > left (n = 1)	American	g.1871A > G
		Anxiety, apathy	PPA			
		Parkinsonism	PD			
López de Munain et al., 2008 [19]	53,57; 2 patients	N/A	FTLD, CBS	N/A	Basque Country	g.1872G > A
	51,71; 2 patients	N/A	FTLD, CBS	N/A	Basque Country	g.1873G > A
	65; 2 patients	N/A	FTLD, CBS	N/A	Basque Country	g.1874G > A
	60; 2 patients	N/A	FTLD, CBS	N/A	Basque Country	g.1875G > A
	63–70; 4 patients	N/A	FTLD, CBS	N/A	Basque Country	g.1876G > A
	52; 2 patients	N/A	FTLD, ALS	N/A	Basque Country	g.1877G > A
Benussi et al., 2009 [5]	60–71; 5 patients	Language dysfunction	PPA	right > left	Italian	g.1977_1980delCACT
		Parkinsonism	CBS			
Kelley et al., 2009 [6]	N/A; 6 patients	N/A	FTLD, PD	symmetrical	American	g.2273_2274insTG
	N/A; 6 patients	N/A	FTLD, PD	right > left	American	g.2597delC
Pietroboni et al., 2011 [7]	47–79; 5 patients	Memory impairment, Acalculia	FTLD, AD	right > left (n = 1) symmetrical (n = 1) N/A (n = 3)	Italian	g.63_64insC
		Language impairment				
Rossi et al., 2011 [8]	47–80; 6 patients	Behavioural abnormality	FTLD Dementia	Left > right	Italian	g.1761_1762delCA
		Language dysfunction				
		Attention impairment				
The present case	75,62; 2 patients	Language dysfunction	PPA	left > right	Japanese	g.1118_1119delCCinsG
		Limb apraxia	CBS			

AD Alzheimer's disease, *ALS* amyotrophic lateral sclerosis, *CBS* corticobasal syndrome, *FTLD* frontotemporal lobar degeneration, *GRN* progranulin gene, *N/A* not available, *PD* Parkinson's disease, *PPA* primary progressive aphasia

analysis. Table 1 provides a summary of known cases of *GRN* mutations that have been associated with familial phenotypic heterogeneity. The presence of familial phenotypic heterogeneity with respect to symptoms such as cognitive dysfunction and motor impairment has been reported in 17 families with *GRN* mutations [4–10, 12–19]. These studies reported significant variations in age of onset and mutation site, and motor neuron diseases were relatively uncommon. Families have also been reported with differing symptom laterality and different regions of brain atrophy. In a genetic analysis of 48 Japanese families with FTLD, PSP, or CBS [10], only one FTLD case with a *GRN* mutation was identified. Therefore, familial FTLD associated with *GRN* mutations is very rare. Furthermore, our report is the first to describe in detail distinct phenotypes within a family. Additional investigations of *GRN* mutations mediating different clinical phenotypes of neurodegeneration within a family are necessary.

As mentioned above, haploinsufficiency is thought to underlie the mechanism of *GRN* mutation-associated FTLD. Haploinsufficiency is a cause of autosomal genetic conditions when the protein expressed by a single allele is not sufficient to maintain its normal function (loss of function) [20]. On the other hand, in many autosomal dominant conditions, toxic gain of function or toxicity of excessive proteins are the cause of disease [21, 22]. In fact, an approximate 50% decrease in mRNA and 33% decrease in progranulin protein was reported in one *GRN* mutation carrier [1, 2]. It has thus been suggested that an effective therapeutic strategy would be to increase progranulin levels in patients [1]. The relationship between *GRN* genetic variability and the risk of developing a neurodegenerative disease such as AD or MND has been reported [1]. Yet, the exact functions of progranulin in the brain remain unclear, and its pathogenic involvement in neurodegenerative disorders is not known. Therefore, the accumulation of new cases of *GRN* mutations that display distinct clinical phenotypes within a family may be helpful not only for the elucidation of progranulin function, but also for the development of replacement therapies in FTLD and other neurodegenerative diseases due to *GRN* mutations.

Abbreviations

AD: Alzheimer's disease; ALS: Amyotrophic lateral sclerosis; bvFTLD: Behavioral variant frontotemporal lobar degeneration; CBD: Corticobasal degeneration; CBS: Corticobasal syndrome; CJD: Creutzfeldt–Jakob disease; DNA: Deoxyribonucleic acid; FTLD: Frontotemporal lobar degeneration; *GRN*: Progranulin gene; *MAPT*: Microtubule-associated protein tau gene; MND: Motor neuron disease; MRI: Magnetic resonance imaging; PCR: Polymerase chain reaction; PD: Parkinson's disease; PPA: Primary progressive aphasia; PSP: Progressive supranuclear palsy; RNA: Ribonucleic acid; RT-PCR: Reverse transcriptase–polymerase chain reaction

Acknowledgements

The authors thank the patient and her family for providing clinical data and allowing the publication of this case report. The authors would also like to thank Dr. N. Takegami for clinical assistance, and Ms. Y. Ishii, A. Kijima, S. Sugimoto and K. Takabe for technical assistance.

Funding

The genomic DNA and mRNA analyses in this study were supported by the Practical Research Project for Rare/Intractable diseases, Japan Agency for Medical Research and Development (AMED).

Authors' contributions

TH and KI collected the clinical data, interpreted the data, and wrote the manuscript. KI recruited the patients and designed the manuscript. AT and KI performed the clinical data analysis and evaluation. TM, NM, KK, and TI analyzed genomic DNA and mRNA of the patient's blood sample. All authors read and approved the final version of manuscript.

Competing interests

The authors declare that they have no competing interests.

Author details

[1]Department of the Neurology, Division of Clinical Medicine, Faculty of Medicine, University of Tsukuba, 1-1-1 Ten'noudai, Tsukuba, Ibaraki 305-8575, Japan. [2]Department of Molecular Genetics, Brain Research Institute, Niigata University, 1-757 Asahimachi, Niigata 951-8585, Japan. [3]Department of Neurology, Brain Research Institute, Niigata University, 1-757 Asahimachi, Niigata 951-8585, Japan.

References

1. Petkau TL, Leavitt BR. Progranulin in neurodegenerative disease. Trends Neurosci. 2014;37:388–98.
2. Baker M, Mackenzie IR, Pickering-Brown SM, Gass J, Rademakers R, Lindholm C, et al. Mutations in progranulin cause tau-negative frontotemporal dementia linked to chromosome 17. Nature. 2006;442:916–9.
3. Cruts M, Gijselinck I, van der Zee J, Engelborghs S, Wils H, Pirici D, et al. Null mutations in progranulin cause ubiquitin-positive frontotemporal dementia linked to chromosome 17q21. Nature. 2006;442:920–4.
4. Beck J, Rohrer JD, Campbell T, Isaacs A, Morrison KE, Goodall EF, et al. A distinct clinical, neuropsychological and radiological phenotype is associated with progranulin gene mutations in a large UK series. Brain. 2008;131:706–20.
5. Benussi L, Ghidoni R, Pegoiani E, Moretti DV, Zanetti O, Binetti G. Progranulin Leu271LeufsX10 is one of the most common FTLD and CBS associated mutations worldwide. Neurobiol Dis. 2009;33:379–85.
6. Kelley BJ, Haidar W, Boeve BF, Baker M, Graff-Radford NR, Krefft T, et al. Prominent phenotypic variability associated with mutations in Progranulin. Neurobiol Aging. 2009;30:739–51.
7. Pietroboni AM, Fumagalli GG, Ghezzi L, Fenoglio C, Cortini F, Serpente M, et al. Phenotypic heterogeneity of the GRN Asp22fs mutation in a large Italian kindred. J Alzheimers Dis. 2011;24:253–9.
8. Rossi G, Piccoli E, Benussi L, Caso F, Redaelli V, Magnani G, et al. A novel progranulin mutation causing frontotemporal lobar degeneration with heterogeneous phenotypic expression. J Alzheimers Dis. 2011;23:7–12.
9. Rohrer JD, Guerreiro R, Vandrovcova J, Uphill J, Reiman D, Beck J, et al. The heritability and genetics of frontotemporal lobar degeneration. Neurology. 2009;73:1451–6.
10. Ogaki K, Li Y, Takanashi M, Ishikawa K, Kobayashi T, Nonaka T, et al. Analyses of the MAPT, PRGN, and C9orf72 mutations in Japanese patients with FTLD, PSP, and CBS. Parkinsonism Relat Disord. 2013;19:15–20.
11. Mesulam MM. Primary progressive aphasia. Ann Neurol. 2001;49:425–32.
12. Skoglund L, Brundin R, Olofsson T, Kalimo H, Ingvast S, Blom ES, et al. Frontotemporal dementia in a large Swedish family is caused by a progranulin null mutation. Neurogenetics. 2009;10:27–34.
13. Spina S, Murrell JR, Huey ED, Wassermann EM, Pietrini P, Grafman J, et al. Corticobasal syndrome associated with the A9D Progranulin mutation. J Neuropathol Exp Neurol. 2007;66:892–900.
14. McDade E, Boeve BF, Burrus TM, Boot BP, Kantarci K, Fields J, et al. Similar clinical and neuroimaging features in monozygotic twin pair with mutation in progranulin. Neurology. 2012;78:1245–9.
15. Rovelet-Lecrux A, Deramecourt V, Legallic S, Maurage CA, Le Ber I, Brice A, et al. Deletion of the progranulin gene in patients with frontotemporal lobar degeneration or Parkinson disease. Neurobiol Dis. 2008;31:41–5.
16. Randemakers R, Baker M, Gass J, Adamson J, Huey ED, Momeni P, et al. Phenotype variability associated with progranulin haploinsufficiency in patients with the common 1477C>T(Arg493X) mutation: an international initiative. Lancet Neurol. 2007;6:857–68.
17. Masellis M, Momeni P, Meschino W, Heffner R Jr, Elder J, Sato C, et al. Novel splicing mutation in the progranulin gene causing familial corticobasal syndrome. Brain. 2006;129:3115–23.
18. Leverenz JB, Yu CE, Montine TJ, Steinbart E, Bekris LM, Zabetian C, et al. A novel progranulin mutation associated with variable clinical presentation and tau, TDP43 and alpha-synuclein pathology. Brain. 2007;130:1360–74.

19. López de Munain A, Alzualde A, Gorostidi A, Otaegui D, Ruiz-Martínez J, Indakoetxea B, et al. Mutations in progranulin gene: clinical, pathological, and ribonucleic acid expression findings. Biol Psychiatry. 2008;63:946–52.
20. Cook DL, Gerber AN, Tapscott SJ. Modeling stochastic gene expression: implications for haploinsufficiency. Proc Natl Acad Sci U S A. 1998;95:15641–6.
21. Davis JA, Naruse S, Chen H, Eckman C, Younkin S, Price DL. An Alzheimer's disease-linked PS1 variant rescues the developmental abnormalities of PS1-deficient embryos. Neuron. 1998;20:603–9.
22. Qian S, Jiang P, Guan XM, Singh G, Trumbauer ME, Yu H. Mutant human presenilin 1 protects presenilin 1 null mouse against embryonic lethality and elevates Abeta1-42/43 expression. Neuron. 1998;20:611–7.

Anatomic mapping of molecular subtypes in diffuse glioma

Qisheng Tang[1†], Yuxi Lian[2†], Jinhua Yu[2*], Yuanyuan Wang[2*], Zhifeng Shi[1*] and Liang Chen[1]

Abstract

Background: Tumor location served as an important prognostic factor in glioma patients was considered to postulate molecular features according to cell origin theory. However, anatomic distribution of unique molecular subtypes was not widely investigated. The relationship between molecular phenotype and histological subgroup were also vague based on tumor location. Our group focuses on the study of glioma anatomic location of distinctive molecular subgroups and histology subtypes, and explores the possibility of their consistency based on clinical background.

Methods: We retrospectively reviewed 143 cases with both molecular information (IDH1/TERT/1p19q) and MRI images diagnosed as cerebral diffuse gliomas. The anatomic distribution was analyzed between distinctive molecular subgroups and its relationship with histological subtypes. The influence of tumor location, molecular stratification and histology diagnosis on survival outcome was investigated as well.

Results: Anatomic locations of cerebral diffuse glioma indicate varied clinical outcome. Based on that, it can be stratified into five principal molecular subgroups according to IDH1/TERT/1p19q status. Triple-positive (IDH1 and TERT mutation with 1p19q codeletion) glioma tended to be oligodendroglioma present with much better clinical outcome compared to TERT mutation only group who is glioblastoma inclined (median overall survival 39 months VS 18 months). Five molecular subgroups were demonstrated with distinctive locational distribution. This kind of anatomic feature is consistent with its corresponding histological subtypes.

Discussion: Each molecular subgroup in glioma has unique anatomic location which indicates distinctive clinical outcome. Molecular diagnosis can be served as perfect complementary tool for the precise diagnosis. Integration of histomolecular diagnosis will be much more helpful in routine clinical practice in the future.

Keywords: Glioma, Molecular diagnosis, Anatomic location

Background

Glioma is the most common malignant brain tumor with heterogeneous growth pattern which can be found in different cerebral lobes [1, 2]. This kind of locational variety has been demonstrated to be of great importance in patient diagnosis and prognosis which can reflect the tumor cells origin as well [3]. Many studies have been performed to prove relationship between molecular biomarkers and tumor location. [2, 4–6]. Recently, new WHO classification of cerebral diffuse gliomas was revised with complementary of three molecular biomarkers (IDH1/1p19q/H3F3A) integrated into comprehensive pathological diagnosis [7]. It demonstrated that glioma-related biomarkers have been playing much more important role in precise medicine. Robert B.Jenkins et al. has successfully used three major biomarkers to classify glioma into five principal molecular subsets represent distinctive clinical significance and germline variants. This finding hallmarked the development of molecular pathology in glioma which was published on New England Journal of Medicine [8]. In our study, we plan to use same stratification system in our patients cohort and delineate tumor locational tendency within different molecular subtypes. Furthermore, we will explore the consistency of tumor location between histological subtypes and their molecular counterparts to identify the complementary effect of molecular diagnosis in cerebral diffuse glioma, especially in outcome prediction.

* Correspondence: jhyu@fudan.edu.cn; yywang@fudan.edu.cn; 13917793493@139.com
†Equal contributors
[2]Department of Electronic Engineering, Fudan University, Shanghai, China
[1]Department of Neurosurgery, Huashan Hospital, Fudan University, Shanghai, China

Methods

Patients and tissue samples

We searched for Molecular Database and Image Bank in Department of Neurosurgery, Huashan Hospital and retrospectively selected 143 glioma samples for further study. H&E slides of all cases were reviewed by 2 individual neuropathologists to confirm the diagnosis of glioma according to WHO 2016 brain tumor guideline. Every patient has molecular diagnostic information. 140 out of 143 patients got complete follow-up. This research work was approved by Ethic Committee of Huashan Hospital and informed consents signed. Patients characteristic are listed in Table 1.

Molecular profiles of IDH1/TERT/1p19q

Paraffin blocks of each case were prepared. Four 4um slides and six 10um slides were sectioned. DNA extraction was performed by commercial DNA extraction kit (Qiagen, Shanghai) using 10um slides. IDH1 and TERT mutational analysis were done by Sanger Sequencing with method reported previously [9]. The status of 1p19q was determined by FISH (fluorescence in situ hybridization). A case of 50% tumor cells present with reference probe signal ratio to target probe signal more than 2:1 was considered 1p19q codeletion, otherwise we called 1p19q intact [10]. Molecular information will be integrated into regular pathological diagnosis.

Tumor location analysis

Image segmentation is an important pre-processing step for location analysis. Convolutional neural network (CNN) was proved to be an effective method for medical image segmentation [11]. In our research, an approach based on CNN was adopted to extract brain tumors on MR images, which got satisfactory performance in the Brain Tumor Segmentation Challenge 2013 and 2015. (http://www.braintumorsegmentation.org/).

In order to study the location features in same coordinate system, the segmentation results were registered to MNI152 (Montreal Neurological Institute (MNI)) brain atlas [12]. A research platform also provided by MNI, SPM12, was used to accomplish this procedure. Both MNI152 and SPM12 were widely used in brain tumor registration [13].

Statistical analysis

Correlation coefficient was calculated to figure out the location relation between specific histology stratification and molecular phenotype. IBM SPSS statistic 20.0 software (SPSS, Chicago, IL, USA) was chosen as the analysis tool. A strong association would be found out with r value closed to 1. Median overall survival time (OS) was defined as the duration from the diagnosis and death or the last follow-up. Kaplan-Meier method was used to draw survival curve and analyzed by Log-rank test.

Results

The molecular combination of IDH1/TERT/1p19q has unique distribution among distinctive histological subtypes in glioma

The information of histology diagnosis and WHO grade among 143 glioma patients can been found in Table 1. Accordance with WHO 2016 instruction, oligoastrocytoma

Table 1 Characteristics of all patients

Characteristic	Total number	Sex		Age		
	143	Male	Female	0–35	36–60	>60
Molecular subtype						
Triple-positive	41 (29%)	23	18	9	32	0
TERT and IDH mutation	7 (5%)	3	4	4	3	0
IDH mutation only	37 (26%)	25	12	19	18	0
Triple-negative	27 (19%)	14	13	7	17	3
TERT mutation only	30 (21%)	21	9	5	13	12
Other	1 (1%)	1	0	1	0	0
WHO grade						
Grade II	82 (57%)	45	37	34	45	3
Grade III	27 (19%)	17	10	6	21	0
Grade IV	34 (24%)	25	9	5	17	12
Pathological Diagnosis						
Astrocytoma	69 (48%)	43	26	29	37	3
Oligodendroglioma	40 (28%)	19	21	11	29	0
Glioblastoma	34 (24%)	25	9	5	17	12

was subdivided into oligodendroglioma or astrocytoma according to 1p19q status [7]. By using panel of IDH1/TERT/1p19q, we divided the whole case cohort into 5 molecular subgroups according to NEJM paper [8]. There are 41 Triple-positive and 27 triple-negative tumors. Proportion of TERT and IDH1 mutation, IDH1 mutation only and TERT mutation only subgroup accounts for 26%, 19% and 21% respectively. Similar to previous studies, IDH1 mutation only tumors were more likely to be seen in astrocytoma with the ratio of 49.3%, while 82.5% triple-positive gliomas belong to oligodendroglioma. 64.7% glioblastomas have TERT mutation only. (Fig. 1).

Different survival outcomes among distinctive molecular subgroups based on IDH1/TERT/1p19q classification system

We have completely follow-up in 140 patients, among whom 43 patients were dead and the other patients were still alive. Patients diagnosed as oligodendroglioma have the best clinical outcome with median overall survival 37.9 months (P < 0.01). Median overall survival are 33 months for astrocytoma and 20.5 months for glioblastoma (Fig. 2a). Regarding to molecular stratification, patients in triple-positive subgroup have the best survival outcome with 39 months of median overall survival compared to IDH1/TERT mutation subgroup (36.9 months), IDH1 mutation only subgroup (34 months), triple-negative subgroup (27.6 months) and TERT mutation only subgroup (19.9 months) (P < 0.0001) (Fig. 2b).

Patients with different anatomic position have unique survival outcome

Previous to studying anatomic preference to special molecular subgroups, we analyzed survival outcome between different tumor location. Herein, we found tumor located in frontal lobe indicated longer overall survival time of 66.1 months compared to tumors located in other cerebral regions (P < 0.01). Tumors located in hemisphere demonstrate better clinical outcome than those in central region even though no significance exists (Fig. 3).

Locational pattern is different among distinctive molecular subgroups

For triple-positive gliomas, tumor location tends to aggregate in bilateral frontal lobes. On the contrary, triple-negative tumors were more likely to locate in bilateral basal ganglia regions. In spite of that, IDH1/TERT mutation subgroup inclined to grow in left frontal lobe close to midline region. IDH1 mutation only subgroup was commonly seen in left frontal lobe and bilateral insular lobes. TERT mutation glioma apparently present with non-midline distribution while sitting in right frontal-insular lobe and left basal ganglia region. Meanwhile, TERT mutation only glioma has deep-seated location than triple-positive cases (Fig. 4).

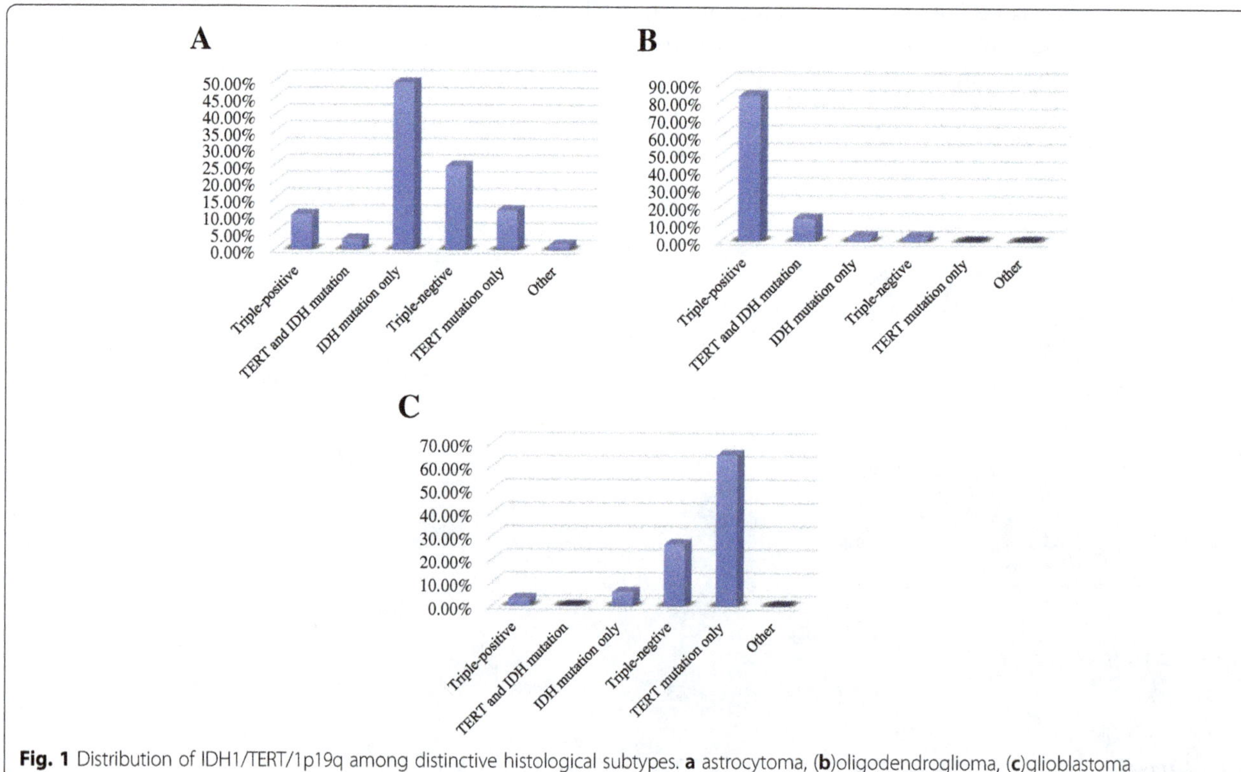

Fig. 1 Distribution of IDH1/TERT/1p19q among distinctive histological subtypes. **a** astrocytoma, (**b**)oligodendroglioma, (**c**)glioblastoma

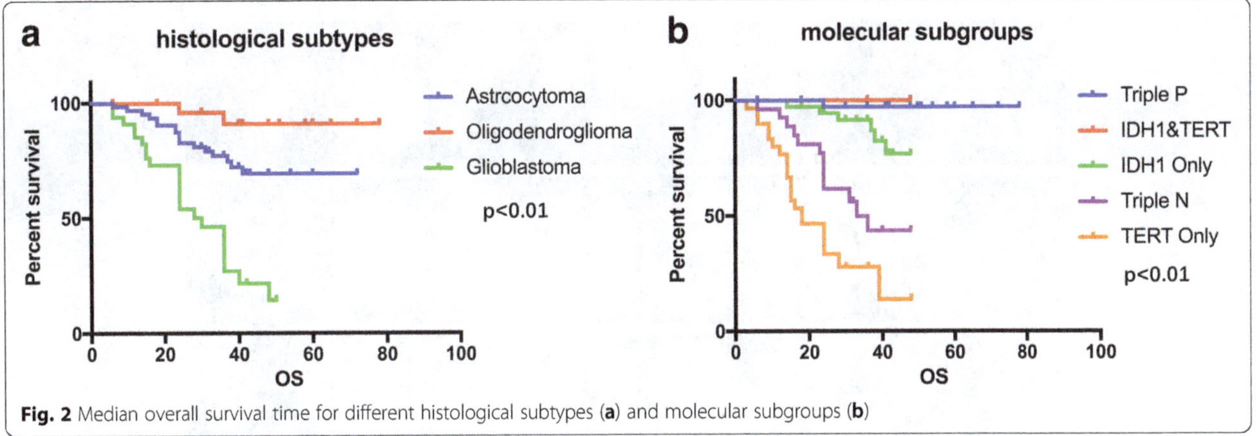

Fig. 2 Median overall survival time for different histological subtypes (**a**) and molecular subgroups (**b**)

Tumor location remains consistently between histological subtype and its corresponding molecular subgroup

Thus glioma histology stratification strongly associated with molecular phenotype, we investigate whether anatomic distribution remains consistent within these two classification systems. We compared triple-positive samples with oligodendroglioma, IDH1 mutation only subgroup with astrocytoma and TERT mutation only tumors with glioblastoma since these genetic events highly represent histological diagnosis. It's interested to find out that the tumor location and growth pattern is quite similar to each other based on MR images. The location correlation coefficients are 0.97, 0.94 and 0.85 accordingly (Fig. 5a–c).

Dissimilarity in molecular background results in different tumor location within mixed diffuse glioma

In 2016 revised WHO diffuse glioma classification, the diagnosis of oligoastrocytoma was gone due to 1p19q can help clearly subdivide tumor into oligo-lineage or astroglial family. We have 14 oligoastrocytoma cases, 10 of them showed 1p19q codeletion with tumor likely to locate in bilateral frontal lobe which is similar to

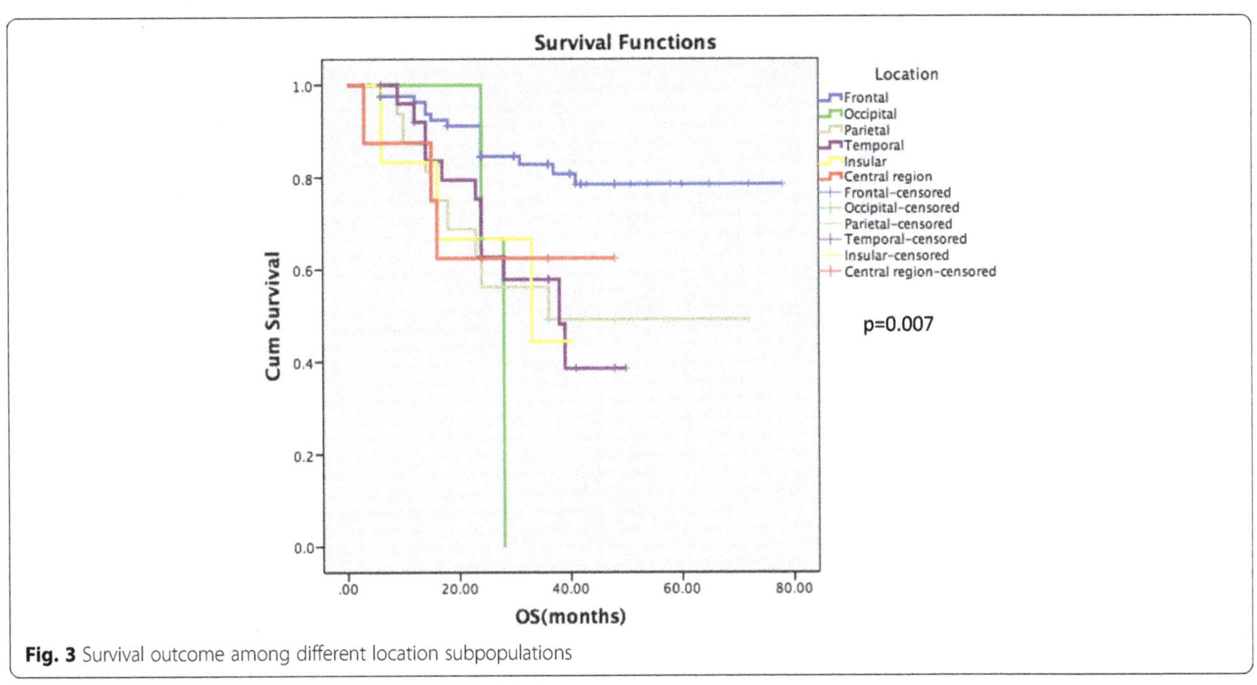

Fig. 3 Survival outcome among different location subpopulations

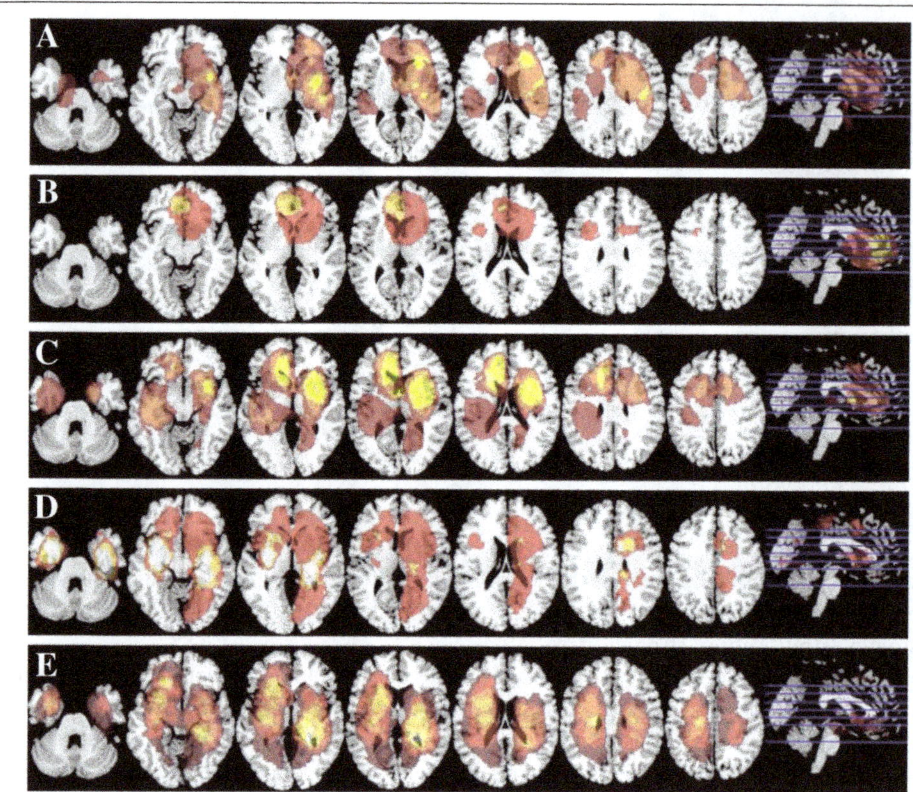

Fig. 4 Distribution of tumor location according to IDH1/TERT/1p19q stratification regimen. **a** Triple-positive, (**b**) TERT and IDH mutation, (**c**) IDH mutation only, (**d**)Triple-negative, (**e**)TERT mutation only

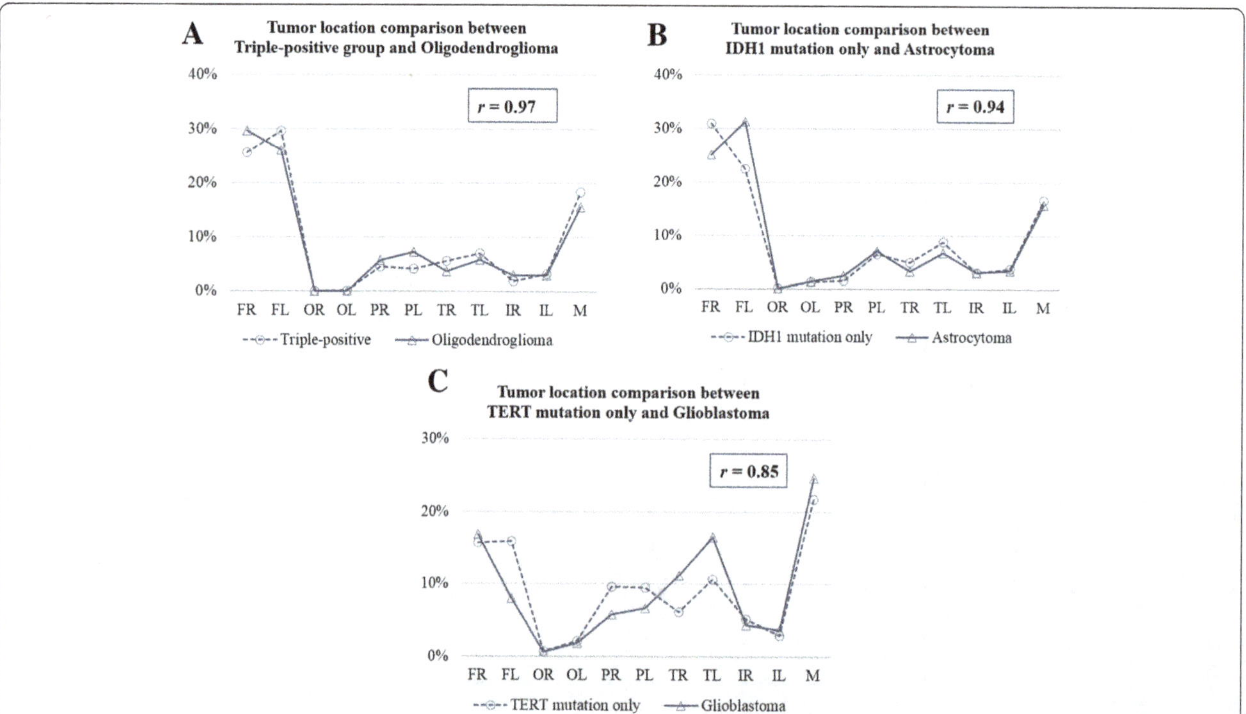

Fig. 5 Tumor location correlation analysis between histological subtype and its corresponding molecular subgroup with (**a**) triple-positive group vs. oligodendroglioma, (**b**) IDH1 mutation only vs. astrocytoma, (**c**) TERT mutation only vs. glioblastoma

oligodendroglioma. On the other hand, tumor with 1p19q intact tends to grow in left insular lobe where is commonly seated by astrocytoma (Fig. 6).

Discussion

Cerebral diffuse glioma is a biological heterogeneous tumor [1]. Patient clinical outcome was affected by many factors including age, anatomic location, tumor size, extent of resection, genetic alteration [14]. Among them, anatomic location plays a crucial role not only for prognosis prediction but also for treatment strategy. It was widely acknowledged that prognosis is poor in midline glioma than non-midline tumor [10]. Regarding to hemispheric glioma, patient with tumor located in frontal lobe tends to be younger, IDH1 mutation and longer survival time [15]. This conclusion is accordance with our result. Furthermore, in our cohort, occipital lobe glioma implied negative impact on clinical outcome which is similar to Liu et al. [16]. The reason might be larger tumor size commonly seen in this area. Meanwhile, anatomic location somehow determines the extent of resection, for example, midline or deep-seated glioma is hard to get gross total resection due to preservation of functional structure or complex surgical corridor [17]. On the contrary, non-eloquent area tumor, especially superficial to the cortex is amendable to completely remove. For the same reason, longer survival time is strongly associated with gross total resection [18]. On the other hand, based on huge amounts of exploration of glioma genetic alteration in the recent years, a panel of classic biomarkers begins to exert great impact on glioma precise diagnosis and prognostic assessment [1]. IDH1/1p19q/H3F3A are the representatives introduced into newly revised 2016 WHO glioma guideline [7]. In our previous study, 4 biomarkers were used to stratify lower grade glioma into 4 subgroups predicting better clinical outcome than the roles of histological diagnosis and WHO grade [19]. The current findings firmly validate the great prognostic value of biomarkers in glioma. Similar to our findings, Jenkins et al. used a genetic combination of IDH1/1p19q/TERT to classify glioma into 5 subpopulations with unique clinical features and germline variants respectively which is highly recognized in the world [8]. We referred to this 3-biomarkers scheme in our study, and drew the same conclusion Triple-positive and IDH1/TERT double-mutation cases are more likely to be oligo-lineage. IDH1 mutation only cases are astrocytoma with maximal possibility. IDH1 wild type and TERT mutation tumors are commonly seen in glioblastoma. According to this scheme, survival outcome in our patient cohort is distinctive among all the subgroups. All these data demonstrate integration of molecular and histology diagnosis being helpful in prognostic and predictive value for glioma patients. Nevertheless, the perfect integration of these two systems still calls for huge efforts like large cohort clinical validation on many aspects, such as image features. Thus, we hypothesized anatomic location, genetic biomarkers and histology diagnosis are highly correlated and intertwined.

In order to verify our hypothesis, we tried to study the interconnection between anatomic location and genetic biomarkers in our patient cohort. Beforehand, many papers published have put forward the cell origin theory underlying possible relationship between these two factors [20, 21]. Many groups have successfully developed computational methods to predict glioma genetic alterations based on location features [18, 22, 23]. For example, IDH1 mutation was commonly seen in left frontal lobe, where TERT mutation only exists as well[2, 5, 23]. Such investigations were performed in the context of MGMT and TP53[24, 25]. In our study, we used a panel composed of IDH1/1p19q/TERT which is worldwide recognized in the precise diagnosis of glioma to demonstrate the anatomic distribution of different molecular subsets. Our data showed similar results to previous research works such as IDH1 mutation prefers to localize in left frontal lobe[2, 15]. Interestingly, we also found that triple-positive tumor located more superficial to cortex than TERT mutation only tumor. This finding may explain the differences in survival outcome and extent of resection. In spite of that,. highly consistency of

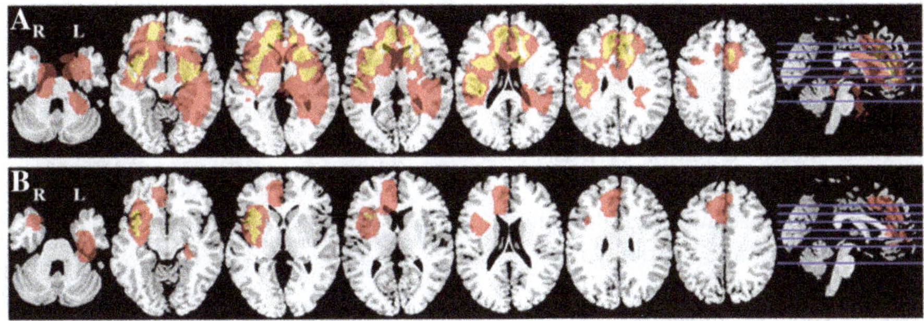

Fig. 6 1p19q status of oligoastrocytoma decide tumor location, (**a**) Oligoastrocytoma with1p19q codeletion, (**b**) Oligoastrocytoma with 1p19q retain

location feature was observed between histological subpopulations and its corresponding molecular counterparts. For example, triple-positive tumor appears to have similar anatomic location with oligodendrogliomas. That means the axis of molecule-cell-tissue depicts the growth pattern of glioma which is additional evidence supporting the cell origin theory. Another interesting finding is that 1p19q codeletion oligoastrocytoma possessing different anatomic location with 1p19q intact oligoastrocytoma which is supportive to new 2016 WHO classification that the diagnosis of oligoastrocytoma is eliminated [7]. Since now, the diagnosis of oligoastrocytoma converts to either oligodendroglioma or astrocytoma according to molecular biomarkers [26]. These findings demonstrate definite molecular feature restricted to precise histological diagnosis. It strongly proved that molecular diagnosis can help clinicians make exactly right diagnostic decision facilitating to tailor personalized treatment.

On the other aspect, methods by using MR images to predict molecular biomarkers are popular recently, which was so-called Radiomics study. Ellingson et al. compared tumor volume ratio of T2 hyperintensity to contrast enhancement and central necrosis to differentiate mesechymal and non-mesenchymal molecular subtype in glioblastoma [27]. His research team also used perfusion and diffusion MRI signatures to successfully stratify lower grade glioma into three subpopulations as IDH1 mut/1p19q codel, IDH1 mut/1p19q non-condel and IDH1 wt [28]. MRS is another popular detectable technology to realize Radiomics study due to unique metabolic features inside glioma. It has been widely applied to predict IDH1 mutational status and medulloblastoma subgrouping [29, 30]. Compared to these methods, our team used anatomic location as basic tumor feature to predict biomarkers like IDH1/1p19q/TERT, which is more simple, cost effective and visualized. The raw materials we need are only T2 flair and T1 contrast MR images without sophisticated computation process. However, our method has its own limitations, like rough estimation accuracy. In general, our team illustrated a simple method to predict molecular biomarkers and reveal anatomic location among different molecular subgroups which offered an alternative in Radiomics study.

Conclusion

Although molecular biomarkers are getting involved in routine pathological diagnosis of cerebral diffuse gliomas, more evidence should be provided to validate perfect match between molecular subtypes and classic histological diagnosis. Our study showed distinct anatomic distribution among different molecular phenotypes which is consistent with corresponding histological subtypes. Integration of molecular biomarkers with histology diagnosis will not only contribute to precise diagnosis but also predict patient clinical outcome. This kind of pathological diagnosis system was highly recommended in future clinical practice. Moreover, we developed a simple and cost-effective method to predict biomarkers which was supposed to be widely used in Radiomics study in glioma.

Abbreviations

CNN: Convolutional neural network; MNI: Montreal Neurological Institute

Acknowledgements

We would like to thank graduate student Yusheng Tong, Zeju Li, Yuan Gao for collecting and preprocessing the data.

Funding

This work is supported by the National Basic Research Program of China (2015CB755500), Natural Science Foundation and Major Basic Research Program of Shanghai (No. 16JC1420100), Shanghai Sailing Program (16YF1415200).

Authors' contributions

QT, YL, JY and ZS conceived of the project, collected the data, performed the analysis of the data and wrote the paper. JY, ZS, WY, and LC provided expert guidance and revised the manuscript critically for important intellectual content. JY, YW, and ZS gave final approval of the version to be published. All authors read and approved the final manuscript.

Competing interests

The authors declare that they have no competing interests.

References

1. Ceccarelli M, Barthel FP, Malta TM, et al. Molecular profiling reveals biologically discrete subsets and pathways of progression in diffuse glioma. Cell. 2016;164(3):550–63.
2. Yu J, Shi Z, Ji C, et al. Anatomical location differences between mutated and wild-type isocitrate dehydrogenase 1 in low-grade gliomas. Int J Neurosci. 2017;6:1–8.
3. Jain R, Poisson L, Narang J, et al. Genomic mapping and survival prediction in glioblastoma: molecular subclassification strengthened by hemodynamic imaging biomarkers. Radiology. 2013;267(1):212–20.
4. Ellingson BM, Lai A, Harris RJ, Selfridge JM, et al. Probabilistic radiographic atlas of glioblastoma phenotypes. AJNR Am J Neuroradiol. 2013;34(3):533–40.
5. Wang Y, Zhang T, Li S, Fan X, Ma J, Wang L, Jiang T. Anatomical localization of isocitrate dehydrogenase 1 mutation: a voxel-based radiographic study of 146 low-grade gliomas. Eur J Neurol. 2015;22(2):348–54.
6. Sonoda Y, Shibahara I, Kawaguchi T, et al. Association between molecular alterations and tumor location and MRI characteristics in anaplastic gliomas. Brain Tumor Pathol. 2015;32(2):99–104.
7. Louis DN, Perry A, Reifenberger G, et al. The 2016 World Health Organization classification of tumors of the central nervous system: a summary. Acta Neuropathol. 2016;131(6):803–20.
8. Eckel-Passow JE, Lachance DH, Molinaro AM, et al. Glioma groups based on 1p/19q, IDH, and TERT promoter mutations in tumors. N Engl J Med. 2015; 372(26):2499–508.
9. Zhang RQ, Shi Z, Chen H, et al. Biomarker-based prognostic stratification of young adult glioblastoma. Oncotarget. 2016;7(4):5030–41.
10. Li YX, Shi Z, Aibaidula A, et al. Not all 1p/19q non-codeleted oligodendroglial tumors are astrocytic. Oncotarget. 2016;7(40):64615–30.
11. Pereira S, Pinto A, Alves V, Silva CA. Brain Tumor Segmentation using Convolutional Neural Networks in MRI Images. IEEE Trans Med Imaging. 2016[Epub ahead of print].
12. Mazziotta J, Toga A, Evans A, et al. A probabilistic atlas and reference system for the human brain: international consortium for brain mapping (ICBM). Philos Trans R Soc Lond Ser B Biol Sci. 2001;356(1412):1293–322.

13. Ellingson BM, Cloughesy TF, Pope WB, et al. Anatomic localization of O6-methylguanine DNA methyltransferase (MGMT) promoter methylated and unmethylated tumors: a radiographic study in 358 de novo human glioblastomas. NeuroImage. 2012;59(2):908–16.
14. Reni M, Mazza E, Zanon S, Gatta G, Vecht CJ. Central nervous system gliomas. Crit Rev Oncol Hematol. 2017;113:213–34.
15. Chen N, Yu T, Gong J, Nie L, Chen X, Zhang M, Xu M, Tan J, Su Z, Zhong J, Zhou Q. IDH1/2 Gene hotspot mutations in central nervous system tumours: analysis of 922 Chinese patients. Pathology. 2016;48(7):675–83.
16. Liu TT, Achrol AS, Mitchell LA, Du WA, Loya JJ, Rodriguez SA, Feroze A, Westbroek EM, Yeom KW, Stuart JM, Chang SD, Harsh GR 4th, Rubin DL. Computational identification of tumor anatomic location associated with survival in 2 large cohorts of human primary glioblastomas. AJNR Am J Neuroradiol. 2016;37(4):621–8.
17. Eisenstat DD, Pollack IF, Demers A, Sapp MV, Lambert P, Weisfeld-Adams JD, Burger PC, Gilles F, Davis RL, Packer R, Boyett JM, Finlay JL. Impact of tumor location and pathological discordance on survival of children with midline high-grade gliomas treated on Children's cancer group high-grade glioma study CCG-945. J Neuro-Oncol. 2015;121(3):573–81.
18. Jungk C, Scherer M, Mock A, Capper D, Radbruch A, von Deimling A, Bendszus M, Herold-Mende C, Unterberg A. Prognostic value of the extent of resection in supratentorial WHO grade II astrocytomas stratified for IDH1 mutation status: a single-center volumetric analysis. J Neuro-Oncol. 2016; 129(2):319–28.
19. Chan AK, Yao Y, Zhang Z, Shi Z, Chen L, Chung NY, Liu JS, Li KK, Chan DT, Poon WS, Wang Y, Zhou L, Ng HK. Combination genetic signature stratifies lower-grade gliomas better than histological grade. Oncotarget. 2015;6(25):20885–901.
20. Sreedharan S, Maturi NP, Xie Y, Sundström A, Jarvius M, Libard S, Alafuzoff I, Weishaupt H, Fryknäs M, Larsson R, Swartling FJ, Uhrbom L. Mouse models of pediatric Supratentorial high-grade glioma reveal how cell-of-origin influences tumor development and phenotype. Cancer Res. 2017;77(3):802–12.
21. Alcantara Llaguno SR, Parada LF. Cell of origin of glioma: biological and clinical implications. Br J Cancer. 2016;115(12):1445–50.
22. Gutman DA, Dunn WD Jr, Grossmann P, Cooper LA, Holder CA, Ligon KL, Alexander BM, Aerts HJ. Somatic mutations associated with MRI-derived volumetric features in glioblastoma. Neuroradiology. 2015;57(12):1227–37.
23. Tang C, Zhang ZY, Chen LC, Sun Z, Zhang Y, Qin Z, Yao Y, Zhou LF. Subgroup characteristics of insular low-grade glioma based on clinical and molecular analysis of 42 cases. J Neuro-Oncol. 2016;126(3):499–507.
24. Wang YY, Zhang T, Li SW, Qian TY, Fan X, Peng XX, Ma J, Wang L, Jiang T. Mapping p53 mutations in low-grade glioma: a voxel-based neuroimaging analysis. AJNR Am J Neuroradiol. 2015;36(1):70–6.
25. Kanas VG, Zacharaki EI, Thomas GA, Zinn PO, Megalooikonomou V, Colen RR. Learning MRI-based classification models for MGMT methylation status prediction in glioblastoma. Comput Methods Prog Biomed. 2017;140:249–57.
26. Sahm F, Reuss D, Koelsche C, Capper D, Schittenhelm J, Heim S, Jones DT, Pfister SM, Herold-Mende C, Wick W, Mueller W, Hartmann C, Paulus W, von Deimling A. Farewell to oligoastrocytoma: in situ molecular genetics favor classification as either oligodendroglioma or astrocytoma. Acta Neuropathol. 2014;128(4):551–9.
27. Naeini KM, Pope WB, Cloughesy TF, Harris RJ, Lai A, Eskin A, Chowdhury R, Phillips HS, Nghiemphu PL, Behbahanian Y, Ellingson BM. Identifying the mesenchymal molecular subtype of glioblastoma using quantitative volumetric analysis of anatomic magnetic resonance images. Neuro-Oncology. 2013;15(5):626–34.
28. Leu K, Ott GA, Lai A, Nghiemphu PL, Pope WB, Yong WH. Liau LM. Ellingson BM. Perfusion and diffusion MRI signatures in histologic and genetic subtypes of WHO grade II-III diffuse gliomas. J Neurooncol: Cloughesy TF; 2017. [Epub ahead of print]
29. Blüml S, Margol AS, Sposto R, Kennedy RJ, Robison NJ, Vali M, Hung LT, Muthugounder S, Finlay JL, Erdreich-Epstein A, Gilles FH, Judkins AR, Krieger MD, Dhall G, Nelson MD, Asgharzadeh S. Molecular subgroups of medulloblastoma identification using noninvasive magnetic resonance spectroscopy. Neuro-Oncology. 2016;18(1):126–31.
30. Leather T, Jenkinson MD, Das K, Poptani H. Magnetic Resonance Spectroscopy for Detection of 2-Hydroxyglutarate as a Biomarker for IDH Mutation in Gliomas. Metabolites. 2017, 7(2).

10

Headache symptoms from migraine patients with and without aura through structure-validated self-reports

Jiawei Wang[1], Bingren Zhang[1], Chanchan Shen[1], Jinhua Zhang[2] and Wei Wang[1*]

Abstract

Background: Headache symptoms self-reported by migraine patients are largely congruent with the clinician-used diagnostic criteria, but not always so. Patients' self-reports of headache symptoms might offer additional clues to characterize migraine with (MA) and without (MO) aura more precisely.

Methods: Firstly, we invited 324 participants with a life-long headache attack to answer an item-matrix measuring symptoms of primary headaches, then we performed both exploratory and confirmatory factor analyses to their answers and refined a headache symptom questionnaire. Secondly, we applied this questionnaire to 28 MA and 52 MO patients.

Results: In participants with a life-long headache, we refined a 27-item, structure-validated headache symptom questionnaire, with four factors (scales) namely the Somatic /Aura Symptoms, Gastrointestinal and Autonomic Symptoms, Tightness and Location Features, and Prodromal/Aggravating Symptoms. Further, we found that MA patients reported higher than did MO patients on the Somatic/Aura Symptoms and Tightness and Location Features scales.

Conclusions: Compared to MO, MA was conferred with more prominent tightness and location features besides its higher somatic or aura symptoms. Patients' self-reports of headache symptoms might offer more clues to distinguish two types of migraine besides their clinician-defined criteria.

Keywords: Factor analysis, Headache symptom, Migraine with aura, Migraine without aura, Patients' self-reports

Background

Migraine is a common disabling primary headache disorder with head pain and autonomic and neurological symptoms [1]. Its diagnosis relies largely on the symptomatology due to the lack of clearly detectable biological markers and explicit radiological features [2]. It is then actually among the most under-recognized and under-treated neurological disorders [3]. The generally accepted diagnostic criteria for primary headaches are those published by the International Headache Society, such as the International Classification of Headache Disorders [4]. These criteria are comprehensive but still need to be further improved. Moreover, the effective application of these criteria requires trained professionals with experience and knowledge and it is not feasible to take a physical exam and medical history in large population-based studies. Besides, physicians' diagnoses depend more on their clinical experience and inconsistent interpretations of these criteria in clinical practices, to some extent that personal description of patients has been neglected.

Besides the overlap of neurological symptoms and nonmutual exclusivity of aura symptoms, there has been long-standing controversy about obligatory characteristics for migraine with (MA) and migraine without aura (MO). According to the definition of the International Headache Society, migraine aura is the reversible focal neurological symptoms that arise before or during a migraine attack. However, clinicians have found that aura might occur before or during a migraine attack, occur without any associated headache, or occur with

* Correspondence: drwangwei@zju.edu.cn; wangmufan@msn.com
[1]Department of Clinical Psychology and Psychiatry/School of Public Health, Zhejiang University College of Medicine, Hangzhou, China

many other types of headache [5–7]. In addition, MO and MA displayed different clinical symptom patterns during pregnancy [8]. Whether the two migraine types are distinct entities in etiology and clinical pattern or they just differ in degree rather than in pathophysiology remains unclear [9].

Further, the reduced parasympathetic activity with sympathetic predominance, and the increased frequency of anxiety and depressive symptoms were found in migraine, especially in MA [10, 11]. One pharmacological study has shown that MA attacks were more severe and the treatment was less effective [12]. One functional magnetic resonance imaging study [13] has demonstrated that there were abnormalities in the cortical and subcortical pain processing networks in MO rather than in MA; during the interictal period, the functional connection between the occipital lobe and the frontal insula of MA was reduced than that of MO. Tedeschi et al. [14] also have found that the functional connection between gyrus lingualis and visual cortex was enhanced during interictal period, which might imply that the central sensitization effect and cortical hyperactivity is a unique pathogenesis of MA [15, 16].

On the other hand, there has been an increasing academic interest in investigating the clinical, epidemiological, and genetic problems of primary headaches, especially about the most common ones – the tension-type headache and migraine. In most studies of migraine, the methods of data acquisition include personal interview, telephone interview and self-administered questionnaire reports [3]. Symptoms reported by patients using a structure-validated symptom questionnaire are limited, most symptom studies however, were from the hospital-based medical records, professional physician interviews in clinics [17]. The distinction between these methods is not always as straight forward as it may be [3]. Differences in screening procedure (e.g., wording differences) may have significant influences on the estimation of headache disorders [2]. The self-reported questionnaire, which can be easily implemented to large samples, is an effective measure to access many diseases and explore constructs that would be difficult to obtain through behavioral or physiological measures. Fortunately, in a migraine study of Women's Health Study sub-cohort, the self-reported migraine and the migraine classified based on the International Classification of Headache Disorders-II revealed a satisfactory agreement [18].

Thus, in the current study, we have invited a group of headache patients to report their complaints of before, during and after a headache attack, since in clinics, a complete migraine includes the prodromal, aura, and headache phases [19]. Patients were also invited to report their knowledge about headache, treatment-seeking behavior, and family history of headache, which might serve as the contextual headache information. Based on the reported symptoms and the statements of the International Classification of Headache Disorders, we developed an item-MATRIX measuring symptoms of primary headaches. The purposes of the present study were (1) to obtain a structure-validated headache symptom questionnaire from the item-MATRIX, and (2) to look for the different aspects of headache symptom between MA and MO through the questionnaire self-reporting. We have hypothesized that both MA and MO patients report their headache symptoms fitting to a time sequence, and MA patients report more intensified headache symptoms than MO patients do apart from the aura.

Methods

The present study contained two stages (see Fig. 1). Firstly, we used the exploratory factor analysis and confirmatory factor analysis on a headache item-MATRIX to develop a structure-validated headache symptom questionnaire, following the scale development guidelines proposed by DeVellis [20]. Secondly, we applied the headache symptom questionnaire to both MA and MO patients.

Questionnaire development

Participants

In total, 324 participants (131 men, age range 16–65 years, mean age 22.16 years ±7.87 S.D.; 193 women, age range 14–75, mean age 24.32 ± 11.26) were recruited from undergraduate students, medical staff-members and clinical outpatients. All participants had a complaint of headache during their life-long period, but did not suffer from any psychiatric or neurological (including neuroinflammatory) disorders, had no prior history of head injury, no alcohol or tobacco abuse, and no substance abuse. The study was approved by a local Ethics Committee, and all participants gave their written informed consents to participate.

Procedure

The headache item-MATRIX included the qualitative dimensions of headache: the headache characteristics, headache-related symptoms, aura symptoms, triggers, aggravating and relieving factors, health-seeking behaviors, etc. Considering the importance of every components and dimensions, 71 items were carefully constructed using the statements of the interviewees. The Likert rating scales, 1 - very unlike me, 2 - moderately unlike me, 3 - somewhat like and unlike me, 4 - moderately like me, 5- very like me, were chosen for the questionnaire.

Statistical analysis

The answers to the 71 items from the 324 subjects were submitted to a principal component analysis, using the Predictive Analytics Software Statistics, Release Version 18.0.0 (SPSS Inc., 2009, Chicago, IL). The factor loadings

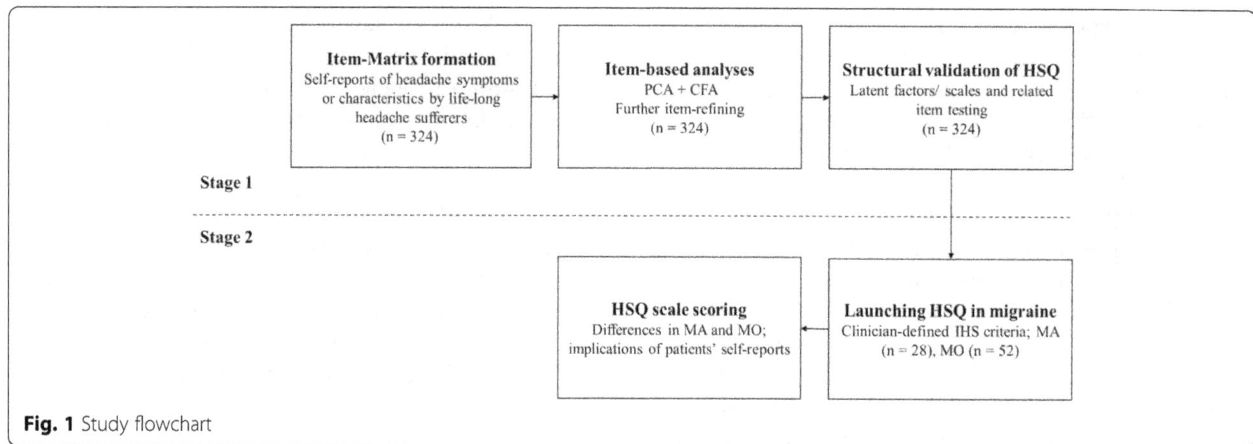

Fig. 1 Study flowchart

were rotated orthogonally using the varimax normalized method. Items which were loaded less heavily (loading ≤ .40) on a target factor, or cross-loaded heavily (cross-loading ≥ .35) on more than one factor were removed from subsequent analyses one-by-one. The procedure continued until no further item was needed to be removed. Afterwards, based on the latent factors, the fit of the structural equation modeling was evaluated by the confirmatory factor analysis using Analysis of Moment Structures (AMOS) version 17.0 (AMOS Development Corp., 2008, Crawfordville, FL). We used the following parameters to identify the model fit: the χ^2/df, the goodness of fit index (GFI), the adjusted goodness of fit index (AGFI), the comparative fit index (CFI), the Tucker-Lewis index (TLI), the root mean square error of approximation (RMSEA), and the standardized root mean square residual (SRMSR). When the optimal model fit was established, the headache symptom questionnaire was developed based on the emerged factors (scales) and their high-loading items. The internal reliability (the Cronbach alpha coefficient) of each scale was then calculated. After both exploratory and confirmatory factor analyses, the structure-validated questionnaire was formed and then used in the second stage of the study.

Application of the structure-validated questionnaire in migraine

Participants

Afterwards, the questionnaire was tested in migraine patients. Altogether, we invited 28 MA (code 1.2., 14 men, age range 16–65 years, mean age 19.43 years ±1.62; 14 women, age range 18–68, mean age 23.81 ± 10.00), and 52 MO (code 1.1., 7 men, age range 18–23, mean age 19.43 ± 1.62; 45 women, age range 14–64, mean age 23.81 ± 10.00) patients who were diagnosed according to the third beta edition of the International Classification of Headache Disorders (ICHD-3 beta; International Headache Society, 2013). There was no statistically significant difference in age distribution between two groups (t = −1.58, p = .12). Data about the headache attack frequency, headache attack duration, and headache intensity were also collected and used to confirm either MA or MO diagnosis. Patients were verified to receive no prophylactic therapy and had been drug-free for at least 24 h prior to the test. They did not suffer from any psychiatric or neurological (including neuroinflammatory) disorders, had no prior history of head injury, no alcohol or tobacco abuse, and no substance abuse. The study was approved by a local Ethics Committee, and all participants gave their written informed consents to participate.

Procedure

Patients were asked to complete the structure-validated questionnaire in a quiet room under supervision of a co-author of the paper (BZ).

Statistical analysis

The scale scores of the structure-validated questionnaire in MA and MO groups were submitted to two-way ANOVA (i.e., group x scale score) plus the independent Student t test. A p value inferior to .05 was considered to be significant.

Results

Questionnaire development

The principal component analysis extracted 20 factors with eigenvalues larger than 1.0. The screen plot and parallel analysis results suggested a seven-factor solution, and the first seven factors accounted for 41.90% of the total variance. When scrutinizing these latent factors and their items, four of which clearly described headache symptoms, and the remaining three described the knowledge about headache, treatment-seeking behavior, and family history of headache. Because the main purpose of the current design, we finally chose the four factors describing headache symptoms, which accounted for 37.03% of the total variance. Using the factor loading of .40 as a cutoff value, we constructed a fit modeling, with

27 items which were distributed in the four factors, and named the questionnaire as the Headache Symptom Questionnaire (HSQ, Fig. 2). In addition, the structural equation modeling confirmed that the four-factor modeling was a suitable solution ($\chi 2/df = 2.00$, GFI = .87, AGFI = .84, TLI = .87, CFI = .88, RMSEA = .057, SRMSR = .060).

The first HSQ factor with 7 items, e.g., "I felt my vision blurred when headache attacked", and "I lost physical balance control when headache attacked", is a mixture of somatic and aura symptom descriptions. The second factor with 6 items, e.g., "I had a poor appetite when headache attacked", and "I looked pale when headache attacked", narrates the gastrointestinal and autonomic symptoms. The third factor with 8 items, e.g., "I felt that my head was hooped by a ribbon when headache attacked", and "Headache location migrated during my headache period", describes the characteristics and location of headache. The fourth factor with 6 items, e.g., "I felt fatigue for a period before headache attacked", describes prodromal or aggravating symptoms before or during headache attacks. The four HSQ factors were then named as the Somatic/ Aura Symptoms (Factor 1, with an internal reliability of .79), the Gastrointestinal and Autonomic Symptoms (Factor 2, internal reliability .79), Tightness and Location Features (Factor 3, internal reliability, .81), and Prodromal/ Aggravating Symptoms (Factor 4, internal reliability .80), respectively (Table 1).

Questionnaire application

The mean HSQ scale scores were significantly different between the two groups (F [1, 78] = 9.90, $p = .002$, mean square effect = 522.32). The t test showed that MA patients scored significantly higher than did MO patients on Somatic/Aura Symptoms ($p < .01$, 95% confidence interval

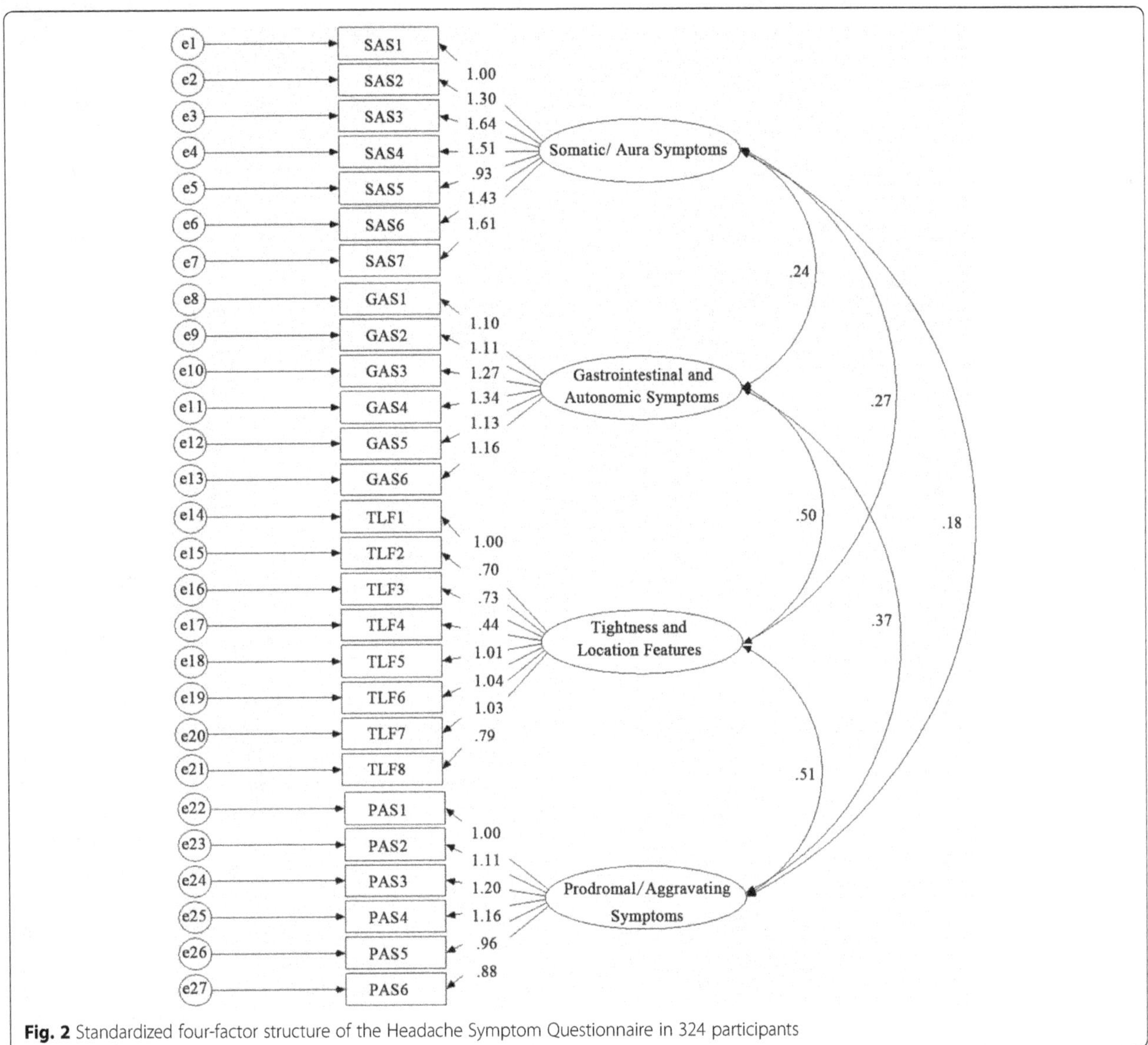

Fig. 2 Standardized four-factor structure of the Headache Symptom Questionnaire in 324 participants

Table 1 Factor loadings on the four factors in 324 participants

	Items	Factor			
		1	2	3	4
Somatic/Aura Symptoms	I felt my vision blurred when headache attacked.	**.71**	.10	.15	.10
	There were black spots in my vision when headache attacked.	**.70**	.16	.08	.12
	I talked less frequently when headache attacked.	**.68**	.15	.10	.00
	I lost physical balance control when headache attacked.	**.64**	.22	.11	.20
	I lost consciousness when headache attacked.	**.63**	.01	.24	−.16
	I was sensitive to strong sound when headache attacked.	**.49**	.22	.11	.17
	I felt abdominal pains when headache attacked.	**.49**	.23	.06	.24
Gastrointestinal and Autonomic Symptoms	I had a poor appetite when headache attacked.	.10	**.82**	.05	.08
	I looked pale when headache attacked.	.24	**.71**	.26	−.01
	I felt weak when headache attacked.	.16	**.60**	.18	.31
	I felt nausea when headache attacked.	.27	**.57**	.18	.18
	I was sensitive to strong light when headache attacked.	.21	**.47**	.31	.20
	I sweated a lot when headache attacked.	.34	**.41**	.19	.19
Tightness and Location Features	I felt that my head was hooped by a ribbon when headache attacked.	.22	.16	**.75**	.05
	I once felt that my head was hooped.	.07	.13	**.75**	.14
	I felt that my head was pressed by a big stone when headache attacked.	.31	.09	**.65**	.21
	I felt I was wearing a hat when headache attacked.	.28	.26	**.64**	.08
	My whole head was extremely painful when headache attacked.	−.03	.15	**.57**	.24
	Headache location migrated during my headache period.	.16	.09	**.41**	.10
	I felt throbbing over my head when headache attacked.	.00	.24	**.41**	.39
	My neck was also painful when headache attacked.	.33	−.05	**.41**	.36
Prodromal/Aggravating Symptoms	I felt fatigue for a period before headache attacked.	.11	.16	.08	**.78**
	I had difficulty in concentrating for a period before headache attacked.	.19	.15	.08	**.76**
	I yawned repetitively for a period before headache attacked.	.23	.05	−.03	**.72**
	I was often upset about my life or study/work.	−.01	.10	.26	**.56**
	I was easily irritated when headache attacked.	.11	.10	.30	**.55**
	Insomnia intensified my headache.	−.08	.20	.36	**.55**

Loadings higher than 0.40 are presented in bold for clarity

(CI) = [5.76, 10.65]) and Tightness and Location Features (p = .01, 95% CI = [.89, 6.31]) (Table 2).

Discussion

After both exploratory and confirmatory factor analyses, we have developed a structure-validated Headache Symptom Questionnaire, with four scales: Somatic/Aura Symptoms, Gastrointestinal and Autonomic Symptoms, Tightness and Location Features, and Prodromal/Aggravating Symptoms. According to the self-reports, MA patients scored higher on the Somatic/Aura Symptoms and the Tightness and Location Features scales than MO patients did.

Table 2 Scale scores (mean ± S.D.) of the Headache Symptom Questionnaire in migraine with (n = 28) and without aura (n = 52) groups

	Migraine with aura	Migraine without aura
Somatic/Aura Symptoms	21.64 ± 5.60	13.44 ± 5.04*
Gastrointestinal and Autonomic Symptoms	20.11 ± 5.45	20.83 ± 4.43
Tightness and Location Features	28.25 ± 5.43	24.65 ± 6.00*
Prodromal/Aggravating Symptoms	23.71 ± 6.65	24.08 ± 5.48

*p < .05 vs Migraine with aura

The first scale Somatic/Aura Symptoms, which describes vision, speech, motor control and some brainstem functions, is the complaints frequently reported from patients during the aura and headache phases [21]. It is stated that the aura normally disappears as the headache starts [4]. However, some scholars are wondering the role of aura in the initiation of headache when referring to its timing in relation to the headache and the prodromal symptoms [7, 22, 23]. Our results also suggest that the aura precedes or accompanies the onset of headache. Interestingly, Schürks et al. [18] have reported MA patients do not always report aura symptoms, while MO patients sometimes do so instead. The higher score of the Somatic/Aura Symptoms in our MA group suggest that it is the severity, frequency and complexity of aura symptoms that distinguishes the two types of migraine, rather than the simple presence of the aura.

The second scale embraces two aspects regarding gastrointestinal and autonomic symptoms, such as the nausea, pale face and hyperhidrosis. It is generally accepted that nausea is the main feature which characterizes migraine [4]. Previous studies do have demonstrated that the reduced parasympathetic activity with sympathetic predominance in patients with migraine [11].

The third scale describes the headache location and quality, which is included by the International Headache Society [4] to characterize tension-type headaches. However, patients with migraine, especially MA, also present bilateral head and neck pains [24]. Drummond [25] noted that tension-type headache patients had bilateral head pain but had few or no features of migraine. Our results showed that migraine had more complex manifestations than the headache criteria currently describe, which sends an appeal that headache specialists consider more about patients' self-reports when diagnosing migraine. Furthermore, the higher score of the Tightness and Location Features scale we found was in line with that the MA manifestations varied more widely than those of MO did [26].

The fourth scale describes physical fatigues and psychiatric concerns related to the head pain. One population-based study found that some psychiatric comorbidities, particular mood and anxiety disorders, were common in migraine patients [27]. Other scholars suggested that the psychiatric comorbidities might be a risk factor for migraine chronification, i.e., for the progression from episodic form to chronic one [28]. Several studies have suggested that the prodromal dysfunctions might act as a primary trigger for a migraine attack [21, 29]. Our results indicate that the prodromal or aggravating symptoms reflecting the respective physical and psychiatric alterations reported by patients generally characterize the two types of migraine.

There were however, at least two limitations of our study design which should be considered. First, we did not enroll patients with other primary or secondary headaches. Second, our sample sizes of both MA and MO groups were relatively small. Future studies might include more headache controls and compare descriptions from patients' self-reports and the clinical criteria.

Conclusions

Through two series of study, we have demonstrated a structure-validated headache questionnaire for patients' self-reports, and found that the two types of migraine might be distinguished by the Somatic/Aura Symptoms and the Tightness and Location Features scales. Patients' self-reports of head pain symptoms might offer more clues to distinguish different headache types than do the clinician-defined criteria.

Abbreviations

HSQ: The Headache Symptom Questionnaire; ICHD: The International Classification of Headache Disorders; MA: Migraine with aura; MO: Migraine without aura

Acknowledgements

None.

Funding

The study was supported by the grants from the Natural Science Foundation of China (No. 81571336) to the correspondent author (Dr. W. Wang).

Authors' contributions

Study concept and design: WW. Acquisition, analysis and interpretation of data: JW, BZ, CS, JZ and WW. Draft written of the manuscript: JW and WW. All authors read and approved the final manuscript.

Competing interests

Regarding research work described in the paper, each one of our co-authors, Jiawei Wang, Bingren Zhang, Chanchan Shen, Jinhua Zhang, and Wei Wang, declares that there is no conflict of interest, and has conformed to the Helsinki Declaration concerning human rights and informed consent, and has followed correct procedures concerning treatment of humans in research.

Author details

[1]Department of Clinical Psychology and Psychiatry/School of Public Health, Zhejiang University College of Medicine, Hangzhou, China. [2]Department of Neurology, Zhejiang Provincial People's Hospital, Hangzhou, China.

References

1. Pressman A, Jacobson A, Eguilos R, Gelfand A, Huynh C, Hamilton L, Avins A, Bakshi N, Merikangas K. Prevalence of migraine in a diverse community-electronic methods for migraine ascertainment in a large integrated health plan. Cephalalgia. 2016;36:325–34.
2. Ligthart L, Boomsma DI, Martin NG, Stubbe JH, Nyholt DR. Migraine with aura and migraine without aura are not distinct entities: further evidence from a large Dutch population study. Twin Res Hum Genet. 2006;9:54–63.
3. Stovner LJ, Hagen K, Jensen R, Katsarava Z, Lipton RB, Scher AI, Steiner TJ, Zwart JA. The global burden of headache: a documentation of headache prevalence and disability worldwide. Cephalalgia. 2007;27:193–210.
4. Headache Classification Committee of the International Headache Society. The international classification of headache disorders, 3rd edition (beta version). Cephalalgia. 2013;33:629–808.
5. Kunkel RS. Migraine aura without headache: benign, but a diagnosis of exclusion. Cleveland Clin. J Med. 2005;72:529.
6. Aiba S, Tatsumoto M, Saisu A, Iwanami H, Chiba K, Senoo T, Hirata K. Prevalence of typical migraine aura without headache in Japanese ophthalmology clinics. Cephalalgia. 2010;30:962–7.
7. Hansen JM, Lipton RB, Dodick DW, Silberstein SD, Saper JR, Aurora SK, Goadsby PJ, Charles A. Migraine headache is present in the aura phase a prospective study. Neurology. 2012;79:2044–9.
8. Torelli P, Allais G, Manzoni GC. Clinical review of headache in pregnancy. Neurol Sci. 2010;31:55–8.
9. Ranson R, Igarashi H, MacGregor EA, Wilkinson M. The similarities and differences of migraine with aura and migraine without aura: a preliminary study. Cephalalgia. 1991;11:189–92.

10. Radat F, Swendsen J. Psychiatric comorbidity in migraine: a review. Cephalalgia. 2005;25:165–78.
11. Matei D, Constantinescu V, Corciova C, Ignat B, Matei R, Popescu CD. Autonomic impairment in patients with migraine. Eur Rev Med Pharmacol Sci. 2015;19:3922–7.
12. Hansen JM, Goadsby PJ, Charles A. Reduced efficacy of sumatriptan in migraine with aura vs without aura. Neurology. 2015;84:1880–5.
13. Hadjikhani N, Ward N, Boshyan J, Napadow V, Maeda Y, Truini A, Caramia F, Tinelli E, Mainero C. The missing link: enhanced functional connectivity between amygdala and visceroceptive cortex in migraine. Cephalalgia. 2013;33:1264–8.
14. Tedeschi G, Russo A, Conte F, Corbo D, Caiazzo G, Giordano A, Conforti R, Esposito F, Tessitore A. Increased interictal visual network connectivity in patients with migraine with aura. Cephalalgia. 2016;36:139–47.
15. Datta R, Aguirre GK, Hu S, Detre JA, Cucchiara B. Interictal cortical hyperresponsiveness in migraine is directly related to the presence of aura. Cephalalgia. 2013;33:365–74.
16. Brighina F, Bolognini N, Cosentino G, Maccora S, Paladino P, Baschi R, Vallar G, Fierro B. Visual cortex hyperexcitability in migraine in response to sound-induced flash illusions. Neurology. 2015;84:2057–61.
17. Viana M, Sprenger T, Andelova M, Goadsby PJ. The typical duration of migraine aura: a systematic review. Cephalalgia. 2013;33:483–90.
18. Schürks M, Buring JE, Kurth T. Agreement of self-reported migraine with ICHD-II criteria in the Women's health study. Cephalalgia. 2009;29:1086–90.
19. Blau JN. Migraine prodromes separated from the aura: complete migraine. Br Med J. 1980;281:658–60.
20. DeVellis RF. Scale development: theory and applications. New York: Sage publications; 2016.
21. Charles A, Hansen JM. Migraine aura: new ideas about cause, classification, and clinical significance. Curr Opin Neurol. 2015;28:255–60.
22. Agostoni E, Aliprandi A. The complications of migraine with aura. Neurol Sci. 2006;27:s91–5.
23. Manzoni GC, Stovner LJ. Epidemiology of headache. Handbook Clin Neurol. 2010;97:3–22.
24. Tepper SJ, Tepper DE. The Cleveland Clinic manual of headache therapy. Berlin: Springer; 2011.
25. Drummond PDA. Quantitative assessment of photophobia in migraine and tension headache. Headache. 1986;26:465–9.
26. Jürgens TP, Schulte LH, May A. Migraine trait symptoms in migraine with and without aura. Neurology. 2014;82:1416–24.
27. Jette N, Patten S, Williams J, Becker W, Wiebe S. Comorbidity of migraine and psychiatric disorders—a National Population-Based Study. Headache. 2008;48:501–16.
28. Ashina S, Serrano D, Lipton RB, Maizels M, Manack AN, Turkel CC, Reed ML, Buse DC. Depression and risk of transformation of episodic to chronic migraine. J head Pain. 2012;13:615–24.
29. Rossi P, Ambrosini A, Buzzi MG. Prodromes and predictors of migraine attack. Funct Neurol. 2005;20:185–91.

11

EEG dynamical correlates of focal and diffuse causes of coma

MohammadMehdi Kafashan[1,4], Shoko Ryu[1], Mitchell J. Hargis[2,5], Osvaldo Laurido-Soto[2], Debra E. Roberts[2,6], Akshay Thontakudi[1], Lawrence Eisenman[2], Terrance T. Kummer[2*] and ShiNung Ching[1,3*]

Abstract

Background: Rapidly determining the causes of a depressed level of consciousness (DLOC) including coma is a common clinical challenge. Quantitative analysis of the electroencephalogram (EEG) has the potential to improve DLOC assessment by providing readily deployable, temporally detailed characterization of brain activity in such patients. While used commonly for seizure detection, EEG-based assessment of DLOC etiology is less well-established. As a first step towards etiological diagnosis, we sought to distinguish focal and diffuse causes of DLOC through assessment of temporal dynamics within EEG signals.

Methods: We retrospectively analyzed EEG recordings from 40 patients with DLOC with consensus focal or diffuse culprit pathology. For each recording, we performed a suite of time-series analyses, then used a statistical framework to identify which analyses (features) could be used to distinguish between focal and diffuse cases.

Results: Using cross-validation approaches, we identified several spectral and non-spectral EEG features that were significantly different between DLOC patients with focal vs. diffuse etiologies, enabling EEG-based classification with an accuracy of 76%.

Conclusions: Our findings suggest that DLOC due to focal vs. diffuse injuries differ along several electrophysiological parameters. These results may form the basis of future classification strategies for DLOC and coma that are more etiologically-specific and therefore therapeutically-relevant.

Keywords: Coma, Classification, Electroencephalogram, Depressed level of consciousness

Background

A depressed level of consciousness (DLOC) is a near universal result of acute severe brain injury, and disorders of consciousness are among the most feared long-term sequelae of such injuries. Coma, a state of complete loss of spontaneous or stimulus-induced arousal, is the most severe form, but all forms of DLOC have substantial impacts on patient outcomes [1, 2]. A DLOC can result from diffuse brain injuries, or from focal insults to brain regions with widespread projections that secondarily induce global alterations in cerebral function [3]. For example, diffuse axonal injury may induce a diffuse DLOC through widespread cortical deafferentation, while a small brainstem hemorrhage may induce a focal DLOC via an injury to the ascending reticular activating system. Formulating an accurate differential is crucial to the clinical management of patients with DLOC, as diagnoses drive the approach to treatment and prognosis [2–4]. Diagnostic formulation often begins with distinguishing between focal and diffuse etiologies.

In some cases a careful history, paired with a basic laboratory workup and screening neuroimaging tests, are all that are required to determine the cause of coma or other DLOC. Often, however, these standard assessments prove inadequate to determine DLOC etiology during acute, therapeutically-relevant windows. There are several common scenarios in which such ambiguity exists: A patient may have a DLOC that exceeds expectations from modest structural brain injury evident on imaging; or a patient's DLOC may result from a focal

* Correspondence: kummert@neuro.wustl.edu; shinung@wustl.edu
[2]Department of Neurology, Washington University School of Medicine, 660 S Euclid Ave. Campus Box 8111, St. Louis, MO 63110, USA
[1]Department of Electrical and Systems Engineering, Washington University in St. Louis, 1 Brookings Dr. Campus Box 1042, St. Louis, MO 63130, USA

process that, due to its nature, acuity, location, or size, is not apparent on screening imaging studies.

More specialized testing, such as expanded laboratory assessments, specialized neuroimaging studies, and invasive procedures, may help to establish a diagnosis. These tests, however, carry risk and expense and are only useful in restricted circumstances. Similarly, highly specialized interventions including specific medications and even surgical procedures are effective in some cases, but are rarely used empirically. A non-invasive, bedside screening test that can help classify DLOC acutely could be of significant utility in guiding both advanced diagnostic strategies and, ultimately, management approaches [5, 6]. Although the differentiation of focal from diffuse DLOC may not be clinically-actionable on its own, it may help distinguish between more specific diagnoses that are, or suggest a more targeted work-up. A strong suggestion of a focal etiology in the absence of initial imaging findings, for example, might prompt more advanced neuroimaging. Similarly, a strong suggestion of a diffuse etiology, even in the presence of distracting structural brain lesions, might prompt a more extensive toxic-metabolic work-up, or a more aggressive correction of known toxic-metabolic abnormalities.

All DLOC, and in particular coma, are characterized by pathological alterations in brain electrical activity [7]. These electrical alterations may provide valuable etiological insight. Consistent with this, in addition to its well-established role in seizure detection, the EEG has been shown to have utility in the monitoring of non-epileptic, large-scale alterations of neurological function. Examples include EEG monitoring of delirium [8, 9], burst suppression [10, 11], and cerebral ischemia [12–14]. Thus, EEG can provide non-invasive, highly temporally-resolved data at the bedside on both structural and non-structural brain injury that may not be apparent on screening neuroimaging studies.

Visual inspection of raw EEG data requires advanced training and cannot easily capture the full complexity of electrical dynamics that are potentially encoded in the EEG signal. In contrast, quantitative EEG methods use computer-assisted analysis of EEG patterns to derive quantitative metrics that are not immediately apparent upon review of raw EEG data. The use of quantitative EEG analysis in the clinical setting has seen significant recent growth, particularly in the domains of sleep [15], epilepsy [16], and general anesthesia [17]. In these scenarios, progress has been made towards translational applications including seizure detection [16, 18], classification of sleep stages [19, 20], and quantification of depth of anesthesia [21, 22].

While a DLOC is expected to entail widespread network dysfunction regardless of injury type, secondary network dysfunction resulting from focal injuries may exhibit temporal or other EEG features distinct from those of primarily diffuse injuries. The goal of this study is to evaluate quantitative EEG analysis for classifying focal and diffuse DLOC [23, 24] with a particular focus on the *temporal* dynamics of the EEG. In other words, do focal injuries give rise to different temporal dynamics as compared to diffuse injuries? This approach contrasts spatial analyses that overtly characterize inter-region relationships (e.g., inter-hemispheric symmetry) with respect to a particular temporal signature (see also Discussion). If successful, such strategies may eventually become applicable to more specific, clinically-actionable DLOC etiological subtypes.

Common treatments of temporal dynamics in EEG involve spectral analysis, which decomposes a given signal into constituent frequencies [25], typically aggregated into the standard EEG 'bands' (i.e., alpha, delta, etc.) [26]. In this context, severe brain injuries and DLOC are classically associated with concentration of EEG power into low frequencies (<1 Hz) [27]. However, while approaches based on spectral analysis are commonplace, this form of analysis only captures sinusoidal harmonic structure in the underlying signal. Other forms of spatio-temporal time series analysis, such as measures of signal entropy and complexity, are available that may complement and augment spectral methods [28], and have been applied to EEG data from limited cohorts of patients with DLOC [29, 30]. We investigated these and other temporal markers to determine their potential for classifying focal and diffuse DLOC.

Methods

Study population and data collected

We retrospectively collected EEG data, EEG reports, and complete medical records from 62 patients who underwent EEG for routine monitoring purposes related to a diagnosis of coma or less-severe DLOC, which we define as a Glasgow Coma Scale (GCS) ≤ 9 at the time of EEG, in the Neurological and Neurosurgical Intensive Care Unit at Barnes-Jewish Hospital and Washington University School of Medicine (St. Louis, MO, USA). GCS was inferred for intubated patients [31]. Table 1 summarizes the study population and clinical determinations. Additional file 1: Table S1.

gives further clinical features for each subject included in this study. There were 62 patients considered and 70 total EEG studies (6 patients underwent EEG monitoring twice and one patient underwent EEG monitoring three times). In all cases EEG was performed for the detection of non-convulsive seizures in patients with otherwise inadequately explained DLOC. Only cases in which seizures were not detected at any point in the hospitalization were analyzed. For each of the 62 patients, two neurointensivists (TTK and either DER or

Table 1 Summary of study population

Classification	Diffuse	Focal
	N = 19 (47%)	N = 21 (53%)
Male	6 (32%)	12 (57%)
Female	13 (68%)	9 (43%)
Age	58.32 (23, 90)	58.42 (18, 87)
GCS at time of EEG	5.74 (3, 8)	5.6 (3, 9)
Injuries Observed		
Vascular	7	14
Diffuse structural	3	0
Brainstem lesion	0	6
Traumatic	2	1
Toxic/Metabolic	7	0

MJH and OLS) examined all diagnostic data available including imaging to assign a focal or diffuse classification. Importantly, these assessments benefited from diagnostic data not available to the team at the time of the initial EEG. Thus in most cases we were able to determine DLOC etiology to a reasonable degree of clinical certainty despite the diagnostic ambiguity that resulted in EEG testing early on. Imaging data was given the greatest weight in etiological determinations. Evidence of herniation or direct injury to brainstem reticular activating structures resulted in assignment to a focal etiology. Less severe structural lesions were interpreted in the context of historical data and coexisting toxic-metabolic influences to determine the etiology of the DLOC. Cases were included in the analysis only when the ultimate etiology (focal vs. diffuse) was apparent from clinical data. In cases of disagreement, the case was re-reviewed and discussed until a consensus was reached (most such cases classified as indeterminate). In total 40 subjects (21 focal and 19 diffuse) were used in the analysis (23 focal and 21 diffuse EEGs, with total 44 studies analyzed). Twenty eight of 40 subjects (70%) had some evidence of more than one potential DLOC contributor, but in all included cases secondary causes were felt to be minor. To examine the utility of traditional clinical EEG metrics, the clinical EEG reports were separately scrutinized to identify reported features that could assist in the classification of cases as focal or diffuse in etiology. Specifically, any focal or lateralized abnormalities in the report were flagged as supportive of a focal as opposed to diffuse etiology. All studies were conducted with approval from the institutional review board at Washington University in St. Louis.

EEG sampling and parsing

Recordings are collected at a sampling frequency of either 250 or 500 Hz using the standard 10–20 system of electrode placement. The 500 Hz data were downsampled to 250 Hz prior to analysis. In our analyses, we used a bipolar montage with 18 bipolar channels (FP1-F7, F7-T7, T7-P7, P7-O1, Fp1-F3, F3-C3, C3-P3, P3-O1, Fz-Cz, Cz-Pz, Fp2-F4, F4-C4, C4-P4, P4-O2, Fp2-F8, F8-T8, T8-P8, and P8-O2). Records were visually analyzed for quality control, with sections of the record containing large-amplitude artifacts excluded from analysis. Each bipolar channel was normalized to zero-mean, unit variance. They were then filtered using a 10th order Chebyshev Type I lowpass filter with cutoff frequency of 50 Hz before further analysis.

Feature extraction and classification

Feature extraction

We considered the 25 features listed in Table 2 for discrimination of focal and diffuse DLOC. These features are related to the dynamical (including spectral) properties of time-series data. Secondary statistics (e.g., higher order moments) of the features were not considered in this analysis. All signal processing and feature extractions were performed in MATLAB (Natick, MA), and feature selection and evaluation of classifiers were computed in R (version 3.1.2).

Definition of trials and analysis epochs

We divided each patient's bipolar montaged EEG data into separate, non-overlapping trials for the purpose of analysis (Fig. 1). Dividing the EEG data into trials results

Table 2 List of features. List of 25 features extracted from EEG data

Feature ID	Description
1–2	Maximum, minimum eigenvalues of the estimated **A** matrix from MVAR fitting of EEG data with unit order; see Eq. (1)
3	Number of absolute eigenvalues of matrix **A** larger than Threshold = 0.95; see Eq. (1)
4–6	Statistical properties: variance, skewness, and kurtosis
7–11	Power in the delta, theta, alpha, beta, and gamma bands
12	Ratio of power in beta and gamma bands to total power
13	Ratio of power in delta and theta bands to total power
14	Hurst exponent [33]
15	Hjorth parameters [33]
16–19	Equidistant mutual information, Equiprobable mutual information, and the first minimums of both types of mutual information [33]
20	Bicorrelation
21	Median frequency [33]
22–24	Spearman autocorrelation, Pearson autocorrelation, and partial autocorrelation
25	Composite permutation entropy index (CPEI) [62]

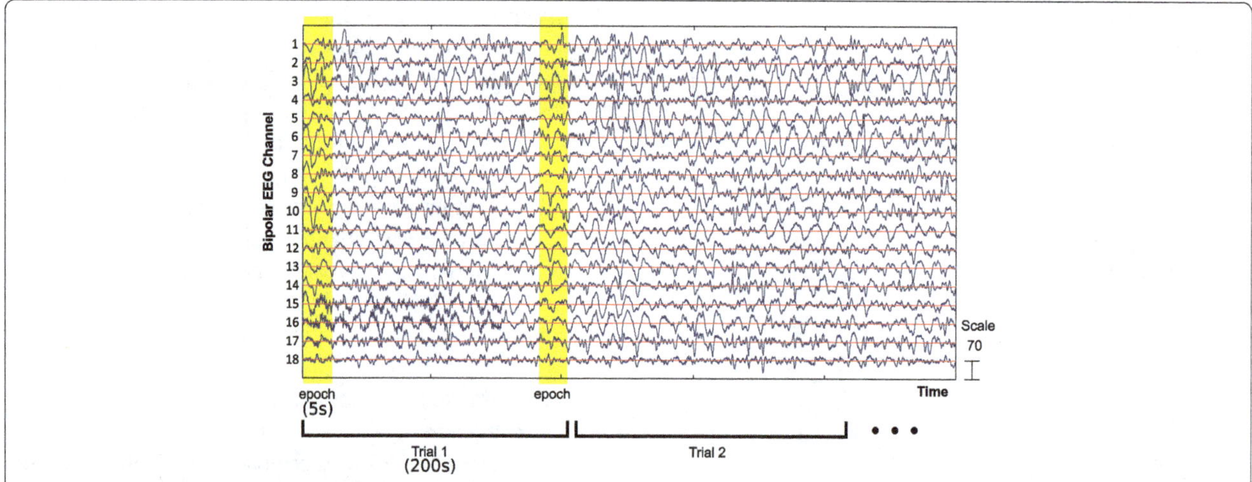

Fig. 1 Schematic illustrating sliding window to define epoch and trial in EGG data with bipolar montage. The EEG channel number on the vertical axes are ordered as: FP1-F7, F7-T7, T7-P7, P7-O1, Fp1-F3, F3-C3, C3-P3, P3-O1, Fz-Cz, Cz-Pz, Fp2-F4, F4-C4, C4-P4, P4-O2, Fp2-F8, F8-T8, T8-P8, P8-O2

in multiple predictions for each subject, thus yielding an empirical probability of focal/diffuse for each subject. Each trial was further subdivided for analysis purposes into epochs (Fig. 1). Specifically, one 25-dimensional feature vector for each trial by averaging feature vectors over all epochs of that trial. In our analysis, we considered trial lengths of 200 s, with epoch lengths of 5 s (i.e., 40 epochs per trial), except as noted when evaluating the robustness of our obtained features. It is important to note that all the trials for a given subject were allocated to either the training or testing set, thus training and testing sets are fully independent (i.e., no subject contributed trials to both the training and testing sets; see also below).

Classification and training/testing separation

We specified a support vector machine (SVM) to function as a binary classifier to discern a patient's DLOC etiology (i.e., focal or diffuse). The SVM approach uses a portion of data as support vectors to create a decision boundary (i.e., threshold) [32, 33]. To train the classifier, we applied principal component analysis (PCA) to the primary feature vectors over trials. Only the first 20 most important principal components (PCs) of feature vectors were kept. The first 20 PCs explain more than 98% of the variance in the original feature vectors (data not shown). We used the *train.R* routine in the Caret toolbox [34], implemented in the R programming language, to rank the features/PCs by importance by evaluating a family of linear vector quantization (LVQ) models. A 10-fold cross validation is used within this feature selection step which is resampled 50 times. We then selected a set of predictive PCs based on their importance (i.e., quantified in terms of their ensuing LVQ classification performance) to train a SVM with a linear kernel according to different clinically-adjudicated DLOC etiologies. Within this cross-validation paradigm, the importance of a feature/PC was obtained as a normalized quantity that characterizes the relative improvement in the region under the receiver operating characteristic (provided by the feature in question). In other words, the extent to which that feature improves accuracy within the cross-validation paradigm.

All classification analysis was performed using strictly independent training and testing sets. Two testing paradigms were considered. In the first paradigm, we partitioned the data into two groups: two-thirds of the total subjects were selected randomly and defined as the training set and one-third of subjects were defined as the testing set. This process was repeated within a cross-validation paradigm in order to evaluate average classification performance. In the second paradigm, we withheld 14 patients (1/3 of the data) as a dedicated test set, and trained strictly on the remaining 2/3 of the patients (i.e., one-time training and testing, with no re-sampling and averaging).

Evaluation of classifier performance

Classification performance was evaluated in two ways: (i) Hard accuracy, wherein each trial from a subject was independently classified, with the overall classification being made on the basis of the majority of trials; (ii) Soft accuracy, wherein each trial was independently classified with no overall classification rendered.

Multivariate autoregressive model of EEG data

Features 1–3 in Table 2 use a multivariate autoregressive model wherein the (multivariate) EEG signal is modeled as a linear sum of previous samples. For a multivariate N-channel process$\mathbf{x}(t) = [\mathbf{x}_1(t), \mathbf{x}_2(t), \cdots, \mathbf{x}_N(t)]^T$, a Multivariate

Autoregressive (MVAR) Model of order p takes the following form:

$$\mathbf{x}(t) = \sum_{k=1}^{p} \mathbf{A}_k \mathbf{x}(t-k) + \mathbf{w}(t), \qquad (1)$$

where $\mathbf{w}(t) \in \mathbb{R}^N$ are additive noise vectors (innovation process) and $\mathbf{A}_k \in \mathbb{R}^{N \times N}$ are the MVAR model coefficients. Here, we used a standard Least-Squares approach to implement the model fit [35].

Statistical evaluation

We used a two-sample t-test to compare feature distributions. Our goal was to generate hypotheses regarding which of the screened features were informative with respect to the considered coma subtypes (focal and diffuse). Since the PCs of the primary features are uncorrelated (see Results), we compared subtype distributions of each PC independently to a nominal significance level of $p = 0.05$.

Results

Several time-series metrics, including non-spectral features, discriminate focal from diffuse DLOC

Correlation of primary features

We first screened and ranked the importance of the primary features, i.e., without applying PCA (Fig. 2a) using testing paradigm 1, i.e., with resampling and cross-validation. As illustrated in Fig. 2b, these primary features exhibit substantial correlation, particularly in the entropic features (i.e., features 15–24 in Table 2). This observation indicates a degree of redundancy in the discriminative power of these features. We also note substantial anti-correlation between spectral and entropic features (i.e., 10–13 and 15–24). Recall that the importance of a feature measures its relative ability to improve classification performance, where an importance of 1 means that the feature in question can alone lead to perfect accuracy. Thus, we transformed the primary features into their uncorrelated principal components, then ranked these PCs (Fig. 3a).

Dichotomy of entropic and spectral features

We observed that the most informative PCs dichotomized into two categories (Fig. 3a): (i) components comprised mostly of entropic time series analyses (i.e., PC1) and higher order statistical signal properties (PC4); and (ii) components comprised mostly of spectral analyses (i.e., band-limited power, (delta, alpha, theta) and delta/theta ratio PC2). This observation is in agreement with the anti-correlation between these categories observed in Fig. 2b. Subsequent PCs, while informative, are comprised of a more random combination of analyses. The composition of these PCs is notable since by definition these components are uncorrelated, meaning that they provide distinct information regarding DLOC subtype. It is interesting to observe that the least informative PC (PC7) has a strong contribution from the median frequency, so that this feature is not particularly useful for discriminating focal and diffuse etiologies.

Variability in diffuse cases

Figure 3b compares the distribution of the three most informative PCs (distributions of focal/diffuse cases are most significantly different). We observed a positive contribution of entropic features (PC1) and higher order statistical signal properties (PC4) to focal cases, versus PC2 which has a positive contribution for diffuse cases. Further, we observed greater variance associated with diffuse cases, which may be suggestive of heterogeneity across channels or trials in these cases (see Discussion). Changing the feature epoch lengths (1, 10, 20 s) had no qualitative effect on the overall results (data not shown).

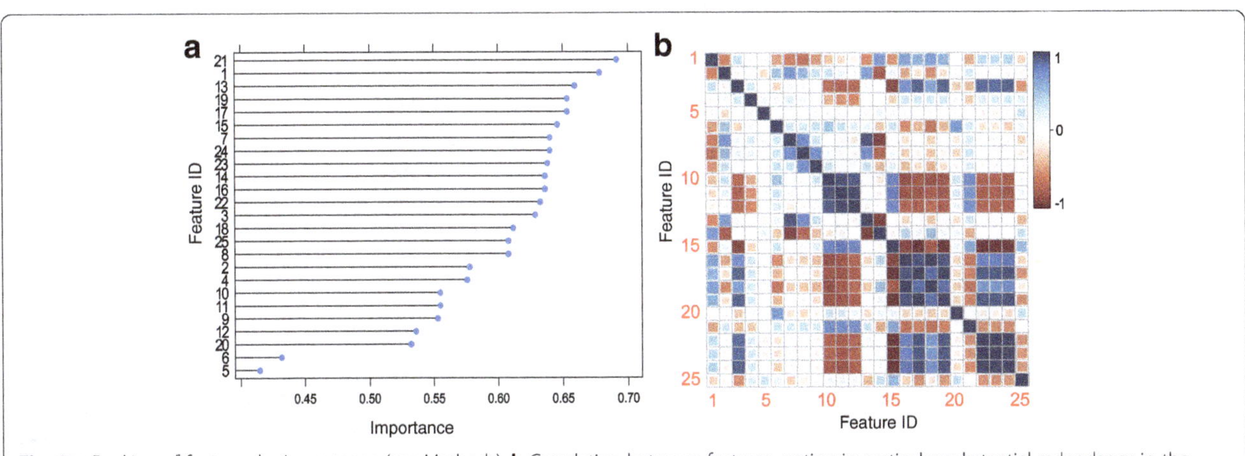

Fig. 2 **a** Ranking of features by importance (see Methods). **b** Correlation between features, noting in particular substantial redundancy in the entropic features 15–24

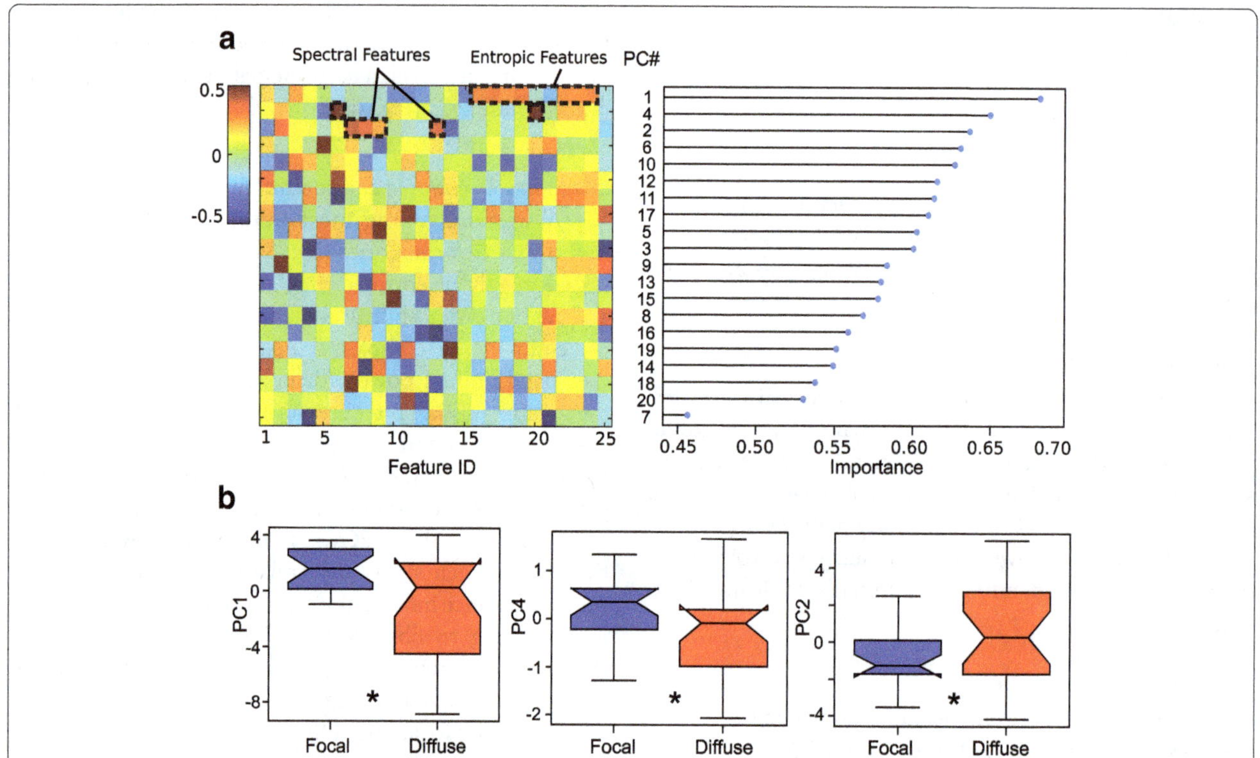

Fig. 3 a (left) Principal component decomposition of primary features. Each row in the matrix depicts the composition of a PC. The colorbar references the weight of each primary feature to the respective PCs. (right) Rows are ranked according to PC importance. **b** Box plots comparing the distributions of PC1 (entropic features), PC4 (kurtosis, bicorrelation) and PC2 (delta, alpha, theta, delta/theta ratio) for focal and diffuse cases

Focal and diffuse DLOC are classified using a limited number of PCA features

We next designed a classifier for focal versus diffuse DLOC on the basis of first the primary features and then the PCs. Table 3 shows the classifier performance using the primary features only (i.e., without applying PCA) for different epoch lengths and number of epochs in a trial. In this analysis, the classifier is trained based on the 10 most informative features on two thirds of the subjects (27 subjects), and then tested on the remaining

Table 3 Averaged classification performance before applying PCA on initial features

Epoch length	Number of epochs in a trial	Accuracy (Hard)	Accuracy (Soft)	Specificity	Sensitivity
1 s	10	0.51	0.52	0.42	0.66
	20	0.53	0.54	0.45	0.68
	40	0.53	0.53	0.41	0.69
	100	0.53	0.53	0.41	0.70
	All	0.57	0.57	0.49	0.69
5 s	10	0.50	0.49	0.44	0.67
	20	0.50	0.50	0.41	0.68
	40	0.52	0.51	0.44	0.67
	100	0.58	0.54	0.51	0.66
	All	0.57	0.57	0.46	0.72
20 s	10	0.51	0.51	0.41	0.69
	20	0.52	0.51	0.38	0.70
	40	0.53	0.53	0.51	0.64
	All	0.59	0.59	0.46	0.77

Classification results are for different epoch length (1 s, 5 s, and 20s) and different number of epochs in a trial (10, 20, 40, 100, and all epochs). All the results are averaged classifier performance over 500 random training and testing sets. In each realization, the subjects in training and testing sets are different patients (13 subjects). We performed training and testing for 500 repetitions (each repetition, subjects in the training set are totally separate from subjects in testing set). The values reported in this table are averaged over repetitions. The classifier exhibits higher sensitivity (true positives; here 'positive' is defined as a focal etiology) compare to specificity (true negatives, i.e., diffuse trials that were classified as diffuse). In this analysis, false positives (misclassification of diffuse as focal etiology) constitute the predominant source of inaccuracy. This Table shows that classifying on the basis of primary features alone is inadequate since performance is not significantly above chance, and particularly poor in correctly identifying diffuse cases.

Thus, we redesigned the classifier using the PCs, after which the performance reported in Table 4 was obtained. Only the first six most informative PCs are used for classification. Working with the PCs results in substantial improvement to the overall classifier performance. Specifically, it can be seen in this table that the false positive rate is improved on average by 0.14, and average performance approaches 68% for many parameterizations.

Finally, we performed a final test of the classifier by withholding 13 subjects as a dedicated testing set, and trained the classifier on only the remaining cases. That is, we trained a classifier on 2/3 of the data, then evaluated it on a separate, withheld patient cohort (paradigm 2). Table 5 reports the classification performance in this scenario, where performance approaches 76% with high sensitivity, but only moderate specificity. It is important to emphasize that within these classification regimes, the feature extraction step is performed on only the (independent) training set.

Clinical EEG interpretation

Lastly, we examined the EEG reports for our study population to determine whether a similar classification performance could be achieved from a more straightforward clinical decision process. Specifically, we catalogued observations of focal or lateralized abnormalities in the EEG reports (lateralized or otherwise focal slowing or epileptiform discharges), an indication of a spatially local electrophysiological phenomenon correlating with focal injury. Of the 21 patients with focal injury in our study, a report of focal/lateralized slowing was only present in seven instances (i.e., corresponding to a sensitivity of 7/21 = 0.33), demonstrating that the clinical EEG report was a poor indicator of focal etiology. Generalized slowing was observed in all study patients.

Discussion

Disambiguating focal and diffuse DLOC etiologies using EEG time series analysis

Our results demonstrate proof-of-concept for EEG-based segregation of focal versus diffuse DLOC subtypes based on time-series analysis and support-vector machine classification. We evaluated the performance of this system by segmenting our data into separate training and testing sets and then using cross-validation to minimize model overfitting. The results demonstrate performance up to 76% accuracy in focal identification, but less robust performance in detecting diffuse cases. In many cases, including all those studied for this report,

Table 4 Averaged classification performance after applying PCA on initial features

Epoch length	Number of epochs in a trial	Accuracy (Hard)	Accuracy (Soft)	Specificity	Sensitivity
1 s	10	0.63	0.63	0.57	0.68
	20	0.64	0.62	0.59	0.68
	40	0.65	0.62	0.59	0.68
	100	0.65	0.63	0.59	0.69
	All	0.62	0.62	0.55	0.67
5 s	10	0.63	0.61	0.57	0.67
	20	0.65	0.64	0.60	0.68
	40	0.65	0.62	0.60	0.69
	100	0.68	0.65	0.57	0.71
	All	0.65	0.62	0.61	0.66
20 s	10	0.63	0.59	0.55	0.66
	20	0.63	0.59	0.56	0.65
	40	0.64	0.61	0.59	0.68
	All	0.64	0.60	0.61	0.67

Classification results are for different epoch length (1 s, 5 s, and 20s) and different number of epochs in a trial (10, 20, 40, 100, and all epochs). All the results are averaged classifier performance over 500 random training and testing sets. In each realization, the subjects in training and testing sets are different

Table 5 Classification performance after applying PCA on initial features with first 13 subjects as testing set

Epoch length	Number of epochs in a trial	Accuracy (Hard)	Accuracy (Soft)	Specificity	Sensitivity
1 s	10	0.69	0.69	0.66	0.71
	20	0.76	0.68	0.65	0.69
	40	0.69	0.71	0.66	0.73
	100	0.69	0.69	0.66	0.73
	All	0.69	0.67	0.52	0.77
5 s	10	0.76	0.69	0.62	0.73
	20	0.69	0.71	0.70	0.73
	40	0.76	0.70	0.66	0.71
	100	0.69	0.69	0.66	0.73
	All	0.61	0.61	0.52	0.73
20 s	10	0.61	0.61	0.51	0.71
	20	0.69	0.65	0.63	0.69
	40	0.61	0.67	0.66	0.71
	All	0.61	0.61	0.62	0.60

Classification results are for different epoch length (1 s, 5 s, and 20s) and different number of epochs in a trial (10, 20, 40, 100, and all epochs)

the ultimate cause of the DLOC only becomes clear in retrospect, hence the clinical decision to order an EEG to rule out seizures as a contributor to a DLOC. Thus even in cases where a clinical diagnosis can eventually be made, an EEG-based diagnostic method could assist with the timely delivery of care.

The design of our classifier reveals that potentially clinically-useful information regarding DLOC subtype may be embedded in both spectral and non-spectral features of the EEG signals of patients with DLOC. Our results further suggest that spectral analysis alone (e.g., band-limited power) may not capture all clinically-meaningful aspects of the underlying neuronal dynamics.

Other potentially useful approaches for detecting focal versus diffuse pathology from the EEG include the brain symmetry index (BSI), which examines inter-hemispheric symmetries in the power-spectral density (i.e., band limited power) [36, 37]. This method has been used in the detection of focal seizures and hemispheric strokes [38, 39]. EEG-based synchronization indices, also derived from the power-spectrum, have also been suggested as a means of detecting diffuse electrophysiological phenomena [40]. It stands to reason that such methods may be sensitive to injury focality, though to our knowledge none of these methods has been used in the context of DLOC or coma. Moreover, while approaches that focus on the spatial distribution of EEG power may be informative, we chose here to focus our attention on the EEG in terms of temporal dynamics only since we were interested in whether focal and diffuse injuring give rise to differing temporal patterns, without overt regard for their spatial distribution. Thus, our results are likely complementary to approaches such as the BSI and comparing the performance of the classifier reported herein with these indices, separately and in combination, is an important future goal. The incorporation of active stimuli to assess EEG reactivity may also provide additional information about DLOC [41, 42], and is a further target of future work.

Significant effort has been directed at the EEG-based analysis of chronic DLOC in rehabilitative settings, such as minimally conscious and persistent vegetative states [43, 44], wherein a large number of EEG analyses have been screened for their potential to disambiguate these subtypes [45]. While these studies have yielded insights into the mechanisms of these conditions, the analyses rely on high-density research grade EEG/MEG instrumentation [43, 46] that is generally unavailable in the acute setting, wherein electrode spatial density and placement precision is limited. It furthermore remains unclear whether insights gleaned from these studies will prove informative in the acute setting, though a recent study did identify several acute electrophysiological correlates of outcome in coma [47], demonstrating the prognostic potential of EEG-based approaches.

Limitations

The main limitation in the development of our algorithm is the lack of a true gold standard upon which to train our classifier. Our cases were independently diagnosed by at least two neurointensivists on the basis of all available retrospective data, including neuroimaging, and only cases in which both felt a clear diagnosis was evident were included.

In this retrospective study we relied on the GCS for identification of patients with DLOC. The GCS is an imperfect measure of DLOC: its measurement is incomplete in intubated patients and many features that are likely to be clinically significant are not assessed. Several other metrics such as the Full Outline of UnResponsiveness (FOUR) score [48] and the JFK Coma Recover Scale, Revised [49] are likely to provide superior differentiation of patients with DLOC. Unfortunately our data did not permit such assessments retrospectively, though a prospective trial is underway including assessment of these metrics in addition to GCS.

A common challenge in the paradigm we pursued here is ensuring independent validation of classifier performance. We used two separate validation paradigms to separate training and testing sets (see Methods). Ongoing studies will test the performance of this classifier on additional independent, prospective cohorts of DLOC patients with clinically-obvious focal or diffuse DLOCs for whom EEG would not otherwise be clinically-indicated.

A drawback of our framework is that direct mechanistic interpretation from descriptive time-series analysis is lacking. The support vector machine approach aggregates all of the data/features (because the best predictors are combinations of the primary features), and then generates a set of predictors that may or may not be overtly linked to an underlying circuit mechanism. However, the decomposition of our PCs into distinct, uncorrelated feature sets (e.g., signal entropy and band-limited power) is suggestive of systematic circuit-level disruption in these patients.

Lastly, this analysis does not include specific steps to manage confounds introduced by the administration of medications such as antiepileptic drugs, including benzodiazepines, on the brain's electrical activity. It is well-established that these medications, among other factors such as sleep [50, 51], can lead to confounding effects on the EEG. In the absence of a much larger trial matched for specific agents or classes of agents, it will be challenging to fully understand the impact of such confounds. It is likely that the confounding effects of these drugs constitute a substantial source of classification error in our dataset. In a future prospective trial it may be feasible to more specifically characterize the effect of classes of medications on the discriminatory power of our classification scheme in individual subjects.

Design considerations

The feature selection framework reported above requires no manual specification of thresholds or other detection rules. The only user-specified design parameter is a desired confidence interval [52]. The method can be applied to any number of EEG channels. However, it should be noted that a pervasive challenge with any clinical EEG recording is overall signal quality and presence of artifacts (e.g., due to patient motion), which is expected to be compounded with added channels.

It is important to note that with this feature selection scheme, any change to the design parameters may lead to a different set of PCA features being chosen. Nevertheless, we found that across a range of design parameterizations (e.g., changing the trial length from 5 min to 10 min) the set of best predictors was largely comprised of the same descriptive time-series statistics. Thus it seems likely that these particular PCA features are robustly informative with respect to the two DLOC variants under investigation.

Conclusions

The use of automatic classifiers in EEG is most well-developed in the detection of seizures [53–60]. A host of additional potential application domains have been considered, however, especially in the development of brain-machine interface technology [61]. Our results demonstrate the potential of using such techniques to assist in the diagnosis of DLOC in the acute setting. Moreover, the methods and algorithms used in our study run in minutes on standard hardware and, thus, could potentially enable real-time assessment of the EEG. If they are further validated on larger patient cohorts, they may form an important component of the overall assessment of acute DLOC.

Abbreviations

BSI: Brain symmetry index; DLOC: Depressed level of consciousness; EEG: Electroencephalogram; FOUR: Full outline of unresponsiveness; GCS: Glasgow coma scale; LVQ: Linear vector quantization; MEG: Magnetoencephalogram; PC: Principal component; PCA: Principal components analysis; SVM: Support vector machine

Acknowledgements

Not applicable.

Funding

This work was supported by grants 1R21NS096590 and CTSA UL1 TR000448 from the US National Institutes of Health. This work was partially supported by the University Strategic Alliance (URSA) program as Washington University in St. Louis. S.C. Holds a Career Award at the Scientific Interface from the Burroughs-Wellcome Fund. T.T.K. is supported by an American Heart Association Scientist Development Grant and a US National Institutes of Health K12 grant (ICTS UL1 TR000448 and KL2 TR000450). Funding agencies were not involved in study design, nor in the collection, analysis or interpretation of data.

Authors' contributions

The study was conceived by TTK and SC. TTK, LE, DER, MJH and OL-S acquired the data. Analysis and statistics were designed and performed by MK, SC and TTK. All authors aided in analysis and interpretation of data. MK, SR, TTK and SC drafted the manuscript. All authors read and approved the final manuscript.

Competing interests

All authors declare that they have no competing interests.

Author details

[1]Department of Electrical and Systems Engineering, Washington University in St. Louis, 1 Brookings Dr. Campus Box 1042, St. Louis, MO 63130, USA. [2]Department of Neurology, Washington University School of Medicine, 660 S Euclid Ave. Campus Box 8111, St. Louis, MO 63110, USA. [3]Division of Biology and Biomedical Science, Washington University in St. Louis, St. Louis, MO 63110, USA. [4]Present Address: Harvard Medical School, Boston, USA. [5]Present Address: Department of Neurology, Novant Health Forsyth Medical Center, Winston-Salem, USA. [6]Present Address: Department of Neurology, University of Rochester, Rochester, USA.

References

1. Godbolt AK, et al. Disorders of consciousness after severe traumatic brain injury: a Swedish–Icelandic study of incidence, outcomes and implications for optimizing care pathways. J Rehabil Med. 2013;45(8):741–8.
2. Whyte J, et al. Functional outcomes in traumatic disorders of consciousness: 5-year outcomes from the National Institute on Disability and Rehabilitation Research traumatic brain injury model systems. Arch Phys Med Rehabil. 2013;94(10):1855–60.
3. Giacino JT, et al. Disorders of consciousness after acquired brain injury: the state of the science. Nat Rev Neurol. 2014;10(2):99–114.
4. Nakase-Richardson R, et al. Longitudinal outcome of patients with disordered consciousness in the NIDRR TBI model systems programs. J Neurotrauma. 2012;29(1):59–65.
5. Laureys S, Boly M. The changing spectrum of coma. Nat Clin Pract Neurol. 2008;4(10):544–6.
6. Owen AM, Schiff ND, Laureys S. A new era of coma and consciousness science. Prog Brain Res. 2009;177:399–411.
7. Young GB. The EEG in coma. J Clin Neurophysiol. 2000;17(5):473–85.
8. van der Kooi AW, et al. Delirium detection using EEG: what and how to measure. Chest. 2015;147(1):94–101.
9. Jacobson S, Jerrier H. EEG in delirium. Semin Clin Neuropsychiatry. 2000;5(2):86–92.
10. Westover MB, et al. Real-time segmentation and tracking of brain metabolic state in ICU EEG recordings of burst suppression. Conf Proc IEEE Eng Med Biol Soc. 2013;2013:7108–11.
11. Ching S, et al. Real-time closed-loop control in a rodent model of medically induced coma using burst suppression. Anesthesiology. 2013;119(4):848–60.
12. Claassen J, et al. Quantitative continuous EEG for detecting delayed cerebral ischemia in patients with poor-grade subarachnoid hemorrhage. Clin Neurophysiol. 2004;115(12):2699–710.
13. Jordan KG. Emergency EEG and continuous EEG monitoring in acute ischemic stroke. J Clin Neurophysiol. 2004;21(5):341–52.
14. Labar DR, et al. Quantitative EEG monitoring for patients with subarachnoid hemorrhage. Electroencephalogr Clin Neurophysiol. 1991;78(5):325–32.
15. Şen B, et al. A comparative study on classification of sleep stage based on EEG signals using feature selection and classification algorithms. J Medical Syst. 2014;38(3):1–21.
16. Claassen J, et al. Detection of electrographic seizures with continuous EEG monitoring in critically ill patients. Neurology. 2004;62(10):1743–8.
17. Brown EN, Lydic R, Schiff ND. General anesthesia, sleep, and coma. N Engl J Med. 2010;363(27):2638–50.
18. Khan YU, Gotman J. Wavelet based automatic seizure detection in intracerebral electroencephalogram. Clin Neurophysiol. 2003;114(5):898–908.
19. Smith JR, et al. Detection of human sleep EEG waveforms. Electroencephalogr Clin Neurophysiol. 1975;38(4):435–7.
20. Smith JR, Karacan I. EEG sleep stage scoring by an automatic hybrid system. Electroencephalogr Clin Neurophysiol. 1971;31(3):231–7.
21. Katoh T, Suzuki A, Ikeda K. Electroencephalographic derivatives as a tool for predicting the depth of sedation and anesthesia induced by sevoflurane. Anesthesiology. 1998;88(3):642–50.
22. Zhang X-S, Roy RJ, Jensen EW. EEG complexity as a measure of depth of anesthesia for patients. Biomed Eng IEEE Trans On. 2001;48(12):1424–33.
23. Laureys S, Schiff ND. Coma and consciousness: paradigms (re) framed by neuroimaging. NeuroImage. 2012;61(2):478–91.
24. Schiff ND, Nauvel T, Victor JD. Large-scale brain dynamics in disorders of consciousness. Curr Opin Neurobiol. 2014;25:7–14.
25. Schomer DL, da Silva FL. Niedermeyer's electroencephalography: basic principles, clinical applications, and related fields. Philadelphia: Wolters Kluwer Health; 2012.
26. Lehembre R, et al. Electrophysiological investigations of brain function in coma, vegetative and minimally conscious patients. Arch Ital Biol. 2012;150(2–3):122–39.
27. Plum F, Posner JB. The diagnosis of stupor and coma, vol. 19. USA: Oxford University Press; 1982.
28. Stam CJ. Nonlinear dynamical analysis of EEG and MEG: review of an emerging field. Clin Neurophysiol. 2005;116:2266–301.
29. Chan HL, Lin MA, Fang SC. Linear and nonlinear analysis of electroencephalogram of the coma. Conf Proc IEEE Eng Med Biol Soc. 2004;1:593–5.
30. Gosseries O, et al. Automated EEG entropy measurements in coma, vegetative state/unresponsive wakefulness syndrome and minimally conscious state. Funct Neurol. 2011;26(1):25–30.
31. Meredith W, et al. The conundrum of the Glasgow coma scale in intubated patients: a linear regression prediction of the Glasgow verbal score from the Glasgow eye and motor scores. J Trauma Acute Care Surg. 1998;44(5):839–45.
32. Pereira F, Mitchell T, Botvinick M. Machine learning classifiers and fMRI: a tutorial overview. NeuroImage. 2009;45(1):S199–209.
33. Kotsiantis SB. Supervised machine learning: a review of classification techniques. Informatica. 2007;31:249–68.
34. Kuhn M. Caret package. Journal of Statistical Software. 2008;28(5):1–26.
35. Steven MK. Modern spectral estimation: theory and application. Signal Processing Series, 1988.
36. van Putten MJ, et al. A brain symmetry index (BSI) for online EEG monitoring in carotid endarterectomy. Clin Neurophysiol. 2004;115(5): 1189–94.
37. van Putten MJ. The revised brain symmetry index. Clin Neurophysiol. 2007;118(11):2362–7.
38. de Vos CC, et al. Continuous EEG monitoring during thrombolysis in acute hemispheric stroke patients using the brain symmetry index. J Clin Neurophysiol. 2008;25(2):77–82.
39. van Putten MJ, Tavy DL. Continuous quantitative EEG monitoring in hemispheric stroke patients using the brain symmetry index. Stroke. 2004;35(11):2489–92.
40. Cursi M, et al. Electroencephalographic background desynchronization during cerebral blood flow reduction. Clin Neurophysiol. 2005;116(11): 2577–85.
41. Noirhomme Q, et al. Automated analysis of background EEG and reactivity during therapeutic hypothermia in comatose patients after cardiac arrest. Clin EEG Neurosci. 2014;45(1):6–13.
42. Hermans MC, et al. Quantification of EEG reactivity in comatose patients. Clin Neurophysiol. 2016;127(1):571–80.
43. Sitt JD, et al. Large scale screening of neural signatures of consciousness in patients in a vegetative or minimally conscious state. Brain. 2014;137(Pt 8):2258–70.
44. Chennu S, et al. Spectral signatures of reorganised brain networks in disorders of consciousness. PLoS Comput Biol. 2014;10(10):e1003887.
45. Noirhomme Q, Brecheisen R, Lesenfants D, Antonopoulos G, Laureys S. "Look at my classifier's result": disentangling unresponsive from (minimally) conscious patients. NeuroImage. 2017;145:288–303.
46. Salti M, et al. Distinct cortical codes and temporal dynamics for conscious and unconscious percepts. elife. 2015;4.
47. Zubler, F., et al., Prognostic and diagnostic value of EEG signal coupling measures in coma. Clin Neurophysiol, 2015.
48. Wijdicks EF, et al. Comparison of the full outline of UnResponsiveness score and the Glasgow coma scale in predicting mortality in critically ill patients*. Crit Care Med. 2015;43(2):439–44.
49. Giacino JT, Kalmar K, Whyte J. The JFK coma recovery scale-revised: measurement characteristics and diagnostic utility. Arch Phys Med Rehabil. 2004;85(12):2020–9.
50. Parthasarathy S, Tobin MJ. Sleep in the intensive care unit. Intensive Care Med. 2004;30(2):197–206.
51. Cologan V, et al. Sleep in disorders of consciousness. Sleep Med Rev. 2010;14(2):97–105.

52. Kuhn M. Building predictive models in R using the caret package. J Stat Softw. 2008;28(5):1–26.
53. Temko A, et al. EEG-based neonatal seizure detection with support vector machines. Clin Neurophysiol. 2011;122(3):464–73.
54. Greene BR, et al. Classifier models and architectures for EEG-based neonatal seizure detection. Physiol Meas. 2008;29(10):1157–78.
55. Nagaraj SB, et al. Robustness of time frequency distribution based features for automated neonatal EEG seizure detection. Conf Proc IEEE Eng Med Biol Soc. 2014;2014:2829–32.
56. Samiee K, Kovacs P, Gabbouj M. Epileptic seizure classification of EEG time-series using rational discrete short-time fourier transform. IEEE Trans Biomed Eng. 2015;62(2):541–52.
57. Oweis RJ, Abdulhay EW. Seizure classification in EEG signals utilizing Hilbert-Huang transform. Biomed Eng Online. 2011;10:38.
58. Lee SH, et al. Classification of normal and epileptic seizure EEG signals using wavelet transform, phase-space reconstruction, and Euclidean distance. Comput Methods Prog Biomed. 2014;116(1):10–25.
59. Chiang CY, et al. Seizure prediction based on classification of EEG synchronization patterns with on-line retraining and post-processing scheme. Conf Proc IEEE Eng Med Biol Soc. 2011;2011:7564–9.
60. Bajaj V, Pachori RB. Classification of seizure and non-seizure EEG signals using empirical mode decomposition. IEEE Trans Inf Technol Biomed. 2012;16(6):1135–42.
61. Muller KR, et al. Machine learning for real-time single-trial EEG-analysis: from brain-computer interfacing to mental state monitoring. J Neurosci Methods. 2008;167(1):82–90.
62. Olofsen E, Sleigh J, Dahan A. Permutation entropy of the electroencephalogram: a measure of anaesthetic drug effect. Br J Anaesth. 2008;101(6):810–21.

12

Case of convulsive seizure developing during electroretinographic recordings

Yuko Hayashi[1], Gen Miura[1*], Akiyuki Uzawa[2], Takayuki Baba[1] and Shuichi Yamamoto[1]

Abstract

Background: To present our findings in a case of convulsive seizures and loss of consciousness that developed during recording electroretinograms (ERG).

Case presentation: A 34-year-old man had reduced vision in his left eye for about 15 years, and night blindness for about two years. His visual acuity was 20/15 in the right eye and 20/50 in the left eye. The fundus was normal but the sensitivity in the macular region of the left eye was decreased. Optical coherence tomography (OCT) showed partial loss of the interdigitation zone. Upon completion of the flicker ERG recording, a paralysis developed in both upper limbs, then convulsions of the lower limbs followed by a loss of consciousness. The convulsions disappeared after an intravenous injection of diazepam. After that incident, he reported that he had had previous conscious-loss seizures.

Conclusions: Photosensitive epileptic seizures can occur with the light stimuli used for conventional ERG recordings. We recommended that clinicians request information on any prior seizure episodes of the patients and their family members before ERG recordings.

Keywords: Electroretinogram (ERG), Seizure, Epilepsy, Photosensitivity

Background

It is well known that an epileptic seizure can be triggered by exposure to intermittent light stimulation. In Japan, many viewers had epileptic seizures while viewing a television animation program, "Pocket Monster", in 1997. Many individuals visited hospitals because of experiencing seizures after watching a 12 Hz red/cyan blinking image lasting 4 s [1]. Of these cases, 76% were first episodes of seizures, and most were tonic-clonic seizures. A similar phenomenon has been reported not only from viewing TV images but also from viewing video game images, and the guidelines for TV broadcasting in each country have been altered to minimize these potential seizure-eliciting images.

Clinically, ERGs and visual evoked potentials (VEPs) are elicited by intermittent light and pattern-reversal stimuli. However, a search of Medline/PubMed did not extract any publications of convulsive seizures that developed during ERG and VEP recordings.

Thus, the purpose of this report is to present our findings in a case of convulsive seizures and loss of consciousness that developed during ERG recordings.

Case presentation

A 34-year-old man had reduced vision in his left eye for about 15 years, and night blindness for about two years. He had a complete ophthalmic examination including measurements of the best-corrected visual acuity (BCVA) and intraocular pressure, slit-lamp examinations, indirect ophthalmoscopy, Goldmann perimetry (GP), perimetry with Humphrey Field Analyzer (HFA), optical coherence tomography (OCT), MP-3 microperimetry, and full-field ERGs. His visual acuity was 20/15 in the right eye and 20/50 in the left eye. The fundus did not show any obvious abnormalities, but optical coherence tomography showed partial loss of the interdigitation zone (Fig. 1). The retinal sensitivity of the macular region was reduced in both eyes (Fig. 2). His family

* Correspondence: gmiura2@chiba-u.jp
[1]Department of Ophthalmology and Visual Science, Chiba University Graduate School of Medicine, Inohana 1-8-1, Chuo-ku, Chiba 260-8670, Japan
Full list of author information is available at the end of the article

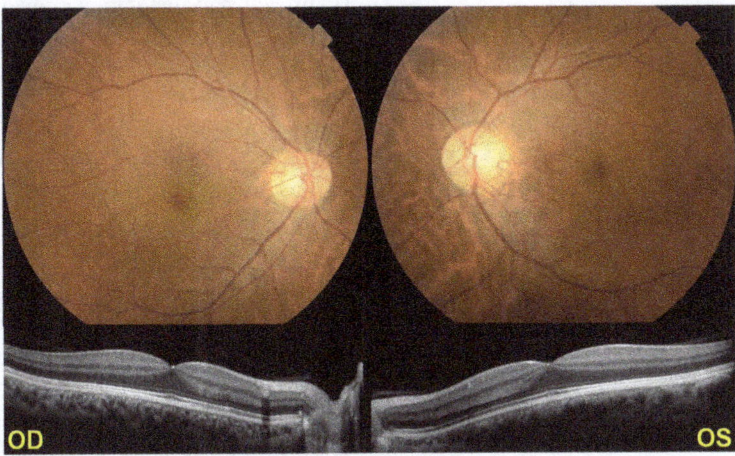

Fig. 1 Color fundus photographs and optical coherence tomographic (OCT) images. Fundus photographs do not show any obvious abnormal findings, and OCT shows partial loss of the interdigitation zone

ocular histories were unknown because both his parents and grandparents were dead.

The ERGs were recorded and analyzed with MEB-9402 (NIHON KOHDEN, Tokyo, Japan) and LS-100 (Mayo, Nagoya, Japan) as light emitting device. Before ERG recordings, we confirmed that the pupils were maximally dilated to approximately 8.0 mm following topical application of a mixture of 0.5% tropicamide and 0.5% phenylephrine (Sandol P; Nitten Pharmaceutical Co. Ltd., Aichi, Japan). ERG recordings performed binocularly with contact lens electrodes.

He was dark-adapted for 20 min, and the dark-adapted 0.01 ERG, dark-adapted 3.0 ERG, and dark-adapted oscillatory potentials were recorded in that order. The eye was then light-adapted for 10 min, and the light-adapted 3.0 ERG, light-adapted 30 Hz flicker (3.0 photopic cd s m^{-2} stimulus luminance) were recorded. Then, ERGs elicited by long-duration stimuli (on and off responses: 63.0 cd/m^2 stimulus intensity with 31.6 cd/m^2 background intensity, 200 ms duration) were recorded. All of the recordings conformed to the International Society for Clinical Electrophysiology of Vision (ISCEV) standard for full-field clinical electroretinography [2].

During the recording of the dark-adapted ERG series elicited by single flashes, there were no changes in the patient's overall condition. However, as soon as the flicker ERG recordings were completed and long-duration flashes began, the patient reported that a paralysis had developed in both upper limbs. Therefore, the examiner immediately stopped the ERG recordings, and soon thereafter, convulsions of the lower limbs developed and he lost consciousness. The convulsions disappeared after an intravenous injection of diazepam. Examinations of the ERG recordings, no apparent decrease in amplitudes or extension of implicit times were observed as compared with the normal waveforms indicated by ISCEV. No abnormality of the a-wave / b-wave ratio at the maximum combined response was observed (Fig. 3). Computed tomography of the head was performed on the same day, and no abnormality was found. Magnetic resonance imaging (MRI) of the head was also performed later, and the findings were normal. There

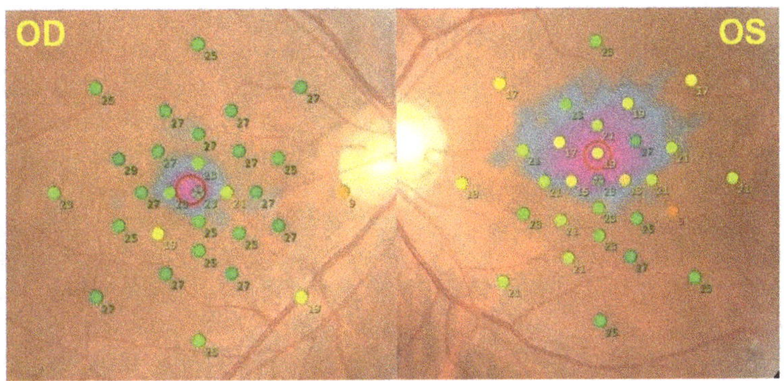

Fig. 2 Retinal sensitivity measured by MP-3 microperimetry. Retinal sensitivity around fovea is decreased of both eyes

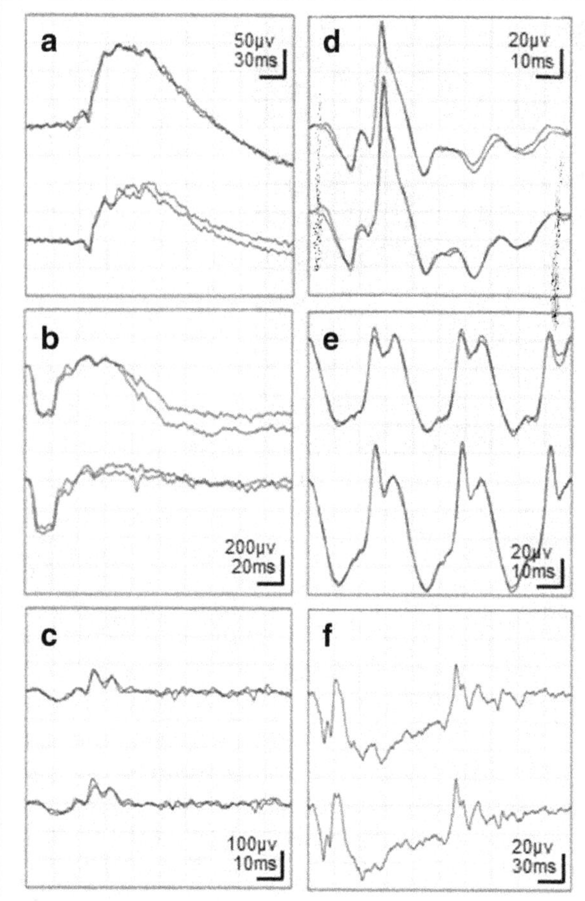

Fig. 3 Electroretinogram (ERG) waveforms. **a** Dark-adapted 0.01; **b** dark-adapted 3.0; **c** dark-adapted oscillatory potentials; **d** light-adapted 3.0 ERG; **e** light-adapted 30 Hz flicker; **f** long-duration flashes (on-off responses). The upper line shows the result of the right eye and the lower line shows the result of the left eye. The recording of the on-off response was interrupted when the patient developed tonic seizure

was no abnormality in the electroencephalogram examination performed after the attack. After that incident, he reported that he had had conscious-loss seizures four years earlier.

Discussion and conclusions

It has been known for more than a century that flickering artificial lighting and sunlight can induce epileptic seizures. It was already reported in 1934 that the electroencephalogram can be changed by photic stimulation [3]. Our patient was diagnosed with a photosensitive epileptic seizure because there were no abnormalities in the head MRI and no signs of partial seizure.

Many investigations have examined the epidemiology of photosensitivity seizures where photosensitivity was defined as a paroxysmal reaction to intermittent photic stimulation (IPS). These electroencephalographic responses are called photo paroxysmal response (PPR). A significant age dependency of PPR has been reported to be between ages 5 and 20 years [4]. Harding et al. reported that photosensitive epilepsy has a prevalence of approximately 1 in 4000 in the general population [5]. They also reported that the prevalence of women with PPR traits was up to 2.5 times higher than in men, and there was no difference in the prevalence of PPR by ethnic origins. Furthermore, the incidence of PPR was relatively high at 8.9% for normal children [6] and 0.5% for normal men [7]. Only 25% of patients lose their photosensitivity in their 20s and 30s, and the photosensitivity in the other patients persists in later life [8]. Therefore, it is necessary to pay attention to the risk of developing photosensitive epilepsy even if the subject is not a young woman as was our case.

Detailed investigations have also been made on the types of stimuli that can induce photosensitive epileptic seizures. Photosensitive seizures can be induced by a range of frequencies with a range of 10 to 30 Hz [9]. Most patients are sensitive to 16 Hz, 49% are sensitive to 50 Hz, and 15% are sensitive to 60 Hz [10]. About 3% of the light-sensitive population have systemic degenerative diseases and are sensitive to IPS of 1 to 3 Hz [11]. In our case, the seizure attack developed when the flicker stimulation ceased, and the on-off response stimulus was beginning to be presented. Thus, we believe that the light stimuli used in the flicker stimulation or the on-off response stimulation was the factor that induced the seizure. The frequency of flicker used in our case was 30 Hz, and the stimulation for the on-off responses was about 2.5 Hz and both used white light. Considering the results of previous studies, it is highly probable that the convulsions were induced by 30 Hz flicker, however the possibility of induction by the stimulation of on-off response cannot be completely be eliminated.

The wavelength of the stimulation light is also related to photosensitivity. Long wavelength red light has been reported to be more provocative even at low luminances [12]. Red light stimulation is sometimes used when investigating the functions of retinal ganglion cells [13, 14], thus attention is required in those cases.

It has been reported that stimulating only the fellow eye with shielding of one eye decreases the incidence of illusion and light sensitive seizures [15]. Therefore, it is assumed that photosensitivity seizures are less likely to occur with VEP, multifocal ERG, and the RETeval system recordings in which the stimuli are presented monocularly. This is in contrast to full-field ERG in which the stimuli are presented binocularly.

Harding et al. also reported that photosensitivity has a strong genetic tendency [8]. Twenty-five percent of mothers with photosensitivity show photosensitivity in the laboratory, and half of them develop photosensitive epileptic seizures. Therefore, it is recommended to confirm not only the patient's past seizure episodes but also family history of seizures before the ERG recording.

In conclusion, there is a possibility of inducing a convulsive seizure with 30 Hz flicker or on-off stimulation. We recommend that clinicians inquire about past seizure episodes of the patients and their family before beginning the ERG recordings, and taking measures such as not conducting flicker or on-off response recording if there are any histories of seizures.

Abbreviations

BCVA: Best corrected visual acuity; ERG: Electroretinogram; GP: Goldmann perimetry; HFA: Humphrey field analyzer; IPS: Intermittent photic stimulation; ISCEV: International Society for Clinical Electrophysiology of Vision; MRI: Magnetic resonance imaging; PPR: Photo paroxysmal response; VEP: Visual evoked potential

Acknowledgements

The authors thank Professor Emeritus Duco Hamasaki, Bascom Palmer Eye Institute, University of Miami, for his critical discussion and editing of the final manuscript.

Authors' contributions

GM has analyzed data, drafted the manuscript and revise. YH has examined the patient and drafted the manuscript. AU, TB and SY attended the cases, analyzed data and critically revised the manuscript. GM and YH had full access to all of the data in this study and take responsibility for the integrity of the data and accuracy of the data analysis. All the authors read and approved the final manuscript.

Competing interests

The authors declare that they have no competing interests.

Author details

[1]Department of Ophthalmology and Visual Science, Chiba University Graduate School of Medicine, Inohana 1-8-1, Chuo-ku, Chiba 260-8670, Japan. [2]Department of Neurology, Graduate School of Medicine, Chiba University, Chiba, Japan.

References

1. Takada H, Aso K, Watanabe K, Okumura A, Negoro T, Ishikawa T. Epileptic seizures induced by animated cartoon, pocket monster. Epilepsia. 1999;40: 997–1002.
2. McCulloch DL, Marmor MF, Brigell MG, Hamilton R, Holder GE, Tzekov R, et al. ISCEV standard for full-field clinical electroretinography (2015 update). Doc Ophthalmol. 2015;130:1–12.
3. Adrian ED, Matthews BHC. The Berger rhythm: potential changes from the occipital lobes in man. Brain. 1934;57:355–85.
4. Shiraishi H, Fujiwara T, Inoue Y, Yagi K. Photosensitivity in relation to epileptic syndromes: a survey from an epilepsy center in Japan. Epilepsia. 2001;42(Suppl 3):393–7.
5. Harding GFA, Jeavons PM. Photosensitivity epilepsy: clinics in development medicine. No.133. London: Mac Keith Press; 1994. p. 28–9.
6. Eeg-Olofsson O, Petersén I, Selden U. The development of the electroencephalogram in normal children from the age of 1 through 15 years. Paroxysmal activity. Neuropadiatrie. 1971;4:375–404.
7. Gregory RP, Oates T, Merry RTG. Electroencephalogram epileptiform abnormalities in candidates for aircrew training. Electroencephalogr Clin Neurophysiol. 1993;86:75–7.
8. Harding GFA, Edson A, Jeavons PM. Persistence of photosensitivity. Epilepsia. 1997;38:663–9.
9. Kasteleijn-Nolst Trenité DGA. Photosensitivity in epilepsy: electrophysiological and clinical correlates. Acta Neurol Scand. 1989; 80(Suppl. 125):1–149.
10. Harding GFA. Mechanism of photosensitive epilepsy. Neurophysiol Clin. 1998;28:360–1.
11. Zifkin BG, Kasteleijn-Nolst Trenité DGA. Reflex epilepsy and reflex seizure of the visual system: a clinical review. Epileptic Disord. 2000;2:129–36.
12. Takahashi T, Tsukahara Y, Kaneda S. EEG activation by use of stroboscope and visual stimulator SLS-5100. Tohoku J Exp Med. 1980;130:403–9.
13. Kondo M, Kurimoto Y, Sakai T, Koyasu T, Miyata K, Ueno S, Terasaki H. Recording focal macular photopic negative response (PhNR) from monkeys. Investig Ophthalmol Vis Sci. 2008;49:3544–50.
14. Kato F, Miura G, Shirato S, Sato E, Yamamoto S. Correlation between N2 amplitude of multifocal ERGs and retinal sensitivity and retinal nerve fiber layer thickness in glaucomatous eyes. Doc Ophthalmol. 2015;131(3):197–206.
15. Wilkins AJ. Visual Stress. Oxford: Oxford University Press; 1995. p. 194.

13

Ventriculoperitoneal shunts in non-HIV cryptococcal meningitis

Jia Liu[1†], Zhuo-lin Chen[1†], Min Li[1†], Chuan Chen[2], Huan Yi[1], Li Xu[1], Feng Tan[3] and Fu-hua Peng[1*]

Abstract

Background: Persistent and uncontrollable intracranial hypertension (ICH) and difficulty in reducing Cryptococcus count are severe problems in cryptococcal meningitis (CM) patients. The therapeutic effects of ventriculoperitoneal shunts (VPS) in non-HIV CM patients are not fully known, and the procedure is somewhat unusual. Here, our study offers a review to investigate the role of VPS in non-HIV CM.

Methods: We retrospectively collected data on 23 non-HIV CM patients with and without ventriculomegaly from 2010 to 2016. Their demographic data, clinical manifestations, cerebrospinal fluid (CSF) features and outcomes were analysed.

Results: We found that non-HIV CM patients without ventriculomegaly were older, had earlier treatment times and had shorter symptom durations than CM patients with ventriculomegaly. In both groups, headache, vomiting, fever and loss of vision were the most common clinical features. CSF pressure and Cryptococcus count were significantly decreased after operation. VPS could provide sustained relief from ICH symptoms such as headache. 13% of patients had poor outcomes because of serious underlying disease, while 87% of patients had good outcomes.

Conclusions: The use of a VPS is helpful in decreasing ICH and fungal overload in non-HIV CM patients, and VPS should be performed before CM patients present with symptoms of severe neurological deficit.

Keywords: Ventriculoperitoneal shunts, HIV, Cryptococcal meningitis, Ventriculomegaly, Intracranial hypertension

Background

Cryptococcus neoformans is an opportunistic pathogen and is an important cause of fungal meningitis associated with high morbidity and mortality rates. It commonly occurs in immunosuppressed patients with HIV infections or transplant conditioning, as well as in previously healthy individuals [1, 2]. There are many patients without a severe immunocompromising illness before the development of cryptococcal meningitis (CM) who have a negative HIV test result. Non-HIV related cryptococcosis is becoming a more significant subpopulation in the developed world, accounting for approximately one-third of cases [3]. Therefore, an increased recognition of CM in immunocompetent hosts has begun to direct more attention towards this infection [4]. Persistent and uncontrollable intracranial hypertension (ICH) is a severe complication in patients with CM and is closely related to the count of Cryptococcus. Delays in treatment of ICH are directly related to poor outcomes, including severe headache, papilledema, loss of vision and hearing, and disturbances in consciousness [5]. ICH is an important risk factor for neurological deficits in CM patients and is associated with early death [6, 7]. It has been documented that reducing ICH to normal levels is essential to improving CM patients' prognosis [6, 8]. Many researchers have previously shown that ventriculoperitoneal shunt (VPS) placement in HIV-infected patients with ICH can result in a good response and a positive outcome [9–11]. In HIV-related CM patients, the uncontrollable ICH could be relieved by VPS [12]. Nevertheless, few studies have examined VPS in non-HIV CM patients. Some researchers have suggested that the effects of VPS in CM patients with hydrocephalus were limited and that this treatment could not be used effectively in comatose patients [7]. However, Po-Chou Liliang et al. proposed that uncontrollable

* Correspondence: pfh93@163.com
[†]Equal contributors
[1]Department of Neurology, the Third Affiliated Hospital of Sun Yat-Sen University, 600# Tianhe Road, Guangzhou 510630, Guangdong, China

ICH in non-HIV CM patients without ventriculomegaly could be resolved by the use of VPS, and the patients' neurological deficits could be improved [13]. Hence, the proposed role of VPS in non-HIV CM patients has also been inconsistent.

Here, our study offers a retrospective review to analyse the difference after VPS between non-HIV CM patients with and without ventriculomegaly. We conducted this study to assess the predictive value of the response to VPS in non-HIV CM patients. An additional aim was to evaluate whether there were differences in the effects of VPS in CM patients with and without ventriculomegaly.

Methods

Clinical data collection

This was a retrospective study. The patients were from the Third Affiliated Hospital of Sun Yat-sen University, Guangzhou, China. From January 2010 to June 2016, the clinical data of 427 non-HIV infected CM patients were reviewed. A total of 378 patients without surgery were excluded. A total of 23 patients satisfied the diagnostic criteria and were recruited into our study. The details of the enrolment process are presented in Fig. 1. The typical brain images of patients with ventriculomegaly or without were shown in Fig. 2.

Patients' definitions

CM patients were identified according to symptomatology along with isolation of *C. neoformans* in cerebrospinal fluid (CSF) culture or a positive result of CSF India ink microscopy [14].

Radiographic diagnosis of ventriculomegaly was made based on enlargement of the temporal horn of the lateral ventricle, without obvious brain atrophy on the initial and/or follow-up CT or MRI [7, 10, 11].

Demographic data, risk factors, time from diagnosis to shunt, clinical features before and after VPS, CSF characteristics, CT/MR findings, antifungal therapy and outcomes were recorded (Tables 1 and 2).

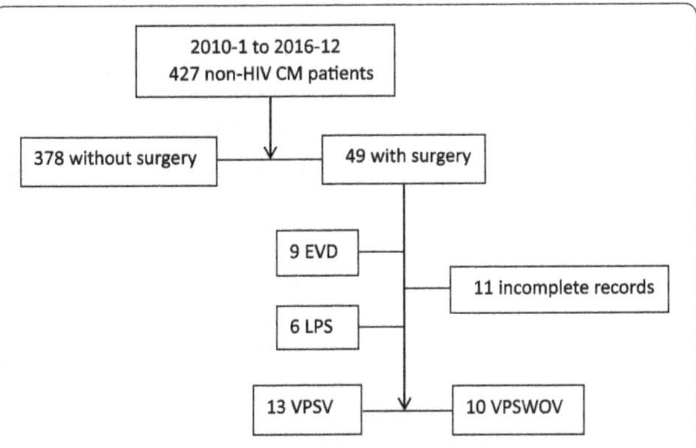

Fig. 1 Enrolment process of patients. CM: cryptococcal meningitis; EVD: external ventricular drainage; LPS: lumboperitoneal shunt; VPS: ventriculoperitoneal shunts; VPSV: VPS with ventriculomegaly; VPSWOV: VPS without ventriculomegaly

Laboratory measurement

Repeated lumbar puncture (LP) was performed in all the patients, and CSF open pressure, differential counts, glucose, protein, chloride, India ink smear and CSF culture were recorded. The CSF sample was subjected to India ink preparation. Cryptococcus count was determined by counting the number of *Cryptococcus neoformans* per millilitre of CSF via microscopic examination after India ink test. Brain computed tomography (CT) and/or magnetic resonance imaging (MRI) was performed before and after operation. All images were analysed by experienced neuroradiologists.

Therapeutic methods

All patients received antifungal therapy with the following methods: amphotericin B (AMB): 0.7–1.0 mg/kg·d, fluconazole (Fluc): 400–800 mg/d, flucytosine (5FC): 100 mg/kg·d [15]. Patients underwent LP three or four times within 1 week, according to their condition. After they had received routine VP operations, LP was performed to dynamically monitor the CSF changes. All patients received follow-up care 1 month after discharge.

Statistical analysis

All statistical analyses in this study were performed using SPSS (version 16.0, Chicago, IL, USA). Numerical variables were presented as the mean ± standard deviation (SD) or median (interquartile range), and categorical variables were expressed as a percentage. Statistical significance was set at $P < 0.05$. Student's t-test was used to analyse normally distributed variables. A mean of repeated-measure ANOVA was used for continuous variables (e.g., CSF parameters). The nonparametric Mann-Whitney *U* test was used for non-normally distributed data. Chi-square or Fisher's exact test was performed for categorical variables.

Results

Subject clinical characteristics

A cohort of 23 non-HIV CM patients who were treated with VPS, including 13 with ventriculomegaly (VPSV) [12 males and 1 female] and 10 without ventriculomegaly (VPSWOV) [6 males and 4 females], were enrolled in our study (Fig. 1 and Table 2). There was no significant difference in gender composition between the groups. The post-operation period was divided into three stages: within 1 week, when discharged from hospital and re-hospitalization 1 month later.

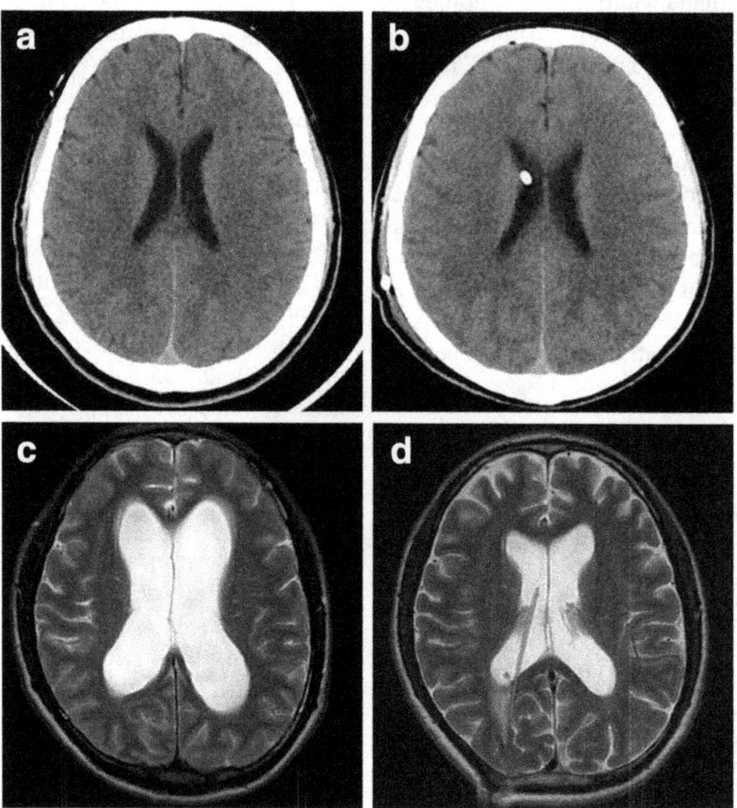

Fig. 2 **a** and **b** Head CT of a 40-year-old VPSWOV patient before and after operation. **a** Pre-operative CT shows no dilation of the cerebral ventricles (**b**) postoperative CT shows no dilation of the cerebral ventricles. **c** and **d** Head MR of a 28-year-old VPSV patient before and after operation. **a** Pre-operative axial T2-weighted image shows dilation of the cerebral ventricles (**b**) postoperative T2-weighted shows narrowing of the cerebral ventricles

The clinical and demographic features of the subjects were summarized in Tables 1 and 2

The male sex was predominant in both groups. Most of the patients had predisposing factors such as liver disease, diabetes mellitus, pulmonary cryptococcosis, malignancy or autoimmune disease. Compared with the VPSV group, those with VPSWOV were older (mean age: 41 years vs. 28 years, $p = 0.032$), and with shorter symptom durations (30 vs. 90 days, $p = 0.019$) and earlier surgical treatments (2 vs. 3.5 months, $p = 0.028$). All the patients had some symptoms of neurological deficit, including headaches, vomiting, vision and hearing loss, loss of consciousness and convulsions. Among these symptoms, headache, vomiting, fever and loss of vision were the most common clinical features in both the VPSV and VPSWOV groups. In our observation period, one male VPSV patient and two VPSWOV patients' conditions deteriorated due to their serious underlying diseases (case 2, 19 and 23).

Comparisons of CSF characteristics between VPSV and VPSWOV groups before operation

As shown in Table 2, in both groups, ICH during LP and CSF assays were abnormal in all patients. High pleocytosis, protein levels, and fungal overload along with low glucose and chloride levels were detected. Higher fungal load was observed in the VPSWOV group than in the VPSV group ($p = 0.001$) in the India ink staining test. However, no intergroup differences were found in CSF cell count or protein, glucose or chloride levels.

Observed clinical and CSF features in VPSV and VPSWOV pre-operation and 1 week post-operation

Within 1 week after VPS, we found that headache, vision, hearing and consciousness were improved to different degrees in both VPSV and VPSWOV patients, and headache had improved significantly ($p < 0.01$). Moreover, ICH in both groups was significantly decreased after operation when compared with pre-operation (153 vs. 330, 180 vs. 330, $p < 0.001$; Table 3). No significant difference was found between the two groups ($p = 0.402$). Patients with VPSV (0 vs. 23) had a significantly lower Cryptococcus count after the operation than before ($p = 0.014$), and patients with VPSWOV also had a lower fungal count after the operation (3.12E2 vs. 1.94E3, $p = 0.337$), although the differences were not statistically significant.

Table 1 Demographic and clinical features in VPSV and VPSWOV patients

No	Age/ gender	Risk factors	Time from diagnosis to shunt (m)	neurological deficit		antifungal therapy	Outcome 1 m
				Before VPS	*After VPS improved*		
				VPSV			
1	38/M	Hepatitis B	4	H,VL,HL	H	AMBisome+Fluc+5FC	better
2	36/M	Hepatitis B, Liver cirrhosis	1.5	H,VL,LOC	H,VL,LOC	AMB + Fluc+5FC	worse
3	40/M	Diabetes mellitus	3	H/V	H	AMB + Fluc+5FC	better
4	17/M		3.5	H/V,VL,LOC	H/V,VL,LOC	AMB + Fluc+5FC	better
5	28/M		1.5	H/V,VL	H,VL	Fluc+5FC	better
6	53/M		6	V, LOC	V, LOC	AMB + Fluc+5FC	better
7	27/M	pulmonary cryptococcosis	3	H/V,VL	H/V	AMB + Fluc+5FC	better
8	21/M		5	H	H	AMB + Fluc+5FC	better
9	31/M	Hepatitis B, Diabetes mellitus	6	H,VL	H,VL	Fluc+5FC	better
10	19/M	AIHA	4	H/V,CO	H/V,CO	AMB + Fluc+5FC	better
11	18/M	Hepatitis B	2	H/V	H/V	AMB + Fluc+5FC	better
12	53/F		3.5	V,LOC	V,LOC	AMB + Fluc+5FC	better
13	50/M	Hepatitis B	6	H,VL	H	Fluc+5FC	better
				VPSWOV			
14	41/F	pulmonary cryptococcosis	4	H/V	H	AMB + Fluc+5FC	better
15	35/M		3	H/V,VL,LOC	H/V,VL,LOC	AMB + Fluc+5FC	better
16	40/M	pulmonary cryptococcosis	3	H/V,VL,HL	H/V,VL	AMB + Fluc+5FC	better
17	51/M	Diabetes mellitus	0.5	H/V,VL	H/V,VL	AMB + Fluc+5FC	better
18	41/M		2	H,VL, CO	H,VL	AMB + Fluc+5FC	better
19	61/F	Malignancy	4	H/V	H/V	Fluc+5FC	worse
20	37/M	Hepatitis B	2	H/V,VL,HL	H/V,VL	AMB + Fluc+5FC	better
21	55/F	SLE	0.5	H/V,VL	H/V,VL	Fluc+5FC	better
22	17/M	pulmonary cryptococcosis	1	H/V,LOC	H/V,LOC	AMB + Fluc+5FC	better
23	45/F	AIHA	1	H,VL,HL,LOC	H,VL	AMB + Fluc+5FC	NA

AIHA autoimmune haemolytic anaemia, *SLE* systemic lupus erythematosus, *H/V* headache and vomiting, *VL* visual loss, *HL* hearing loss, *LOC* loss of consciousness, *CO* convulsions, *NA* Not available, *AMB* Amphotericin B, *5FC* flucytosine, *Fluc* Fluconazole, *M* month, 1–13: VPSV, 14–23: VPSWOV

Outcomes and follow-up

We further assessed outcomes for both groups at discharge and at the follow-up re-hospitalization 1 month later. Details of the clinical characteristics and laboratory examinations are shown in Tables 4 and 5. We were able to observe that VPSV patients had significantly decreased ICH (100 vs. 330, 158 vs. 330, $p < 0.001$) and obviously reduced fungal load (0 vs. 23, $p < 0.01$) regardless of when they were discharged or re-hospitalized 1 month later. Interestingly, we could reach a similar conclusion in the VPSWOV group, where we found that at these same time points, patients also had significantly lower ICH (142 vs. 330, 125 vs. 330, $p < 0.001$) and fungal load (0 vs. 1.94E3, $p < 0.01$). There was no evidence to show that there were differences in ICH and Cryptococcus count between the VPSV and VPSWOV groups.

Of all symptoms, headache was most obviously improved after surgery, and this improvement was stable during our observation period ($p<0.01$). Nevertheless, some patients with vision and hearing symptoms were not reversible due to the long-term ICH. Additionally, we found that most of patients had good outcomes. The exceptions were cases 2, 19 and 23, who had a poor prognosis after the operation, and case 23, which was missing from follow-up.

Analysis of the cases with poor patient outcomes

Case 2, a 36-year-old male with VPSV, presented with vomiting and loss of vision and hearing and was unconscious. Before he received VPS, LP indicated 400 mmH_2O intracranial pressure (ICP) and 7500 mL^{-1} Cryptococcus count. Medical history showed that he had hepatitic cirrhosis. After VPS, his vomiting and consciousness state

Table 2 Clinical and CSF characteristics in VPSV and VPSWOV patients pre-operation

Characteristic	VPSV (*n* = 13)	VPSWOV (*n* = 10)	*P*
Sex(M/F)	12/1	6/4	0.127
Age(Y) median (range)	28(17–53)	41(17–61)	0.032
Symptoms duration, days, median (range)	90 (20–180)	30(10–180)	0.019
headache	11/13 (84.6%)	10(100%)	0.486
fever	7/13(53.8%)	5/10(50%)	>0.999
Vomiting	8/13(61.5%)	8/10(80%)	0.405
Visual symptoms	7/13(53.8%)	7/10(70%)	0.669
Auditory symptom	2/13(15.4%)	3/10(30%)	0.618
Altered mental status	5/13(38.5%)	3/10(30%)	>0.999
Seizure	1/13(7.69%)	2/10(20%)	0.560
Indian ink smear (+)	12/13(92.3%)	10/10(100%)	>0.999
CSF culture positive (+)	8/13(61.5%)	7/10(70%)	>0.999
Time to operation(m)	3.5(1.5–6)	2(0.5–4)	0.028
CSF pressure (mmH2O) median (range)	330(200–1020)	330(204–660)	0.059
WBC count(×106/l) median (range)	60(0–550)	36(1–496)	0.225
Protein, g/L median (range)	0.53(0.12–4.06)	0.8(0.23–1.62)	0.139
Glucose(mmol/l) median (range)	2.33(0.01–5.58)	2.53(0.23–5.7)	0.753
Chloride(mmol/l) median (range)	118(103–133)	120(108–136)	0.150
India ink Cryptococcus count	23(0–1.3E4)	1.94E3(4–1.67E5)	0.001

M male, *F* female, *CSF* cerebrospinal fluid, *P* VPSV versus VPSWOV pre-operation

were improved. Vision and hearing had no obvious improvement. As the illness progressed, his liver function deteriorated and he had poor outcome.

Case 19 was a 61-year-old female with VPSWOV and uterine cervical cancer. After VPS, her headache was improved, but she had a poor outcome because the cancer had metastasized to other parts of the body.

Case 23 was a 45-year-old female VPSWOV patient with autoimmune haemolytic anaemia (AIHA). She had been treated with hormones for a very long time. After VPS, her headache and vomiting were improved, but she had a poor prognosis.

In summary, the poor outcomes for each of these patients were closely related to serious underlying diseases, not shunt-related complications.

Discussion

CM is the most common fungal meningitis in HIV-positive patients. In the absence of HIV, CM patients with underlying immune dysfunction, such as organ

Table 3 Comparison of clinical and CSF characteristics in VPSV and VPSWOV patients within 1 week after the operation

		VPSV (*n* = 13)	VPSWOV (*n* = 10)	P_1	P_2	*P*
symptoms improved	headache	10/11(90.1%)	10/10(100%)	0.001	<0.001	>0.999
	Visual	4/7(57.1%)	5/7(71.4%)	>0.999	0.153	>0.999
	Auditory	1/2(50%)	0/3	0.371	0.07	0.40
	Mental change	4/5(80%)	2/3(66.7%)	0.615	0.510	0.464
CSF	CSF pressure (mmH2O) median (range)	153(55–330)	180(95–330)	<0.001	<0.001	0.402
	WBC count (×106/l) median (range)	70(2–459)	80(25–232)	0.42	0.018	0.868
	Protein, g/L median (range)	1.43(0.3–7.7)	1.61(0.51–3.98)	<0.001	<0.001	0.334
	Glucose(mmol/l) median (range)	1.7(0.03–3.54)	1.17(0.43–7.45)	0.008	0.026	0.526
	Chloride(mmol/l) median (range)	117(103–126)	116(103–126)	0.285	0.020	0.96
	India ink Cryptococcus count	0(0–480)	3.12E2(0–3.01E4)	0.014	0.337	0.003

P_1 pre-operation versus within 1 week post operation in the VPSV group
P_2 pre-operation versus within 1 week post operation in the VPSWOV group
P VPSV versus VPSWOV within 1 week post operation

Table 4 The conditions of VPSV and VPSWOV patients when they were discharged from hospital

		VPSV ($n = 13$)	VPSWOV($n = 10$)	P_1	P_2	P
symptoms improved	headache	11/11(100%)	9/10(90%)	<0.001	<0.001	0.476
	Visual	5/7(71.4%)	6/7(85.7%)	0.374	0.05	>0.999
	Auditory	1/2(50%)	2/3(66.7%)	0.371	0.51	>0.999
	Mental change	4/5(80%)	2/3(66.7%)	0.615	0.510	0.464
CSF	CSF pressure (mmH2O) median (range)	100(50–200)	142(90–330)	<0.001	<0.001	0.064
	WBC count (×106/l) median (range)	26(6–70)	80(25–232)	0.62	0.798	0.281
	Protein, g/L median (range)	1.27(0.18–4.8)	1.61(0.51–3.98)	0.018	0.002	0.325
	Glucose(mmol/l) median (range)	1.61(0.69–5)	1.17(0.43–7.45)	0.04	0.312	0.806
	Chloride(mmol/l) median (range)	124(120–128)	122(115–132)	0.03	0.935	0.166
	India ink Cryptococcus count	0(0–32)	0(0–5)	0.001	<0.001	0.577

P_1 pre-operation versus discharged from hospital in the VPSV group
P_2 pre-operation versus discharged from hospital in the VPSWOV group
P VPSV versus VPSWOV at discharge from hospital

transplantation, corticosteroid medication use and malignancy, account for the majority of cases. In our study, we found that liver disease, diabetes mellitus, malignancy, pulmonary cryptococcosis and autoimmune diseases were the major underlying diseases. These findings had some similar features to a previous study in HIV-negative patients [16, 17] but also showed some differences. In our study, we found that in the VPSV group, 5 of the 13 (38.5%) patients suffered from liver diseases. Five patients (38.5%) had no apparent underlying disease. In the VPSWOV group, 3 of the 10 patients (30%) had pulmonary cryptococcosis. Two patients (20%) had no apparent underlying disease. The male sex was predominant in both groups. VPSWOV patients were obviously older than VPSV, and people with VPSWOV tended to receive surgical treatment earlier, making the symptom duration shorter.

Uncontrollable ICH, a severe complication in patients with CM, is defined as a CSF opening pressure > 250 mmH_2O and is generally considered to relate to high fungal burden in the CSF [18]. Symptoms include headache, papilledema, vomiting, vision and hearing loss, and impaired mentation. Our study showed that headache, vomiting, fever and loss of vision were the most common clinical features in both the VPSV and VPSWOV groups. Headache could continue to ease after VPS operation. On the other hand, impaired eyesight and hearing, as well as altered mental status, were not improved significantly.

An elevated CSF pressure level is significantly linked to increased mortality and poor outcomes [19, 20]. The goal of CM treatment is to reduce fungal burden and to prevent long-term neurological deficits. The decompression is a very important parameter in this management. Ventriculomegaly is an uncommon complication of CM patients. There are multiple treatments to control ICP such as medications, repeated LP, temporary external drainage or permanent VPS [15]. For CM patients with progressive ventriculomegaly, VPS is a favoured method of diversion to relieve the ICH, which is well studied in

Table 5 Follow up with VPSV and VPSWOV patients when they returned to hospital 1 month after the operation

		VPSV ($n = 13$)	VPSWOV ($n = 9$)	P_1	P_2	P
symptoms improved	headache	12/13(92.3%)	8/9(88.9%)	0.001	<0.001	>0.999
	Visual	5/7(71.4%)	5/6(83.3%)	0.374	0.05	>0.999
	Auditory	1/2(50%)	2/3(66.7%)	0.371	>0.999	>0.999
	Mental change	4/5(80%)	1/2(50%)	0.615	0.364	0.333
CSF	CSF pressure (mmH2O) median (range)	158(65–280)	125(50–180)	<0.001	<0.001	0.509
	WBC count (×106/l) median(range)	14.5(8–46)	21(2–86)	0.014	0.185	0.488
	Protein, g/L median (range)	0.95(0.15–3.86)	1.31(0.18–2.16)	0.236	0.096	0.692
	Glucose(mmol/l) median (range)	2.25(1.24–2.89)	2.42(1.27–4.17)	0.384	0.593	0.644
	Chloride(mmol/l) median (range)	124(114–131)	124(112–130)	0.104	0.264	0.742
	India ink Cryptococcus count	0(0–266)	0(0–5)	0.004	<0.001	0.377

P_1 pre-operation versus returned to hospital after 1 month in the VPSV group
P_2 pre-operation versus returned to hospital after 1 month in the VPSWOV group
P VPSV versus VPSWOV when patients returned to hospital 1 month after the operation

HIV-positive [10, 21] and HIV-negative [7, 11] CM patients. However, relevant articles about VPS treatment in non-HIV patients without ventriculomegaly are limited. Available data are limited to case reports [13] and smaller case studies [22]. Comparative data concerning the non-HIV CM population with and without ventriculomegaly are sparse. Here, we present a comprehensive analysis of clinical, CSF characteristics and prognosis in both groups in order to further assess the roles of VPS in non-HIV CM patients.

The mechanisms of the development of elevated ICP with ventriculomegaly in CM are complex. Some reports have shown the following possible pathogenesis pathways: (1) the channels for CSF drainage may be blocked by fungal polysaccharides, or (2) the passage of CSF across the arachnoid villi may be blocked by an inflammatory response [23]. For those CM patients with ICH but without ventriculomegaly, previous research has suggested that (1) deposits of cryptococcal capsular polysaccharides on the brain surface and within the parenchyma tissue could lead to the brain's inability to respond to the increased CSF volume and pressure [7, 24]. (2) The venous stenosis may limit cerebral blood outflow due to an infection-mediated mechanism [21]. In brief, ICH is closely associated with fungal overload. In our study, by comparing the pre-operation CSF characteristics, we found that a higher Cryptococcus count was observed in the VPSWOV group than in the VPSV group via India ink staining tests. There was no significant difference found in CSF cell counts or protein, glucose or chloride levels between the two groups. When compared with pre-operation levels, we found that the CSF pressure in both groups and fungal count in the VPSV group were significantly decreased within 1 week after the operation. Moreover, we presented the status when patients were discharged from hospital and when they returned to hospital after 1 month. Interestingly, we see similar results at these two observation time points. There were significantly decreased ICH and fungal loads after VPS in both the VPSV and VPSWOV groups. VPS helped to reduce ICH and fungal load. However, our results suggest patients would have poor outcomes if they have a serious underlying disease.

Continuous ICH, in CM patients both with and without ventriculomegaly, can lead to irreversible neurological complications and increase morbidity and mortality. Failure to address the consequences of ICH would be significantly detrimental. If the initial treatment, even combined with appropriate antifungal therapy, still fails to control ICH, VPS could be an effective choice. Our study has shown that CSF pressure and Cryptococcus counts were significantly decreased after VPS, and headache could continue to improve.

Conclusions

In summary, our data suggest that early placement of a VPS is helpful in decreasing uncontrollable ICH and fungal overload, regardless of the ventriculomegaly status of non-HIV CM patients. The VPS could not only relieve the symptoms of ICH, but could also improve the clinical features of CM patients. Therefore, early diagnosis and early use of VPS in CM patients, before the onset of severe neurological deficit symptoms, could be beneficial and essential. We look forward to future clinical studies to confirm this result.

Limitations

Our study has some limitations. Due to the exclusion of other surgical methods and some missing data at follow-up, this study had a limited sample size. Further research with a multicentre study and a larger samples size will be more convincing.

Abbreviations

5FC: Flucytosine; AIHA: Autoimmune haemolytic anaemia; AMB: Amphotericin B; CM: Cryptococcal meningitis; CSF: Cerebrospinal fluid; CT: Computed tomography; EVD: External ventricular drainage; Fluc: Fluconazole; ICH: Intracranial hypertension; ICP: Intracranial pressure; LP: Lumbar punctures; MRI: Magnetic resonance imaging; VPS: Ventriculoperitoneal shunts; VPSV: VPS with ventriculomegaly; VPSWOV: VPS without ventriculomegaly

Acknowledgements

The authors would like to thank all the patients' participation and all of the physicians who helped to collect the clinical data.

Funding

The study was supported by National Science Foundation (No. 81271327), Guangdong Science Foundation of Guangdong Province (NO.2015A03013167), Science&technology Project of Guangzhou (NO.201510010251).

Authors' contributions

JL and ML were responsible for the data integrity and the accuracy of the data analysis. LX and ZLC analysed the data of CSF and CT. JL, ML and CC prepared the manuscript. JL, ZLC, HY and FT revised the manuscript. HFP reviewed the whole paper, including the figures and legends. All authors read and approved the final manuscript.

Competing interests

The authors declare that they have no competing interests.

Author details

[1]Department of Neurology, the Third Affiliated Hospital of Sun Yat-Sen University, 600# Tianhe Road, Guangzhou 510630, Guangdong, China. [2]Department of Neurosurgery, the Third Affiliated Hospital of Sun Yat-Sen University, Guangzhou 510630, Guangdong, China. [3]Department of Neurology, Foshan Chinese Medicine Hospital, Foshan 528000, Guangdong, China.

References

1. In: Rapid Advice: Diagnosis, Prevention and Management of Cryptococcal Disease in HIV-Infected Adults, Adolescents and Children. edn. Geneva; 2011.

2. Panackal AA, Wuest SC, Lin YC, Wu T, Zhang N, Kosa P, Komori M, Blake A, Browne SK, Rosen LB, Hagen F, Meis J, Levitz SM, Quezado M, Hammoud D, Bennett JE, Bielekova B, Williamson PR. Paradoxical immune responses in non-HIV Cryptococcal meningitis. PLoS Pathog. 2015;11:e1004884.
3. Pyrgos V, Seitz AE, Steiner CA, Prevots DR, Williamson PR. Epidemiology of cryptococcal meningitis in the US: 1997-2009. PLoS One. 2013;8:e56269.
4. Ou XT, Wu JQ, Zhu LP, Guan M, Xu B, Hu XP, Wang X, Weng XH. Genotypes coding for mannose-binding lectin deficiency correlated with cryptococcal meningitis in HIV-uninfected Chinese patients. J Infect Dis. 2011;203:1686–91.
5. Saag MS, Graybill RJ, Larsen RA, Pappas PG, Perfect JR, Powderly WG, Sobel JD, Dismukes WE. Practice guidelines for the management of cryptococcal disease. Clin Infect Dis. 2000;30:710–8.
6. Vidal JE, Gerhardt J, Peixoto de Miranda EJ, Dauar RF, Oliveira Filho GS, Penalva de Oliveira AC, Boulware DR. Role of quantitative CSF microscopy to predict culture status and outcome in HIV-associated cryptococcal meningitis in a Brazilian cohort. Diagn Microbiol Infect Dis. 2012;73:68–73.
7. Liliang PC, Liang CL, Chang WN, Chen HJ, Su TM, Lu K, Lu CH. Shunt surgery for hydrocephalus complicating cryptococcal meningitis in human immunodeficiency virus-negative patients. Clin Infect Dis. 2003;37:673–8.
8. de Vedia L, Arechavala A, Calderon MI, Maiolo E, Rodriguez A, Lista N, Di Virgilio E, Cisneros JC, Prieto R. Relevance of intracranial hypertension control in the management of Cryptococcus neoformans meningitis related to AIDS. Infection. 2013;41:1073–7.
9. Cherian J, Atmar RL, Gopinath SP. Shunting in cryptococcal meningitis. Journal of neurosurgery. 2016;125:177–86.
10. Liu L, Zhang R, Tang Y, Lu H. The use of ventriculoperitoneal shunts for uncontrollable intracranial hypertension in patients with HIV-associated cryptococcal meningitis with or without hydrocephalus. Bioscience trends. 2014;8:327–32.
11. Park MK, Hospenthal DR, Bennett JE. Treatment of hydrocephalus secondary to cryptococcal meningitis by use of shunting. Clin Infect Dis. 1999;28:629–33.
12. Corti M, Priarone M, Negroni R, Gilardi L, Castrelo J, Arechayala AI, Messina F, Franze O. Ventriculoperitoneal shunts for treating increased intracranial pressure in cryptococcal meningitis with or without ventriculomegaly. Rev Soc Bras Med Trop. 2014;47:524–7.
13. Liliang PC, Liang CL, Chang WN, Lu K, Lu CH. Use of ventriculoperitoneal shunts to treat uncontrollable intracranial hypertension in patients who have cryptococcal meningitis without hydrocephalus. Clin Infect Dis. 2002;34:E64–8.
14. Bahr NC, Boulware DR. Methods of rapid diagnosis for the etiology of meningitis in adults. Biomark Med. 2014;8:1085–103.
15. Perfect JR, Dismukes WE, Dromer F, Goldman DL, Graybill JR, Hamill RJ, Harrison TS, Larsen RA, Lortholary O, Nguyen MH, Pappas PG, Powderly WG, Singh N, Sobel JD, Sorrell TC. Clinical practice guidelines for the management of cryptococcal disease: 2010 update by the infectious diseases society of america. Clin Infect Dis. 2010;50:291–322.
16. Lee YC, Wang JT, Sun HY, Chen YC. Comparisons of clinical features and mortality of cryptococcal meningitis between patients with and without human immunodeficiency virus infection. J Microbiol Immunol Infect. 2011;44:338–45.
17. Liao CH, Chi CY, Wang YJ, Tseng SW, Chou CH, Ho CM, Lin PC, Ho MW, Wang JH. Different presentations and outcomes between HIV-infected and HIV-uninfected patients with Cryptococcal meningitis. J Microbiol Immunol Infect. 2012;45:296–304.
18. Bicanic T, Brouwer AE, Meintjes G, Rebe K, Limmathurotsakul D, Chierakul W, Teparrakkul P, Loyse A, White NJ, Wood R, Jaffar S, Harrison T. Relationship of cerebrospinal fluid pressure, fungal burden and outcome in patients with cryptococcal meningitis undergoing serial lumbar punctures. AIDS. 2009;23:701–6.
19. Husain M, Jha DK, Rastogi M. Angiographic catheter: unique tool for neuroendoscopic surgery. Surg Neurol. 2005;64:546–9.
20. Iwashita T, Kitazawa K, Koyama J, Nagashima H, Koyama T, Tanaka Y, Hongo K. A saccular-like dissecting aneurysm of the anterior cerebral artery that developed 2 years after an ischemic event. Surg Neurol. 2005;64:538–41.
21. Petrou P, Moscovici S, Leker RR, Itshayek E, Gomori JM, Cohen JE. Ventriculoperitoneal shunt for intracranial hypertension in cryptococcal meningitis without hydrocephalus. J Clin Neurosci. 2012;19:1175–6.
22. Wang H, Ling C, Chen C, He HY, Luo L, Ning XJ. Evaluation of ventriculoperitoneal shunt in the treatment of intracranial hypertension in the patients with cryptococcal meningitis: a report of 12 cases. Clin Neurol Neurosurg. 2014;124:156–60.
23. Stevens DA, Denning DW, Shatsky S, Armstrong RW, Adler JD, Lewis BH. Cryptococcal meningitis in the immunocompromised host: intracranial hypertension and other complications. Mycopathologia. 1999;146:1–8.
24. Lee SC, Casadevall A. Polysaccharide antigen in brain tissue of AIDS patients with cryptococcal meningitis. Clin Infect Dis. 1996;23:194–5.

Dose effects of mycophenolate mofetil in Chinese patients with neuromyelitis optica spectrum disorders

Yujuan Jiao[1], Lei Cui[1], Weihe Zhang[1], Chunyu Zhang[2], Yeqiong Zhang[1], Xin Zhang[1] and Jinsong Jiao[1*]

Abstract

Background: Neuromyelitis optica (NMO) spectrum disorder (NMOSD) is a devastating autoimmune inflammatory disorder of the central nervous system, which can result in blindness or paralysis. Currently, there is a dire need for new treatment options in the clinic. Several case series have shown that mycophenolate mofetil (MMF) may be an effective treatment for NMOSD patients. The dosing of MMF in the treatment of NMOSD has been poorly studied. Therefore, we evaluated the efficacy, tolerability, influential factors and optimal dosage of MMF in Chinese patients with NMOSD.

Methods: A case series of 109 NMO or NMOSD (limited forms of NMO with seropositive AQP4-IgG) patients were retrospectively analyzed and followed up. Out of the 109 patients, 86 patients had received MMF for 6 months or longer and were included for efficacy assessment.

Results: When comparing the annualized relapse rate (ARR) of MMF treatment with that of pre-MMF treatment period, MMF was found to significantly reduce ARR in 75 (87%) patients ($p < 0.0001$). The median pre-treatment Expanded Disability Status Scale (EDSS) score in remission decreased from 3 (range, 0–8.5) to 2.5 (range, 0–8) at the last follow-up ($p = 0.006$), yet no significant difference was found in the visual score. The higher doses of MMF (1750 mg/d to 2000 mg/d) significantly lowered the relapse risks compared with lower doses (1000 mg/d or less, $p < 0.0001$) or moderate doses (1250 to 1500 mg/d, $p = 0.031$). Coexisting with systemic autoimmune diseases (HR, 2.418; $p = 0.0345$) and attack number before MMF initiation (HR, 1.117; $p = 0.02$) were important risk factors for relapses. MMF was generally well tolerated with adverse effects occurring in 21 patients (19%). While four patients decreased their daily doses because of the adverse effects, only one patient stopped MMF treatment.

Conclusions: MMF is generally effective and well tolerated in Chinese NMOSD patients. High-dose MMF was more potent than the lower dose for NMOSD patients, with 1750 mg of daily MMF being the recommended dosage for Chinese patients with NMOSD. MMF treatment reduces the frequency of relapses and improves the quality of life for patients with this debilitating disease.

Keywords: Mycophenolate mofetil, Neuromyelitis optica, Neuromyelitis optica spectrum disorders, Efficacy, Tolerability, Dose effects

* Correspondence: jiao_jinsong@163.com
[1]Department of Neurology, China-Japan Friendship Hospital, #2 Yinghuayuan East Street, Chaoyang District, Beijing 100029, China
Full list of author information is available at the end of the article

Background

Neuromyelitis optica (NMO) spectrum disorder (NMOSD) is a devastating autoimmune inflammatory disorder of the central nervous system, which can lead to blindness or paralysis. The risk of developing disabilities increases significantly with the number of relapses [1, 2]. Prevention of relapse is essential for the successful treatment of NMOSD patients. While there have been no placebo-controlled or comparative randomized controlled trials of immunosuppressive therapies conducted in NMO patients, several case series have reported that mycophenolate mofetil (MMF) may be effective for treatment of NMOSD [3–10]. To date, there are no clear recommendations regarding the dosing of MMF. In this study, we aimed to evaluate the efficacy, safety profile and recommendable dosage of MMF in a large cohort of Chinese patients with NMO and NMOSD.

Methods

Patients

This study was approved by the Medical Ethics Committee of China-Japan Friendship Hospital (2016–62). Patient consent forms were obtained from all patients or his/her legal representatives before the study. We performed a retrospective review of the medical records from patients that presented with NMO, using the 2006 revised NMO criteria [11] or the NMOSD (limited forms of NMO with seropositive AQP4-IgG) [12]. From January 2009 to October 2016, 109 patients (96 female and 13 males) received MMF treatment and were enrolled for individual tolerability assessments. Of the 109 patients, 86 received ≥6 months of MMF were included for the efficacy assessment, 22 patients had recently initiated MMF treatment, and one patient stopped MMF before the end of 6 months due to an adverse reaction. Patients who received 1000 mg/d or less of MMF were classified as the low-dose treatment group, while MMF dosages of 1250 mg/d and 1500 mg/d were deemed as the moderate-dose treatment. The highest dosages utilized in this study were 1750 mg/d and 2000 mg/d, which were considered as the high-dose treatment. While receiving MMF treatment, each patient received long-term concomitant oral corticosteroids (10–15 mg every other day) for the first one to two years. At each follow-up appointment, routine blood tests were performed to assess the efficacy of the therapy. The patients were recommended to follow-up every 3 months, and there was a minimum annual follow-up requirement and all of the follow-up appointments were recorded.

Clinical assessment

Data was recorded for the patients, including demographic data, detailed treatment plans (daily dose of MMF and glucocorticoid, date and reason for the initiation or cessation of immunosuppressive agents, and the starting or stopping of any other treatments), clinical course, adverse reactions, modified Expanded Disability Status Scale (EDSS) and corrected visual acuity at remission and each follow-up appointment [1].

Visual acuity was assessed separately for each eye using the following scale: 0 = 20/20; 1 = scotoma, but better than 20/30; 2 = 20/30 to 20/59; 3 = 20/60 to 20/199; 4 = 20/200 to 20/800; 5 = count fingers only; 6 = light perception; 7 = no light perception [1]. The visual outcome in remission was the sum of the visual scores for each eye after each attack and at the follow-up appointments.

A relapse is defined as a sudden worsening of neurological function lasting for more than 24 h that is unknown in origin with no other identifiable causes, such as a fever or infection. Additionally, a relapse will increase the EDSS score by a half point or more, or it may be indicated by a worsening of one point in two of the functional systems or two points in a single functional system. A severe relapse was defined as an EDSS score of six or more, which required a walking aid to travel 100 m with or without resting, at the nadir of the attack. In those patients with baseline EDSS scores ≥6.0, an increase of 0.5 points or more was classified as a severe relapse. In cases of optic neuritis (ON), a severe relapse was defined as a sudden worsening of visual acuity (VA) of 0.1 or less in patients with baseline VA scores of greater than 0.1. When accompanied with MRI evidence of ON, any decrease of VA was regarded as a severe relapse if the baseline vision was light perception, hand motion, or counting fingers [5, 9]. Suboptimal treatment with MMF was defined as 6 months or less of therapy or daily dosages less than the minimal therapeutic dose (1250 mg in adults).

Statistical analyses

Data were analyzed using SAS version 9.3 (SAS institution Inc., NC, USA). A two-sided $p \leq 0.05$ was considered statistically significant. The Wilcoxon signed-rank test was used to compare pre-treatment annualized relapse rates (ARR), EDSS, and visual scores with on-treatment indexes. The number of severe attacks that occurred before and during MMF treatment was compared using the Pearson chi-square test. Characteristics were compared among the different MMF dosage groups (i.e., female and male) using the Pearson chi-square test for categorical data and the Kruskal-Wallis H-test for continuous data. The Kaplan-Meier method was used to determine the time to first relapse among different groups, and were then compared using the log-rank test. Hazard ratios (HR) that pertained to the first relapse after the start of MMF treatment were calculated using the Cox proportional hazard model, as follows:

$$h(t, x) = h_0(t)\ \exp(\beta_1 x_1 + \beta_2 x_2 + \ldots + \beta_m x_m)$$

where t is the first relapse time, and x is the MMF dosage, concomitant with any systemic autoimmune diseases, pre-MMF ARR, pre-MMF EDSS, duration of MMF therapy, duration of pre-MMF, attacks number before MMF initiation, gender, age at onset and serum AQP4-IgG positivity.

Results

Baseline demographic and clinical data

The demographic and clinical characteristics of the cohort are summarized in Table 1. Diagnoses at the initiation of MMF therapy were NMO (64), transverse myelitis (9, recurrent in 7), recurrent optic neuritis (3), and NMOSD with other clinical characteristics (10). Among NMOSD patients receiving different dosages of MMF, there were no significant differences between the baseline characteristics including age, female percentage, complete NMO patient percentage, aquaporin-4 antibody positivity, age at disease onset, duration of MMF treatment, treatment-naïve patients, disease duration, attack number, ARR and EDSS before receiving MMF (Additional file 1: Table S1).

Table 1 Demographic characteristics of patients who received MMF treatment for six months or longer

Characteristic	Value
Number of Patients	$n = 86$
Current age, median (range), y	53 (15–84)
Female sex, No. (%)	77 (90%)
NMO diagnosis, No. (%)	64 (74%)
NMOSD diagnosis, No. (%)	22 (26%)
Aquaporin-4 antibody positivity, No. (%)	74 (86%)
Age at onset, median (range), y	43 (6–68)
Overall disease duration, median (range), mo	71 (7–535)
Disease duration before receiving MMF, median (range), mo	71 (6–444)
Attack number before receiving MMF, median (range)	5 (1–33)
Duration of MMF treatment, median (range), mo	20 (6–89)
Abnormal autoantibodies[a], n (%)	39 (45%)
Coexisting with systemic autoimmune diseases	29 (34%)
Concurrent use of prednisone, n (%)	65 (76%)
treatment-naïve patients, n (%)	21 (24%)
Previous immunosuppressive agents:	
Corticosteroids[b], n (%)	33 (38%)
Azathioprine, n (%)	15 (17%)
Cyclophosphamide, n (%)	4 (5%)
Rituximab, n (%)	2 (2%)
Tacrolimus (FK506)	1 (1%)
Methotrexate	1 (1%)
Previous immunomodulatory therapies:	
β-interferons, n (%)	6 (7%)
hydroxychloroquine sulfate, n (%)	2 (2%)
Mitoxantrones, n (%)	1 (1%)

[a]Autoantibodies refers to rheumatoid factors, antinuclear antibodies, anti-double-stranded DNA antibodies, ribose nuclear proteins, anti-SM antibodies, anti-SSA and anti-SSB antibodies, TPO and TG antibodies
[b]Corticosteroids refers to continuously taking oral prednisone or methylprednisolone for more than 3 months

Efficacy: MMF therapy significantly reduced ARR of NMOSD

During a median course of 20 months (average 27) therapy with MMF, 55 (64%) patients were relapse-free and 75 (87%) of the 86 evaluated patients experienced improvement in their ARR. Among the 31 patients who relapsed during MMF therapy, 7 (23%) patients experienced their first relapse within 6 months of initiating MMF therapy. The median ARR during MMF treatment (0, range 0–2.8) was significantly reduced ($p < 0.0001$, Table 2) compared with the pre-treatment ARR (1.4, range 0.1–11.0). The Kaplan-Meier survival estimated the significant difference between the relapse-free rates of pre-treatment and during treatment periods ($p < 0.001$, Fig. 1a).

Efficacy: MMF therapy significantly decreased the risk of severe relapses

A total of 572 attacks were recorded in 86 patients with NMOSD. Of the 572 attacks, 502 (6 with uncertain severities) of them happened prior to the initiation of MMF therapy, including 200 (40%) attacks rated as severe and 296 attacks rated as mild. During MMF treatment, only 16 (23%) of the 70 relapses were severe. There was a significantly lower risk of patients experiencing severe relapses during MMF treatment when compared with the period prior to MMF therapy initiation ($p = 0.006$).

Disability efficacy: MMF was effectual for improving disabilities in NMOSD

The EDSS scores improved in 36 patients and were unchanged in 39 patients, which was 75 out of the 86 (87%) NMOSD patients. There was a statistically significant decrease between the median EDSS score obtained at the beginning of MMF treatment (in remission) and at the last follow-up ($p = 0.006$, Table 2). The median visual scores obtained at pre-MMF treatment (in remission) and the last follow-up visit were 2 (average 3.0, range, 0–13) and 1 (average 2.7, range, 0–13), respectively. While the visual scores improved in 11 patients and stabilized in 68 patients (total of 79 out of 86 or 92% NMOSD patients), there was no significant difference between values obtained at pre-treatment and the last follow-up ($P = 0.106$).

Table 2 Subanalysis of treatment efficacy in patients treated with MMF

	ARR	p	EDSS	P	On-MMF, Patients, %		
	Median (Range)		Median (Range)		Relapse free	Improved ARR	Improved or Stabilized EDSS
Total patients ($n = 86$)							
Pre-MMF treatment	1.4(0.1–11)	< 0.0001	3(0–8.5)	0.006	64	87	87
on-MMF treatment	0(0–2.8)		2.5(0–8.5)				
Patients with high dose MMF treatment ($n = 52$)							
Pre-MMF treatment	1.5(0.1–11)	< 0.0001	3(0–8.5)	0.511	81	92	89
on-MMF treatment	0(0–2.8)		2.5(0–8.5)				
Patients with moderate dose MMF treatment ($n = 23$)							
Pre-MMF treatment	1.4(0.2–6)	0.0003	3(0–8.5)	0.071	52	78	83
on-MMF treatment	0(0–2.2)		2(0–6.5)				
Patients with low dose MMF treatment ($n = 11$)							
Pre-MMF treatment	1.2(0.5–6)	0.0078	4(0–8.5)	0.438	9	82	91
on-MMF treatment	0.5(0–1.0)		4(0–8.5)				

pre-MMF before initiation of MMF treatment, *on-MMF* during treatment of MMF

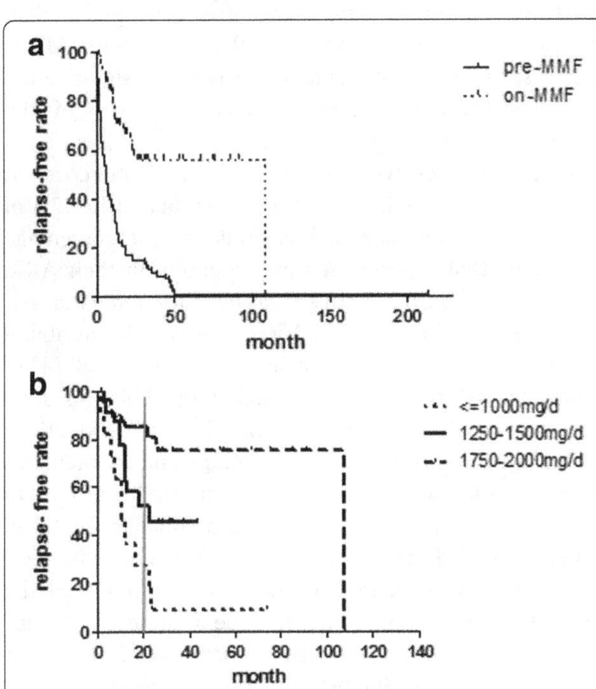

Fig. 1 Kaplan-Meier survival estimates pertaining to probabilities of being free of the occurrence of any relapse (**a**) between during MMF treatment (on-MMF, dashed line) and before MMF treatment initiation (pre-MMF, black line) in NMOSD patients (Log-rank test, $p < 0.001$). The relapse-free rates after 1 year and 2 years therapy with MMF were 72% and 58%, respectively. Those values were much higher than 30% and 14% before initiation of MMF therapy. (**b**) with different dose of MMF therapy. After 20 months of MMF therapy, approximately 68% and 42% of NMOSD patients in the high-dose and moderate-dose groups would remain relapse-free, respectively (Log-Rank test, $p = 0.019$). However, only 9% of the patients receiving low-dose MMF would remain relapse-free, significant lower than the moderate or high-dose groups (Log-Rank test $p = 0.031$, $p < 0.0001$)

Efficacy: High dose MMF was more potent than lower dose for NMOSD

Among 31 NMOSD patients who relapsed during MMF therapy, 10 of the 11 (91%) patients were taking the lowest dosage of 1000 mg/d or less MMF relapsed, 11 of the 23 (48%) patients were on the median dosage of 1250 mg/d or 1500 mg/d, and 10 of the 52 patients (19%) were receiving the highest dosage of 1750 mg/d or 2000 mg/d (Table 2). The proportion of patients on concomitant corticosteroids for more than 1 year and 2 years did not differ among the three doses. Statistically significant differences in relapse-free rates were found between the lower and moderate dosage groups ($p = 0.031$), moderate and higher dosage groups ($p = 0.019$), and the lower and higher dosage groups ($p < 0.0001$, Fig. 1b). The adjusted hazard risks also indicated that the higher dosage of MMF was a protective factor for preventing relapse (Fig. 2). The EDSS scores were improved in 18 patients (35%), 13 patients (57%), and 5 patients (46%) in the lower, moderate, and higher MMF dosage groups, respectively. Additionally, the EDSS scores remained unchanged in 28 patients (54%), 6 patients (26%), and 5 patients (46%) in the lower, moderate, and higher MMF dosage groups, respectively. However, among the three MMF dosage groups, there is no statistically significant difference either in the number of patients with improved EDSS scores or in the number of patients with unchanged EDSS scores ($p = 0.276$).

NMOSD patients coexist with concomitant systemic autoimmune diseases were more prone to relapses

There were 29 (34%) NMOSD patients who had at least one systemic autoimmune disease in this study, which included 20 patients with thyroid disease, 7 patients with Sjögren syndrome, 4 patients with systemic lupus erythematosus, 2 patients with rheumatoid arthritis, 2 patients

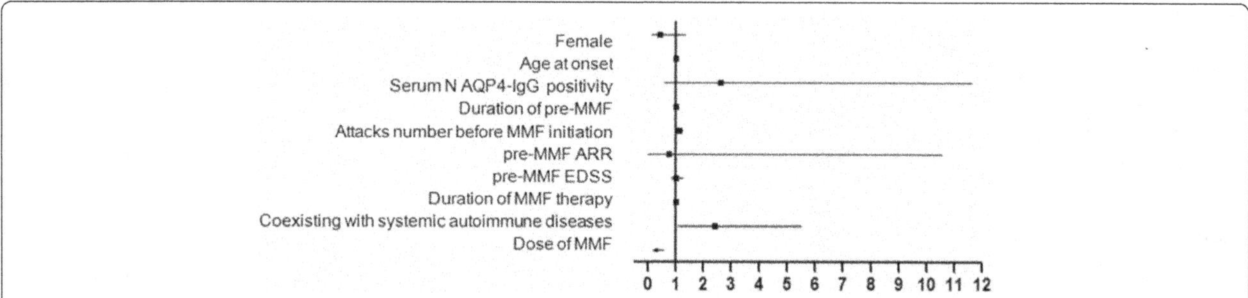

Fig. 2 Adjusted Hazard Risks for relapse after MMF initiation, according to the clinical characteristics and based on patients who received MMF for more than 6 months. NMOSD patients treated with the higher dose of MMF had a significantly lower risk of relapse (HR, 0.291; 95% confidence interval, 0.164–0.516; $p < 0.0001$). Significant risk factors for relapse in NMOSD patients were the presence of any systemic autoimmune disease (HR, 2.418; 95% confidence interval, 1.066–5.481; $p = 0.0345$) and an increased number of relapses before MMF initiation (HR, 1.117; 95% confidence interval, 1.018–1.227; $p = 0.020$). Other factors were determined to have little influence on the effect of MMF treatment

with Castleman disease, 2 patients with psoriasis, 2 patients with interstitial pneumonia and 1 patient with myasthenia gravis. It was found that concomitant systemic autoimmune disease (HR, 2.418; 95% confidence interval, 1.066–5.481; $p = 0.0345$) and relapses numbers before the initiation of MMF treatment (HR, 1.117; 95% confidence interval, 1.018–1.227; $p = 0.02$) were significant risk factors for the relapse in NMOSD patients (Fig. 2).

Side-effects and MMF tolerability

Twenty-one of 109 patients (19%) reported adverse effects with MMF treatment, including hair loss ($n = 5$), increased transaminase levels ($n = 3$), low white blood cell and neutrophil counts ($n = 3$, one of these patients also reported interstitial pneumonia and another reported human papillomavirus type 1 [HPV-1] infection), diarrhea and abdominal pain ($n = 2$), shingles ($n = 2$), herpes simplex infection ($n = 2$), headache ($n = 2$), thrombocytopenia ($n = 1$), constipation ($n = 1$), and chronic dermopathy on the hands and nails (n = 1). Five patients (4.6%) reported moderate to severe adverse effects and among them, two patients treated with MMF 2000 mg/d were admitted to hospital due to increased transaminase levels and interstitial pneumonia, respectively. Of the two patients, one discontinued MMF in the first two months of treatment, while the dosage was decreased from 2000 mg/d to 1250 mg/d for the second patient. The dosage of three additional patients was lowered from 2000 mg/d to 1500 mg/d because of increased transaminase levels, HPV-1 infection, or low neutrophil counts, within six months of initiating MMF treatment. These side effects were mild and symptomatic treatment were effective.

Discussion

In this study, patients received MMF with concomitant low dose oral corticosteroids therapy in the first one to two years of MMF therapy. It was reported that the proportions of relapse-free patients that experienced improved ARR values and EDSS scores did not differ between patients treated with MMF alone and MMF in combination with prednisone [6]. Thus, we discuss the overall treatment of MMF with or without oral corticosteroids as MMF therapy. Similar to previous studies [3–10], MMF therapy significantly reduced ARR in 87% of patients, and 64% were relapse-free during a median course of 20 months (average 27) therapy with MMF. Our results confirmed that MMF therapy significantly decreased the risks of severe relapses, in terms of disability, as recently reported [9, 10, 13].

For patients receiving MMF therapy, EDSS scores at last follow-up were improved and maintained in 87% of the NMOSD patients, which is similar to the percentage of patients that experiencing improvement in their ARR. Hence, MMF is an effective treatment for reducing disabling relapses in NMOSD. We compared the disability status in remission before or at the beginning of MMF treatment with those at the last follow-up. This was done to minimize the influence on EDSS scores reductions caused by corticosteroid impulse therapy and spontaneous recovery in the acute phase. It was reported that 68% to 97% patients experienced improved or unchanged EDSS scores after MMF treatment [4, 9, 12, 14]. This difference in results may be caused by the varying number of the patients in acute phase and treatment duration. In our study, the post-treatment visual scores, which were not mentioned in any of the previous studies, remained statistically unchanged, suggesting that visual deficiency is usually fixed and more difficult to improve than the disability caused by myelitis.

As of now, there are no standard criteria for determining the optimal dosage of MMF for treating NMOSD among treatment centers. As this is a retrospective study based on a review of medical records, the evaluated NMOSD patients were receiving different daily doses of MMF. While all dosage levels of MMF have shown some benefit in reducing relapse rates in NMOSD patients, the lower and moderate dosage carry a much higher risk of relapse. Nearly 9 out of 10 of NMOSD patients taking the lower dosage of MMF experienced a relapse, which was reduced to 5 out of 10 patients in the moderate dosage group. These results verified that 1500 mg/d or less MMF was insufficient for most of the Chinese NMOSD patients. While there were no significant differences in EDSS between the three different treatment groups, longer follow-up times could have revealed different results. Hence, longer follow-up or prospective controlled trials are necessary to validate these findings. Considering that nearly 20% of the patients receiving 1750 to 2000 mg/d of MMF still relapsed, natural history studies infer a stepwise accumulation of attack-related disability for most patients with NMOSD and any treatment failure is potentially devastating for NMOSD patients [2]. Overall, we found that high-dose MMF therapy provided the most benefit to NMOSD patients.

One-third of our NMOSD patients had at least one coexisting systemic autoimmune disease. Any coexisting systemic autoimmune disease was a significant risk factor for relapse. As another point of view, MMF was also effective for Sjögren syndrome, systemic lupus erythematosus, and several other autoimmune disorders [15–17], suggesting that high-dosage MMF may be an optimal treatment for NMOSD patients with coexisting systemic autoimmune diseases. While most of the moderate to severe adverse effects were reported by the patients receiving high-dosage MMF (2000 mg/d) therapy, pharmacokinetic studies may allow for individualization of MMF dosing for NMOSD patients in the future.

In this study, the number of relapses before the initiation of MMF was another risk factor for further relapses in NMOSD patients. This indicated that patients were more prone to relapse if they had several prior attacks. The usage, dosage, and timing of prophylactic agents are still being actively investigated for NMOSD patients. However, these results suggest an adequate immunosuppressant should be recommended for NMOSD patients with a history of relapse.

In terms of tolerability, MMF was generally well tolerated in the 109 Chinese NMOSD patients. Adverse effects were reported by 21 patients, and 5 of the 52 patients receiving high-dosage MMF (2000 mg/d) reported moderate to severe adverse effects that required therapeutic intervention. From this study and other case series and cohort studies published so far [3–10], MMF was administrated alone or in combination with oral corticosteroids in more than 500 NMOSD patients. No serious toxicity concerns, such as malignancies or progressive multifocal leukoencephalopathy, which had been reported in transplant patients when MMF was used in conjunction with other immunosuppressants [14].

The present study was limited by its absent blinding, retrospective design, and the uneven assignment of patients to the different dosage group. Specifically, more recently diagnosed patients were more likely to receive the higher dosage of MMF. Despite these methodological limitations, this study provides useful information on the influence factors and optimal MMF dosage choice for the treatment of NMOSD. In the future, randomized controlled trials will be necessary to further verify the finds from this study.

Conclusion

MMF is a safe and effective oral immunosuppressant for treatment of NMOSD. High-dosage MMF was more potent than the lower dose for treatment of NMOSD, with 1750 mg of daily MMF being the recommended dosage for Chinese patients with NMOSD. As for NMOSD patients with coexisting systemic autoimmune diseases, a higher daily dosage of MMF may be recommended.

Abbreviations

ALT: Alanine aminotransferase; AQP4: Aquaporin-4; ARR: Annualized relapse rate; AST: Aspartate aminotransferase; EDSS: Expanded Disability Status Scale; HPV: Human papillomavirus; HR: Hazard ratio; IgG: Immunoglobulin G; MMF: Mycophenolate mofetil; NMO: Neuromyelitis optica; NMOSD: Neuromyelitis optica spectrum of disorders; ON: Optic neuritis; VA: Visual acuity

Acknowledgements

We would like to thank laboratory technicians, Ying Hao and Jin Zhang, for collecting and processing the serum samples.

Funding

This work was supported by the Research Fund of the China-Japan Friendship Hospital (2013-RC-3) and the Foundation of Capital Characteristic Clinical Application Research (2106-BKJ-004).

Authors' contributions

JJ had full access to all the data in the study and takes responsibility for the integrity of the data and the accuracy of the data analysis. Study concept and design: YJ and JJ. Acquisition of data: YJ, LC, WZ, JJ, YZ and XZ. Analysis and interpretation of data: JJ, YJ, LC, WZ, CZ and XZ. Drafting of the manuscript: YJ. Critical revision of the manuscript for important intellectual content: All authors. Statistical analysis: YJ and CZ. Obtained funding: YJ and JJ. Supervised the study: JJ, YJ, LC and WZ. All authors read and approved the final manuscript.

Competing interests

The authors declare that they have no competing interests.

Author details

[1]Department of Neurology, China-Japan Friendship Hospital, #2 Yinghuayuan East Street, Chaoyang District, Beijing 100029, China. [2]Department of Health Reform and Development, China-Japan Friendship Hospital, Beijing, China.

References

1. Wingerchuk DM, Hogancamp WF, O'Brien PC, Weinshenker BG. The clinical course of neuromyelitis optica (Devic's syndrome). Neurology. 1999;53(5):1107–14.

2. Wingerchuk DM, Pittock SJ, Lucchinetti CF, Lennon VA, Weinshenker BG. A secondary progressive clinical course is uncommon in neuromyelitis optica. Neurology. 2007;68(8):603–5.
3. Mealy MA, Wingerchuk DM, Palace J, Greenberg BM, Levy M. Comparison of relapse and treatment failure rates among patients with neuromyelitis optica: multicenter study of treatment efficacy. JAMA Neurol. 2014;71(3):324–30.
4. Jacob A, Matiello M, Weinshenker BG, Wingerchuk DM, Lucchinetti C, Shuster E, et al. Treatment of neuromyelitis optica with mycophenolate mofetil: retrospective analysis of 24 patients. Arch Neurol. 2009;66(9):1128–33.
5. Huh SY, Kim SH, Hyun JW, Joung AR, Park MS, Kim BJ, et al. Mycophenolate mofetil in the treatment of neuromyelitis optica spectrum disorder. JAMA Neurol. 2014;71(11):1372–8.
6. Chen H, Zhang Y, Shi Z, Feng H, Yao S, Xie J, et al. The efficacy and tolerability of mycophenolate Mofetil in treating Neuromyelitis Optica and Neuromyelitis Optica Spectrum disorder in western China. Clin Neuropharmacol. 2016;39(2):81–7.
7. Xu Y, Wang Q, Ren HT, Qiao L, Zhang Y, Fei YY, et al. Comparison of efficacy and tolerability of azathioprine, mycophenolate mofetil, and cyclophosphamide among patients with neuromyelitis optica spectrum disorder: a prospective cohort study. J Neurol Sci. 2016 Nov 15;370:224–8.
8. Chen H, Qiu W, Zhang Q, Wang J, Shi Z, Liu J, et al. Comparisons of the efficacy and tolerability of mycophenolate mofetil and azathioprine as treatments for neuromyelitis optica and neuromyelitis optica spectrum disorder. Eur J Neurol. 2017;24(1):219–26.
9. Jeong IH, Park B, Kim SH, Hyun JW, Joo J, Kim HJ. Comparative analysis of treatment outcomes in patients with neuromyelitis optica spectrum disorder using multifaceted endpoints. Mult Scler J. 2016;22(3):329–39.
10. Montcuquet A, Collongues N, Papeix C, Zephir H, Audoin B, Laplaud D, et al. NOMADMUS study group and the Observatoire Français de la Sclérose en plaques (OFSEP). Effectiveness of mycophenolate mofetil as first-line therapy in AQP4-IgG, MOG-IgG, and seronegative neuromyelitis optica spectrum disorders. Mult Scler. 2017;23(10):1377–84.
11. Wingerchuk DM, Lennon VA, Pittock SJ, Lucchinetti CF, Weinshenker BG. Revised diagnostic criteria for neuromyelitis optica. Neurology. 2006;66:1485–9.
12. Wingerchuk DM, Lennon VA, Lucchinetti CF, Pittock SJ, Weinshenker BG. The spectrum of neuromyelitis optica. Lancet Neurol. 2007;6(9):805–15.
13. Tackley G, O'Brien F, Rocha J, Woodhall M, Waters P, Chandratre S, et al. Neuromyelitis optica relapses: race and rate, immunosuppression and impairment. Mult Scler Relat Disord. 2016;7:21–5.
14. US Food and Drug Administration. Communication about an ongoing safety review of CellCept (mycophenolate mofetil) and Myfortic (mycophenolic acid). Rockville, MD: US Food and Drug Administration; 2015.
15. Fialho SC, Bergamaschi S, Neves FS, Zimmermann AF, Castro GR, Pereira IA. Mycophenolate mofetil in primary Sjögren's syndrome: a treatment option for agranulocytosis. Rev Bras Reumatol. 2012;52(2):297–9.
16. Alexander S, Fleming DH, Mathew BS, Varughese S, Jeyaseelan V, Tamilarasi V, et al. Pharmacokinetics of concentration-controlled mycophenolate mofetil in proliferative lupus nephritis: an observational cohort study. Ther Drug Monit. 2014;36(4):423–32.
17. Lourdudoss C, Vollenhoven RV. Mycophenolate mofetil in the treatment of SLE and systemic vasculitis: experience at a single university center. Lupus. 2014;23(3):299–304.

15

Ictal asystole: a case presentation

Nirmeen Kishk[1], Amani Nawito[2], Ahmed El-Damaty[3] and Amany Ragab[1*]

Abstract

Background: Epileptic seizures can lead to cardiac arrhythmias. The arrhythmias may be in the form of tachycardia, bradycardia or asystole. Ictal bradycardia and asystole can lead to sudden unexpected death.

Case presentation: A case report of a 40-year-old male with complex partial temporal lobe epilepsy. He has coincident attacks of fall and pallor. The patient underwent simultaneous electrocardiogram (ECG) and video electroencephalogram (EEG) monitoring. The slow activity in EEG coincide with the appearance of bradycardia in ECG then cardiac asystole which clinically correspond to the patient syncope. After insertion of a cardiac pacemaker, only complex partial attacks develop with a marked reduction in frequency and no more fall attacks.

Conclusion: Epileptic seizures can present with cardiac arrhythmias, with ictal asystole leading to sudden unexpected death. Simultaneous EEG and ECG are essential for the diagnosis. A cardiac pacemaker can be lifesaving for patients with ictal arrhythmias.

Keywords: Ictal asystole, Epilepsy, Cardiac arrhythmia, Pacemaker, Simultaneous ECG and EEG

Background

Epileptic seizures can affect the heart rate leading to arrhythmia [1]. The most common arrhythmia associated with epilepsy is ictal tachycardia (80–100% of all seizures) [2]. Ictal bradycardia occurs in fewer than 6% of seizures. This slowing of the heart rate may be severe enough to cause ictal asystole. Ictal asystole defined as the absence of ventricular complexes for more than 4 s, accompanied by electrographic seizure onset [3].

Ictal asystole is found in 0.27–0.4% of patients undergoing video-EEG. Clinically, a loss of epileptic activity occurs due to brain anoxia along with a loss of muscle tone and consciousness [4, 5]. Approximately 80% of cases are associated with temporal lobe epilepsy while 20% of cases occur with extratemporal lobe seizures [6, 7].

Ictal bradycardia and ictal asystole may lead to sudden unexpected death in epilepsy patients (SUDEP) [8, 9].

Case presentation

The patient is a 40- years- old right-handed Egyptian male accountant with a negative perinatal history, no family history of epilepsy, no consanguineous marriage, and no medical comorbidities.

At the age of 23, after graduating from university, his father noticed recurrent nocturnal attacks in the form of right-sided head and neck deviation with tonic movements in both the upper and lower limbs. The episodes lasted for approximately 30–40 s and recurred 2–3 times on the same night with no tongue biting or urinary incontinence.

Conventional EEG showed left temporal epileptiform discharge.

Improvement was observed with carbamazepine (400 mg/day), and the patient became seizure-free for 1 year.

At the age of 32, he started to develop recurrent attacks with the following characteristics: A prodromal sense of dizziness followed by loss of contact with the environment, automatism, and stereotyped motor movement in both the upper and lower limbs (marching movements). He became pale and then experienced a loss of tone, causing him to fall to the ground, lasting 40–60 s. No tongue biting or urinary incontinence were reported, but sometimes self-injuries occurred. Then the patient regained consciousness after approximately 15 min of confusion. Each time he asked, “What day is it today?” and “What time is it?” This episode was followed by a sense of fatigue.

* Correspondence: dr.ahmajd@kasralainy.edu.eg
[1]Neurology Department, Faculty of Medicine, Kasr Alainy Hospital, Cairo University, Cairo, Egypt

These attacks did not occur out of sleep and recurred every 1–2 weeks.

Neurological Examination, conventional EEG, and brain magnetic resonance imaging (MRI) were normal.

The patient was prescribed levetiracetam 2000 mg /day, oxcarbazepine 500 mg/day, clonazepam 0.5 mg /day, and lacosamide 150 mg per day with a partial reduction in the frequency of the attacks.

When patient attended our clinic, he was monitored to ensure that he was compliant with his medications, and the doses were adjusted according to his body weight. We increased the doses and gave him 4 anti-epileptic drugs (AEDs) (Levetiracetam 3000 mg, oxcarbazepine 900 mg, lacosamide 200 mg, clonazepam 0.5 mg/day).

The frequency of events (dizziness, loss of contact, motor automatism) was reduced. However, the attacks of pallor and falling still recurred once per month. Sometimes the attacks were related to psychological or mental stress. Thus, the patient was referred for overnight video-EEG in our unit.

The video- EEG recording was performed overnight using a Nihon Kohden Neurofax 9200 EEG apparatus (Tokyo, Japan). The electrodes were applied according to the 10–20 electrode placement system, in addition to T1 and T2 electrodes. An additional ECG channel was included. Three minutes of hyperventilation and photic stimulation were performed as provocative procedures (Fig. 1).

The patient was awake when his father indicated that the usual seizure had started. The patient had lost contact and began experiencing motor automatism in the form of repetitive movements of the right hand, then the left hand, and finally, the lower limbs. The EEG showed rhythmic alpha frequencies over the left temporal region evolving into theta frequencies that involved both hemispheres. Then, the patient turned his head to the left side and displayed tonic movement in both upper limbs.

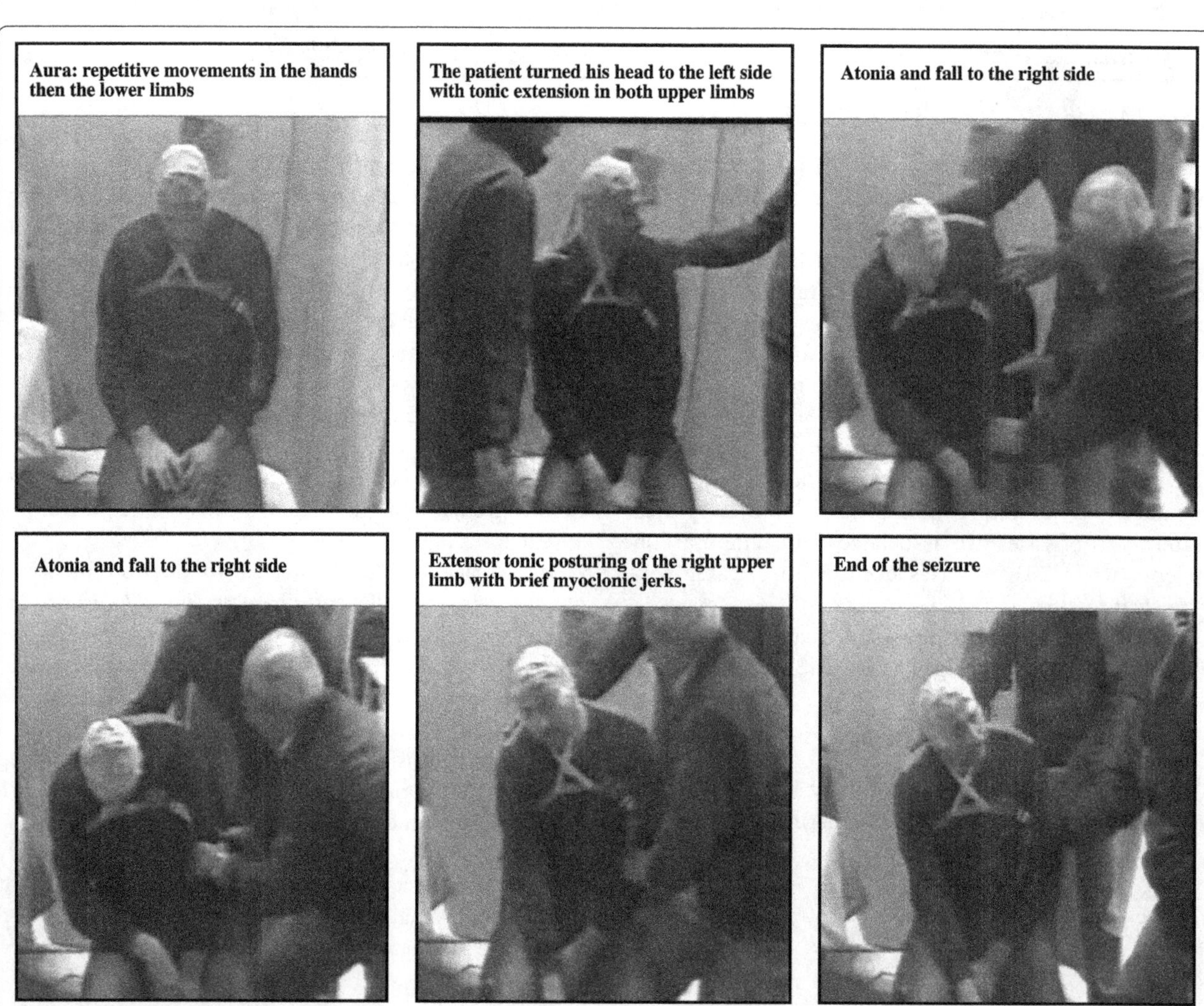

Fig. 1 Screenshots from the video- EEG Results

The simultaneous EEG revealed bilateral, rhythmic temporal theta frequencies. The ECG channel showed 5 s of bradycardia then a 10- s asystole (Fig. 2). Approximately 7 s after the onset of asystole, the patient had atonia and fell to the right side (syncope). The EEG indicated diffuse slowing with amplitude suppression. Next, the patient showed tonic extensor posturing of the right upper limb and brief myoclonic jerks. Here, the EEG was masked by movement and electromyogram (EMG) artifacts. Meanwhile, the ECG revealed bradycardia and then a regular rhythm.

After video EEG ictal recording we decided to stop lacosamide 200 mg to avoid the aggravation of the cardiac arrhythmia. In the same week, the patient was referred for permanent cardiac pacemaker implantation and advised to continue his prescribed antiepileptic medications.

After implantation of a dual chamber pacemaker, only complex partial attacks occurred and did so with a lower frequency. No additional falling attacks followed.

Discussion

A complex relationship exists between seizures and the heart.

Epileptic activity originating in the amygdala, insular cortex, cingulate gyrus, frontopolar region, and frontotemporal region can produce a broad range of cardiac abnormalities, including supraventricular tachycardia, sinus tachycardia, sinus bradycardia, sinus arrest, atrioventricular block, and asystole [4].

Intraoperative stimulation of the human insular cortex reveals that right insular stimulation leads to tachycardia and pressor responses, while left insular stimulation leads to bradycardia and depressor responses [10].

Ictal bradycardia is observed in patients with a long history of epilepsy, especially those with refractory seizures. This may occur because repeated seizures or antiepileptic drugs use impairs the neurocardiac regulatory system [11].

Ictal asystole should be suspected if the typical seizure semiology is associated with syncopal episodes [12, 13].

Simultaneous EEG and ECG recordings are the only methods to differentiate between primary cerebrogenic and cardiogenic causes of arrhythmias. In primary cerebrogenic bradyarrhythmia, EEG seizure activity precedes the onset of bradyarrhythmia. Also, a 24-h Holter ECG is essential to exclude intrinsic cardiac disease, which may be a predisposing factor for ictal asystole [10].

This case is a diagnostic challenge and difficult to be diagnosed unless in a highly specialized integrated epilepsy unit with a rapid and easy referral and effective communication between departments.

Conclusion

Epileptic seizures can present with cardiac arrhythmias and ictal asystole, which may lead to sudden unexpected death. Simultaneous EEG and ECG recordings are essential for diagnosis. A cardiac pacemaker can be lifesaving for patients with ictal arrhythmias.

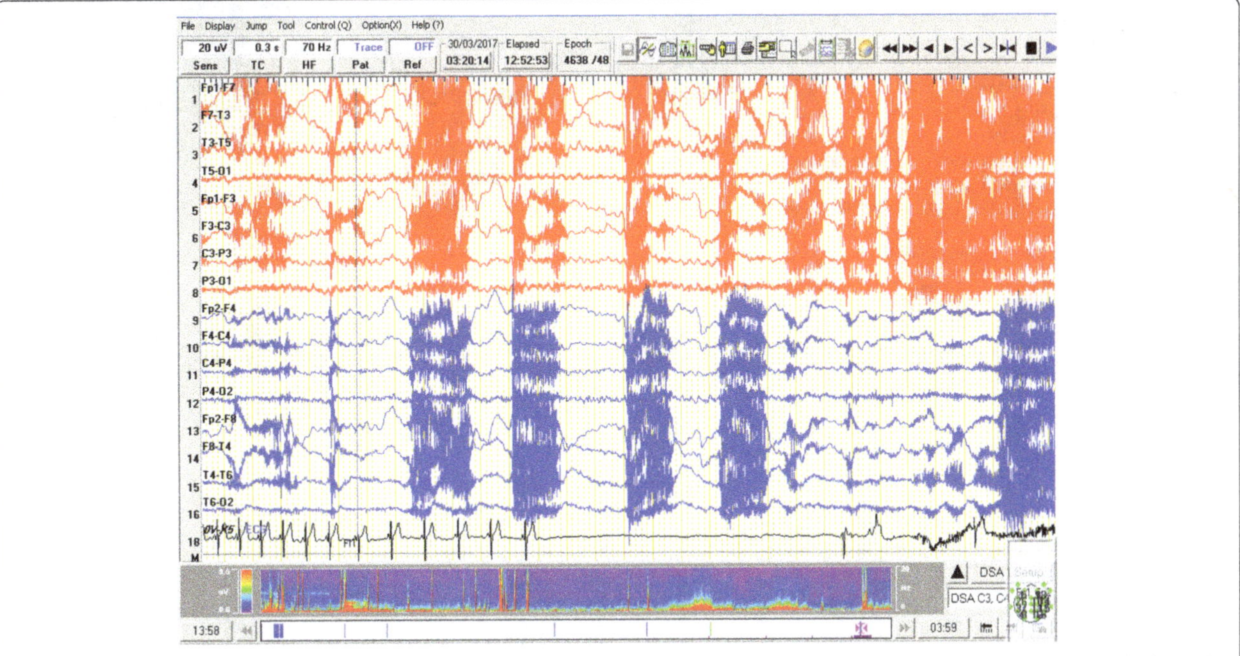

Fig. 2 A compressed EEG segment (30 s) showing bilateral temporal ictal EEG discharges more on the left side followed by the period of asystole

Abbreviations
AEDs: Anti-epileptic drugs; ECG: Electocardiogram;
EEG: Electroencephalogram; EMG: Electromyogram; MRI: Magnetic resonance imaging; SUDEP: Sudden unexpected death in epilepsy patients

Acknowledgments
Many thanks to our cooperative patient, the nurses, the EEG technicians and the operative team and finally to our head of the department for her support and encouragement.
This publication is approved by all authors and explicitly by the responsible authorities where the work was carried out, and that, if accepted, it will not be published elsewhere in the same form, in English or any other language.

Authors' contributions
NK and AR had performed the interview and did the clinical assessment of the patient; AN was responsible for the video EEG and its interpretation; AE was the one who did the cardiac evaluation and inserted the pacemaker. All authors shared in the writing, read and approved the final manuscript.

Competing interests
The authors declare that they have no competing interests.

Author details
[1]Neurology Department, Faculty of Medicine, Kasr Alainy Hospital, Cairo University, Cairo, Egypt. [2]Clinical Neurophysiology Unit, Faculty of Medicine, Kasr Alainy Hospital, Cairo University, Cairo, Egypt. [3]Cardiovascular Department, Faculty of Medicine, Kasr Alainy Hospital, Cairo University, Cairo, Egypt.

References
1. Nei M, Ho RT, Sperling MR. EKG abnormalities during partial seizures in refractory epilepsy. Epilepsia. 2000;41(5):542–8.
2. Sevcencu C, Struijk JJ. Autonomic alterations and cardiac changes in epilepsy. Epilepsia. 2010;51(5):725–37.
3. Moseley BD, Ghearing GR, Munger TM, Britton JW. The treatment of ictal asystole with cardiac pacing. Epilepsia. 2011;52(4):e16–9.
4. Rocamora R, Kurthen M, Lickfett L, Von Oertzen J, Elger CE. Cardiac asystole in epilepsy: clinical and neurophysiologic features. Epilepsia. 2003;44:179–85. https://doi.org/10.1046/j.1528-1157.2003.15101.x.
5. Nguyen-Michel V-H, Adam C, Dinkelacker V, Pichit P, Boudali Y, Dupont S, et al. Characterization of seizure-induced syncopes: EEG, ECG, and clinical features. Epilepsia. 2014;55(1):146–55.
6. Mascia A, Quarato PP, Sparano A, Esposito V, Sebastiano F, Occhiogrosso G, et al. Cardiac asystole during right frontal lobe seizures: a case report. Neurol Sci. 2005;26:340–3.
7. Duplyakov D, Golovina G, Lyukshina N, Surkova E, Elger CE, Surges R. Syncope, seizure-induced bradycardia, and asystole: two cases of clinical and pathophysiological features. Seizure. 2014;S1059-1311(14):00070–3.
8. Hirsh LJ, Hauser WA. Can sudden unexplained death in epilepsy be prevented? Lancet. 2004;364:2157–8.
9. Bergen DC. In a heartbeat: autonomic changes during seizures. Epilepsy Curr. 2005;5:194–6.
10. Lim EC, Lim S, Wilder-Smith E. Brain seizes, heart ceases: a case of ictal asystole. J Neurol Neurosurg Psychiatry. 2000;69:557–9.
11. Jansen K, Lagae L. Cardiac changes in epilepsy. Seizure. 2010;19:455–60.
12. Rubboli G, Bisulli F, Michelucci R, Meletti S, Ribani MA, Cortelli P, et al. Sudden falls due to seizure-induced cardiac asystole in drug-resistant focal epilepsy. Neurology. 2008;70:1933–5.
13. Beal JC, Sogawa Y, Ceresnak SR, Mahgerefteh J, Moshe SL. Late-onset ictal asystole in refractory epilepsy. Paediatr Neurol. 2011;45:253–5.

16

Altered cerebral glucose metabolism normalized in a patient with a pediatric autoimmune neuropsychiatric disorder after streptococcal infection (PANDAS)-like condition following treatment with plasmapheresis

A. H. Nave[1,2*], P. Harmel[1], R. Buchert[3] and L. Harms[1]

Abstract

Background: Pediatric autoimmune neuropsychiatric disorder after streptococcal infection (PANDAS) is a specific autoimmune response to group-A streptococcal infections in children and adolescents with a sudden onset of obsessive-compulsive disorders or tic-like symptoms. Cerebral metabolic changes of patients have not yet been observed.

Case presentation: We present a case of an 18-year old male with a PANDAS-like condition after developing tic-like symptoms and involuntary movements three weeks after cardiac surgery. The patient had suffered from pharyngotonsillitis before the symptoms started. The anti-streptolysin O (ASO) titer was elevated (805 kU/l). Antibiotic therapy did not improve his condition. Intravenous immunoglobulins and high-dose cortisone therapy had minor beneficial effects on his involuntary movements. 18F-Fluorodeoxyglucose positron emission tomography/ computer tomography (18F-FDG PET/CT) demonstrated pronounced hypermetabolism of the basal ganglia and cortical hypometabolism. The patient was treated with five cycles of plasmapheresis. A marked clinical improvement was observed after four months. Cerebral metabolic alterations had completely normalized.

Conclusions: This is the first report of cerebral metabolic changes observed on FDG-PET/CT in a patient with a PANDAS-like condition with a normalization following immunomodulatory treatment. Cerebral FDG-PET/CT might be a promising tool in the diagnosis of PANDAS.

Keywords: PANDAS, PET-CT, Plasmapheresis

Background

Acute neuropsychiatric symptoms in children and adolescents can have multiple causes, including autoimmune reactions following a preceding microbial infection. [1] Pediatric Acute-onset Neuropsychiatric Syndromes (PANS) can be triggered by infection (pediatric infection-triggered autoimmune neuropsychiatric disorders, PITANDS) or have non-infectious metabolic, or environmental triggers. [2] PITANDS are frequently caused by group A beta-hemolytic streptococcal (GAS) infections [3], which has been coined pediatric autoimmune neuropsychiatric disorder after streptococcal infection (PANDAS) by Susan Swedo and colleagues in 1998. [4] In PANDAS, it is hypothesized that antibodies directed against streptococcal antigens cross-react with surface proteins of the basal ganglia activating calcium calmodulin-dependent protein kinase II (CaMKII), hence causing altered central dopamine

* Correspondence: alexander.nave@charite.de
[1]Klinik und Hochschulambulanz für Neurologie, Charité-Universitätsmedizin Berlin, Berlin, Germany
[2]Berlin Institute of Health (BIH), Berlin, Germany

neurotransmission. [5] Additionally, it is thought that specific strains of S. pyogenes causing a strong immune response must meet a genetic predisposition of infected children that lead to autoimmune reactions with cellular and humoral immune responses. [6] Most recently, findings of a large-scale study support the PANDAS hypothesis, demonstrating an increased risk of mental disorders, particular OCD (obsessive-compulsive disorders) and tic disorders, in young individuals with GAS throat infections. [7]

So far, published imaging findings of patients diagnosed with PANDAS are mainly restricted to magnetic resonance imaging (MRI) describing increased volumes of the basal ganglia. [8, 9] One study could demonstrate increased microglia-mediated neuroinflammation in the basal ganglia on positron emission tomography (PET) using a ^{11}C-[R]-PK11195 tracer. [10] To our knowledge, no data exist on the use of fluorodeoxyglucose (FDG) PET in patients with PANDAS. Here, we report the first case with a PANDAS-like condition that received a FDG-PET/CT before and after treatment with plasmapheresis.

Case presentation

A male, 18-year old patient presented at the Department of Neurology at the Charité – University Hospital Berlin, in February 2016 because of involuntary movements and neuropsychiatric symptoms.

Involuntary movements included orofacial dyskinesias and tic-like symptoms, dysarthric voice accompanied by dysphagia, and hyperkinetic movements of the extremities with jerking and dystonic components that were predominantly present on the left side of his body.

Six months earlier, in August 2015, the patient, who had a congenital bicuspid aortic valve with aortic distension, underwent surgical replacement of the aortic valve and the ascending aorta using a cardiopulmonary bypass system and mild hypothermia. The remaining medical history was unremarkable without pre-existing neuropsychiatric conditions.

Precisely 3 weeks after surgery, the patient experienced the acute onset of an emotional dysbalance, hyperactivity, and loss of concentration accompanied by involuntary movements of his left upper extremity, especially his left hand. Because of further deterioration of the involuntary movements, now extending to his left leg and causing gait instability; worsening of his mood state with increasing aggressiveness at home; sleeping problems with frequent nightmares; and a severe decline in school performance the patient was admitted to a clinic in November 2015. He was reported to have had symptoms of pharyngotonsillitis days before symptoms initially started. The anti-streptolysin O (ASO) titer was elevated at 805 kU/l (reference values: < 200 kU/l). Further laboratory tests including anti-basal ganglia antibodies, CSF analysis, and a cranial CT scan showed unremarkable results.

Assuming a post-streptococcal neuropsychiatric disorder, the patient was treated with high-dose penicillin (3 x 1 Mio. I.E./ d) for three days without any clinical effect. An immunomodulatory therapy with intravenous immunoglobulins (IVIG) with a dose of 2 g per kg of bodyweight (105 g in total) was applied showing a minor, short-lasting improvement of his involuntary movements. He was discharged home on a symptomatic, anti-dopaminergic therapy with tiapride 100 mg TID. Tiapride mildly improved his sleep quality, but induced dizziness during daytime.

On presentation at the Charité several weeks later, the patient showed further psychological deterioration revealing depressive moods, attention deficits, and progressive decline in school performance, threatening his graduation. He described having vivid nightmares and a loss of body weight (5 kg in 2 months, i.e. 9% of body weight). The ASO titer was still elevated at 450 kU/l, whereas anti-deoxyribonuclease B (Anti-DNaseB) titer, autoimmunological parameters, and CSF analyses remained unremarkable. In particular, cerebral autoantibodies (a large panel antibodies including anti-NMDA receptor- and anti-TPO-antibodies) could not be detected neither in serum nor in CSF. Immunohistologically, plasmapheresis eluate of the patient did not reveal any specific or unspecific binding on murine brain tissue. Cerebral magnetic resonance imaging (MRI) showed small bicerebellar and left frontal microbleeds, but no focal lesion or specific pattern of atrophy. Electroencephalography (EEG) displayed diffuse brain dysfunction without further implication.

Comprehensive neuropsychological testing identified a dysexecutive syndrome characterized by a decrease in working memory capacity, attention, and concentration deficits, as well as frequent failure of spontaneous speech. Psychosomatic counseling revealed several underlying family-based conflicts. His mother was described as a controlling person who discounted his symptoms and persistently browsed through his personal belongings. He described himself as sad with fears of separation and being lonely. Suicidal thoughts had occurred two months prior to the second admission. The clinical course of the patient is depicted in Fig. 1.

The differential diagnoses at this time were: 1) Sydenham chorea minor (SC), 2) Pediatric Autoimmune Neuropsychiatric Syndrome after Streptococcal infection (PANDAS) or PANDAS-like condition, 3) antibody-mediated autoimmune encephalitis (e. g anti-NMDA receptor encephalitis) 4) Psychosomatic disorder, 5) Post pump chorea. [11]

Diagnostic work-up was expanded and a cerebral FDG positron emission tomography/ computer tomography (PET/CT) demonstrated a moderate to severe hypermetabolism of the basal ganglia, especially of the left

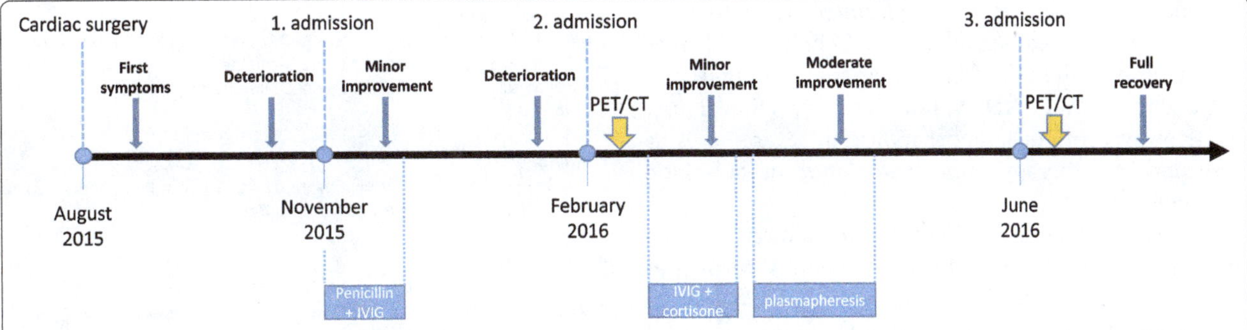

Fig. 1 Timeline of the clinical course of the presented case. First symptoms started three weeks after cardiac surgery. Intravenous immunoglobulin and cortisone treatment resulted in only minor and transient improvement of symptoms. Clinical stabilization was first observed after plasmapheresis. Normalization of impaired cerebral glucose metabolism measured via PET/CT was achieved four months later

striatum, whereas the cortex revealed hypometabolic signals (Fig. 2).

The anti-dopaminergic medication was discontinued and an additional IVIG therapy had marginal effects on his symptoms. A series of high-dose cortisone therapy (1 g i.v.) for five days improved his restlessness, muscle strength of his left arm, and quality of sleep, but symptoms persisted. Subsequently, we initiated five cycles of plasmapheresis, and ASO titer significantly decreased (78 kU/l).

Four months later at follow-up, the patient demonstrated a normalized neurological exam with a minimal fine motor skill deficit in his left hand. Neuropsychological disorders had resolved. Follow-up FDG-PET/CT revealed a complete normalization of cerebral glucose metabolism (Fig. 2). The ASO titer remained at normal levels (197 kU/l). The patient's personality returned to its premorbid state and family-based stress factors had dissolved. He resumed taking psychotherapeutic sessions twice a month.

Discussion and conclusions

We report the case of an adolescent patient diagnosed with a PANDAS-like condition that showed severe striatal hypermetabolism and cortical hypometabolism on FDG PET/CT imaging. Consistent with clinical improvement, glucose metabolism completely normalized four months after immunomodulatory therapy with five cycles of plasmapheresis. To the best of our knowledge, this is the first report of a patient with a PANDAS-like condition demonstrating changes of glucose metabolism before and after treatment.

Opposed to surgical intervention [12], the beneficial effects of immunomodulatory therapies, such as IVIG and plasmapheresis, in OCD/tic disorder patients have been reported previously. [13–15] Although IVIG administration could not demonstrate statistically significant effects compared to placebo in a large clinical trial, the application was safe and well tolerated in all treated patients. [16] We also did not experience any

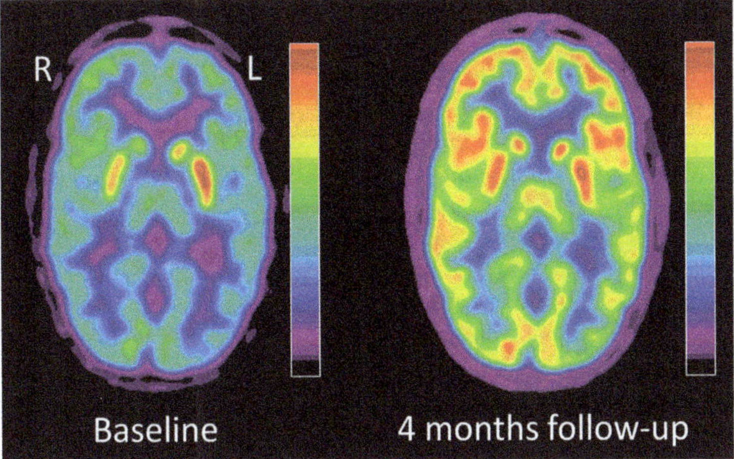

Fig. 2 Images of the cerebral FDG positron emission tomography/ computer tomography (PET/CT). At baseline prior to plasmapheresis, the patient demonstrated a moderate to severe hypermetabolism of the left striatum. The cortex revealed hypometabolic signal. Metabolic changes were completely normalized at follow-up four months later

complication during IVIG or plasmapheresis therapy. Despite the reported benefits, several clinical guidelines do not support the use of immunomodulatory therapies in patients with PANDAS limiting their clinical use. [17] However, others support its use in severe cases as a second-line therapy after inefficiency of antibiotic treatment. [18, 19]

We assume that a PANDAS-like condition was the most appropriate diagnosis for our patient. According to the published diagnostic criteria on PANDAS, patients must meet the following criteria: 1) abrupt onset of OCD/tic-like symptoms or severely restricted food intake, 2) prepubertal onset of symptoms, 3) acute symptom onset and episodic (relapsing-remitting) course, 4) temporal association between Group A streptococcal infection and symptom onset/exacerbations, and 5) association with neurological abnormalities. [20] In our case, the patient experienced an acute onset three weeks after cardiac surgery. Additional to orofacial dyskinesia and tic-like symptoms, he demonstrated neuropsychiatric symptoms including obsessional fears, separation anxiety, depressive mood, sleep and body weight problems as well as dramatic decline in school performance. Because of the age of the patient and the lack of a positive throat culture, a PANDAS diagnosis is not justified. Striatal hypermetabolism was described in SC [21, 22], however, post pump chorea, presenting in children following open-heart surgery, was shown to be associated with hypometabolism of the basal ganglia. [23] In addition, patients described with post pump chorea developed symptoms within the first two weeks after surgery and were much younger (age < 3 years). Other differential diagnoses such as atypical manifestations of an anti-NMDA receptor encephalitis or Hashimoto's encephalitis must be mentioned. However, negative antibody titers in both blood and CSF as well as the absence of immunohistological findings on murine brain tissue, and the cerebral distribution of metabolic changes on FDG-PET/CT make these diagnoses unlikely. [24–26]

In conclusion, PANDAS is a severe disorder that needs appropriate treatment with immunomodulatory therapy, if antibiotic treatment is not effective and symptoms progress. FDG PET/CT seems to be a valuable diagnostic approach to prove cerebral metabolic alterations in PANDAS. Future cohort studies should assess the sensitivity of FDG PET/CT in diagnosed PANDAS patients and investigate the association of metabolic abnormalities with severity of clinical symptoms.

Abbreviations

ASO: anti-streptolysin O; *FDG PET/CT*: FDG positron emission tomography/ computer tomography; *GAS*: group A beta-hemolytic streptococcus; IVIG: intravenous immunoglobulins; OCD: obsessive-compulsive disorders; *PANDAS*: Pediatric Autoimmune Neuropsychiatric Disorder after Streptococcal Infection; SC: Sydenhams's Chorea

Acknowledgments

We thank Ute Scheller for helping us to monitor the clinical course of the patient as detailed as possible. We also thank the Dpt. of Radiology and Nuclear Medicine of the Charité, Campus Mitte for performing the FGD PET/CT examinations.

Funding

Dr. Nave is participant in the BIH-Charité Clinical Scientist Program funded by the Charité and the Berlin Institute of Health.

Authors' contributions

AHN treated the patient and drafted the manuscript. PB and LH treated the patient and critically revised the manuscript. RB performed and rated the FDG PET/CT images and revised the manuscript. All authors read and approved the final manuscript.

Competing interests

The authors declare that they have no competing interests.

Author details

[1]Klinik und Hochschulambulanz für Neurologie, Charité-Universitätsmedizin Berlin, Berlin, Germany. [2]Berlin Institute of Health (BIH), Berlin, Germany. [3]Department of Diagnostic and Interventional Radiology and Nuclear Medicine, University Medical Centre Hamburg-Eppendorf, Hamburg, Germany.

References

1. Benros ME, Waltoft BL, Nordentoft M, Ostergaard SD, Eaton WW, Krogh J, et al. Autoimmune diseases and severe infections as risk factors for mood disorders. JAMA Psychiatry. 2013;70:812.
2. Calaprice D, Tona J, Parker-Athill EC, Murphy TK. A survey of pediatric acute-onset neuropsychiatric syndrome characteristics and course. J. Child Adolesc. Psychopharmacol. 2017;27:607–18.
3. Allen AJ, Leonard HL, Swedo SE. Case study: a new infection-triggered, autoimmune subtype of pediatric OCD and Tourette's syndrome. J Am Acad Child Adolesc Psychiatry The American Academy of Child and Adolescent Psychiatry. 1995;34:307–11.
4. Swedo SE, Leonard HL, Garvey M, Mittleman B, Allen AJ, Perlmutter S, et al. Pediatric autoimmune neuropsychiatric disorders associated with streptococcal infections: clinical description of the first 50 cases. Am J Psychiatry. 1998;155:264–71.
5. Cunningham MW, Cox CJ. Autoimmunity against dopamine receptors in neuropsychiatric and movement disorders: a review of Sydenham chorea and beyond. Acta Physiol. 2016;216:90–100.
6. Cutforth T, DeMille MM, Agalliu I, Agalliu D. CNS autoimmune disease after Streptococcus pyogenes infections: animal models, cellular mechanisms and genetic factors. Future Neurol. 2016;11:63–76.
7. Orlovska S, Vestergaard CH, Bech BH, Nordentoft M, Vestergaard M, Benros ME. Association of Streptococcal Throat Infection with Mental Disorders: testing key aspects of the PANDAS hypothesis in a Nationwide study. JAMA psychiatry. 2017;74:740–6.
8. Perlmutter SJ, Garvey MA, Castellanos X, Mittleman BB, Giedd J, Rapoport JL, et al. A case of pediatric autoimmune neuropsychiatric disorders associated with streptococcal infections. Am J Psychiatry. 1998;155:1592–8.
9. Giedd JN. MRI assessment of children with obsessive-compulsive disorder or tics associated with streptococcal infection. Am J Psychiatry. 2000;157:281–3.
10. Kumar A, Williams MT, Chugani HT. Evaluation of basal ganglia and thalamic inflammation in children with pediatric autoimmune neuropsychiatric disorders associated with streptococcal infection and Tourette syndrome. J Child Neurol. 2015;30:749–56.
11. Du Plessis AJ, Bellinger DC, Gauvreau K, Plumb C, Newburger JW, Jonas RA, et al. Neurologic outcome of choreoathetoid encephalopathy after cardiac surgery. Pediatr Neurol. 2002;27:9–17.
12. Pavone P, Rapisarda V, Serra A, Nicita F, Spalice A, Parano E, et al. Pediatric autoimmune neuropsychiatry disorder associated with group a streptococcal infection: the role of surgical treatment. Int J Immunopathol Pharmacol. 2014;27:371–8.

13. Perlmutter SJ, Leitman SF, Garvey MA, Hamburger S, Feldman E, Leonard HL, et al. Therapeutic plasma exchange and intravenous immunoglobulin for obsessive-compulsive disorder and tic disorders in childhood. Lancet. 1999;354:1153–8.
14. Latimer ME, L'Etoile N, Seidlitz J, Swedo SE. Therapeutic plasma apheresis as a treatment for 35 severely ill children and adolescents with pediatric autoimmune neuropsychiatric disorders associated with streptococcal infections. J Child Adolesc Psychopharmacol. 2015;25:70–5.
15. Vitaliti G, Tabatabaie O, Matin N, Ledda C, Pavone P, Lubrano R, et al. The usefulness of immunotherapy in pediatric neurodegenerative disorders: a systematic review of literature data. Hum Vaccin Immunother. 2015;11: 2749–63.
16. Williams KA, Swedo SE, Farmer CA, Grantz H, Grant PJ, D'Souza P, et al. Randomized, controlled trial of intravenous immunoglobulin for pediatric autoimmune neuropsychiatric disorders associated with streptococcal infections. J. Am. Acad. Child Adolesc. Psychiatry2016;55. 860–7:e2.
17. Cortese I, Chaudhry V, So YT, Cantor F, Cornblath DR, Rae-Grant A. Evidence-based guideline update: plasmapheresis in neurologic disorders: report of the therapeutics and technology assessment Subcommittee of the American Academy of neurology. Neurology. 2011;76:294–300.
18. Cortese I, Cornblath DR. Therapeutic plasma exchange in neurology: 2012. J Clin Apher. 2013;28:16–9.
19. Williams KA, Swedo SE. Post-infectious autoimmune disorders: Sydenham's chorea, PANDAS and beyond. Brain Res. 2015;1617:144–54.
20. E. Swedo S. From Research Subgroup to Clinical Syndrome: Modifying the PANDAS Criteria to Describe PANS (Pediatric Acute-onset Neuropsychiatric Syndrome). Pediatr. Ther; 2012. p. 02.
21. Goldman S, Amrom D, Szliwowski HB, Detemmerman D, Goldman S, Bidaut LM, et al. Reversible striatal hypermetabolism in a case of sydenham's chorea. Mov Disord. 1993;8:355–8.
22. Paghera B, Caobelli F, Giubbini R, Premi E, Padovani A. Reversible striatal hypermetabolism in a case of rare adult-onset Sydenham chorea on two sequential 18F-FDG PET studies. J Neuroradiol. 2011;38:325–6.
23. Medlock MD, Cruse RS, Winek SJ, Geiss DM, Horndasch RL, Schultz DL, et al. A 10-year experience with postpump chorea. Ann Neurol. 1993;34(6):820.
24. Citak EC, Gücüyener K, Karabacak NI, Serdaroğlu A, Okuyaz C, Aydin K. Functional brain imaging in Sydenham's chorea and streptococcal tic disorders. J Child Neurol. 2004;19:387–90.
25. Solnes LB, Jones KM, Rowe SP, Pattanayak P, Nalluri A, Venkatesan A, et al. Diagnostic value of ^{18}F-FDG PET/CT versus MRI in the setting of antibody-specific autoimmune encephalitis. J Nucl Med. 2017;58:1307–13.
26. Kelley BP, Patel SC, Marin HL, Corrigan JJ, Mitsias PD, Griffith B. Autoimmune encephalitis: pathophysiology and imaging review of an overlooked diagnosis. Am J Neuroradiol. 2017;38:1070.

17

The behavioural variant frontotemporal dementia phenocopy syndrome is a distinct entity

E. Devenney[1,2*], T. Swinn[3], E. Mioshi[4], M. Hornberger[4], K. E. Dawson[5], S. Mead[6], J. B. Rowe[5] and J. R. Hodges[1,2]

Abstract

Background: This study aimed to i) examine the frequency of *C9orf72* expansions in a cohort of patients with the behavioural variant frontotemporal dementia (bvFTD) phenocopy syndrome, ii) observe outcomes in a group of phenocopy syndrome with very long term follow-up and iii) compare progression in a cohort of patients with the phenocopy syndrome to a cohort of patients with probable bvFTD.

Methods: Blood was obtained from 16 phenocopy cases. All met criteria for possible bvFTD and were labeled as phenocopy cases if they showed no functional decline, normal cognitive performance on the Addenbrooke's Cognitive Examination-Revised (ACE-R) and a lack of atrophy on brain imaging, over at least 3 years of follow-up. In addition, we obtained very long term follow-up data in 6 cases. A mixed model analysis approach determined the pattern of change in cognition and behaviour over time in phenocopy cases compared to 27 probable bvFTD cases.

Results: All 16 patients were screened for the *C9orf72* expansion that was present in only one (6.25%). Of the 6 cases available for very long-term follow-up (13 - 21 years) none showed progression to frank dementia. Moreover, there was a decrease in the caregiver ratings of behavioural symptoms over time. Phenocopy cases showed significantly slower rates of progression compared to probable bvFTD patients ($p < 0.006$).

Conclusion: The vast majority of patients with the bvFTD phenocopy syndrome remain stable over many years. An occasional patient can harbor the *C9orf72* expansion. The aetiology of the remaining cases remains unknown but it appears very unlikely to reflect a neurodegenerative syndrome due to lack of clinical progression or atrophy on imaging.

Keywords: Frontotemporal dementia, Phenocopy syndrome, Prognosis, Genetics, Cognition, Behaviour

Background

The classical features of behavioural variant Frontotemporal Dementia (bvFTD) syndrome are well established. The current consensus criteria incorporates cognitive, behavioural, neuroimaging, genetic and pathological parameters, to provide a framework to make accurate diagnoses by ranking the level of diagnostic certainty as possible, probable and definite [1]. Although the accuracy of these criteria has been pathologically validated, controversy still exists regarding the aetiology, progression and prognosis of possible bvFTD [2].

* Correspondence: emma.devenney@sydney.edu.au
[1]Brain and Mind Centre, University of Sydney, Sydney, NSW 2050, Australia
[2]ARC Centre of Excellence in Cognition and its Disorders, Sydney, Australia

A recent study which followed FTD patients over a five year period found that a number of possible bvFTD patients remain in this category for many years and appear not to progress on cognitive and behavioural measures [3]. A number of these patients are classified as 'phenocopy syndrome' cases [4–7]. Patients harboring the *C9orf72* expansion may also satisfy criteria for possible, but not probable, bvFTD at first presentation and may be atypical with pervasive psychotic features [3]. Moreover, cases who have been labeled as the 'phenocopy syndrome' have also been reported to carry the *C9orf72* expansion [8, 9]. The question remains, just how many of the phenocopy cases have the expansion?

The present study sought to address this issue by exploring the outcomes in a large and unique cohort of phenocopy patients that have been followed over many years and screened for the *C9orf72* expansion. A mixed model analysis was employed to determine the rate of change in global cognition and behaviour over time in these phenocopy cases compared to a group of patients with probable bvFTD.

Methods

Patients

Patients were assessed at the specialist early-onset dementia clinic at Addenbrooke's Hospital Cambridge between 1993 and 2007. Patients who satisfied criteria for possible bvFTD only, and were seen on at least two occasions; with initial and follow-up evaluation at least 3 years apart, and in whom blood had been obtained for gene screening, were included in the study. Patients were excluded from the study if they progressed to probable bvFTD over the study period. Exclusion criteria also included a current or past medical history of a psychiatric condition, traumatic brain injury, drug or alcohol abuse and cerebrovascular disease. Of note patients who experienced delusions or hallucinations were included in the study.

Of the 16 cases, three were still under regular review in the clinic in 2014. We attempted to contact the remainder and we able to reassess three additional cases. Thus very long term follow-up (ranging from 13 to 21 years) was available in 6 cases.

A group of probable bvFTD patients were included in the study to serve as a comparison group for the mixed model analysis, to determine differences in progression rates. These patients ($n = 27$) were assessed at FRONTIER, a frontotemporal dementia specialist research clinic and met probable diagnostic criteria for bvFTD. They were matched for age, sex and education to the phenocopy cases. Patients with probable bvFTD who were subsequently found to carry the *C9orf72* expansion were not included in this group. None of these patients carried a *GRN* or *MAPT* mutation. The results below relate to the phenocopy cases only unless otherwise stated.

Patients were classified according to the current international diagnostic criteria [1]. Patients were classified as possible bvFTD when they met three of the six core behavioural features of bvFTD, but had normal brain imaging and an absence of typical genetic or pathological findings. Probable bvFTD, criteria was met when patients firstly satisfied possible criteria with additional evidence of functional decline, and frontal or temporal abnormalities on MRI or Fludeoxyglucose (18F)-Positron emission tomography (FDG-PET) [1]. In this study MRI scans were performed in all cases and a validated visual rating scale, assessed atrophy of the orbitofrontal cortex, anterior temporal poles and insular cortex, according to previously published data [10, 11]. Atrophy was rated on a Likert scale by a blinded rater after appropriate training on an independent data set. Intra-class correlation coefficient to assess inter-rater reliability was very high (Cronbach's alpha = .9).

Clinical assessment

A comprehensive clinical assessment was conducted with the patient and behavioural symptoms were explored with the carer using the CBI (Cambridge Behavioural Inventory), [12]; a higher score indicates greater impairment (maximum score – 316). Global cognitive function was measured using the Addenbrooke's Cognitive Examination-Revised (ACE-R) [13]; a normal score > 88/100.

Genetic screening

Blood samples were screened at the Medical Research Council Prion Unit, London, or at NeuRA, Sydney, for the *C9orf72* expansion based on the repeat-primed polymerase chain reaction technique as previously described by Renton [14]. Genomic DNA was extracted from blood according to standard procedures. Samples were scored as expansion-positive if they harbored > 30 repeats. *C9orf72* hexanucleotide repeat non-expansion alleles were detected by polymerase chain reaction amplification and capillary electrophoresis.

Statistical analysis

Data were analyzed using SPSS 22.0 statistical package. Normal distribution was determined by means of Kolmogorov-Smirnoff tests. Parametric variables were compared across groups via independent t-tests and analysis of variance (ANOVA). Non-parametric data were analyzed using Mann-Whitney and Kruskal-Wallis tests, and Chi-Square tests compared categorical data. Linear mixed effect models examined change in performance over time [15]. Such measures are useful in these circumstances as they take into account the variability in follow-up time within the phenocopy and probable bvFTD groups, and the significant difference in follow-up between the two groups.

Results

Patients

Between 1993 and 2007 a total of 89 patients with possible bvFTD were assessed and followed for at least 3 years in the specialist clinic. Of these 89, a diagnosis of probable bvFTD became apparent on follow up in 63 (Fig. 1). The remaining 26 were given a label of phenocopy syndrome on the basis of a lack of progression with relative preservation of activities of daily living, maintained performance on the ACE-R and a normal MRI as assessed by a validated visual rating scale.

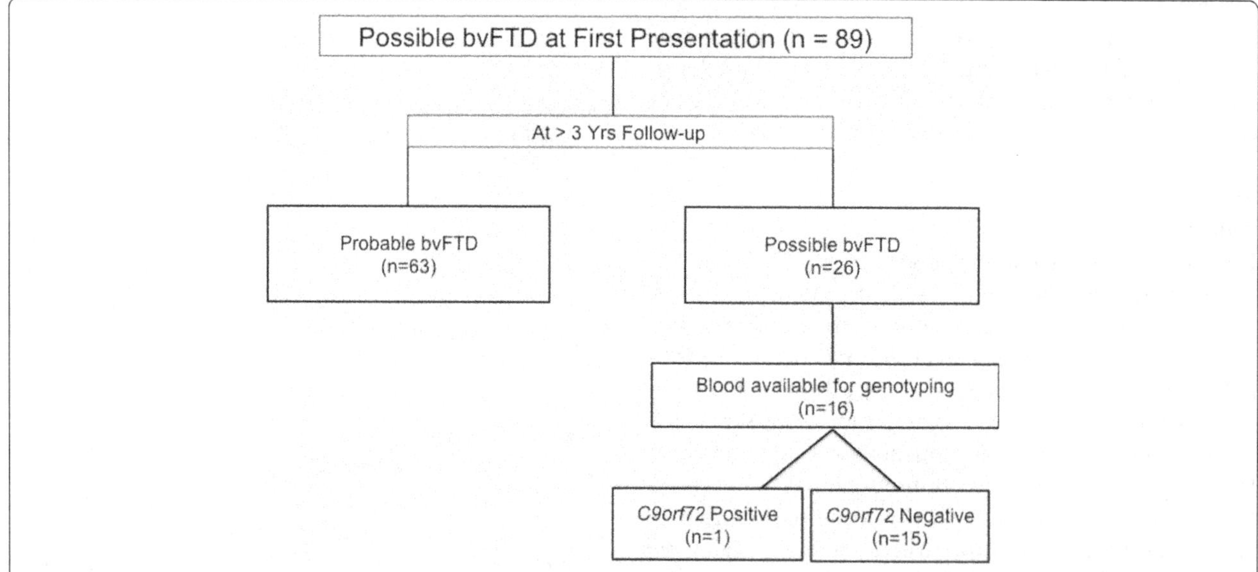

Fig. 1 Longitudinal changes in diagnosis and genetic findings. Flowchart demonstrating the number of patients from the Cambridge cohort at presentation with possible bvFTD, according to diagnostic criteria for bvFTD, and the change in diagnosis and subsequent genetic findings over the follow-up period

Within the comparison bvFTD group, four patients have now come to autopsy and each of these patients showed FTLD pathology including TDP-43 in one, TAU in another and FUS in another.

Blood sampling was obtained in all cases attending the clinic in 2007. In the phenocopy cohort of 26 cases, blood was available in 16 for genotyping.

Genetic testing

The *C9orf72* expansion was present in one of 16 patients who had blood obtained for genotyping, representing 6.25% of the cohort. This patient was male and in his 60's when he presented with a two-year history of behavioural change. At presentation his score on the CBI of 152 was very high and on the ACE-R his score of 81 was just below the cut-off of 88. A MRI scan was normal. When last seen in 2006 scores, had improved with a CBI score of 136 and an ACE-R score of 89. An FDG-PET scan showed no areas of significant brain hypometabolism. He was then lost to follow up in 2008 (11 years after onset) and died of an unrelated condition in 2010. Unfortunately post mortem brain examination was not performed.

Cognitive and behavioural measures at baseline and follow-up

The 16 phenocopy patients with available genotyping comprised 15 men with a mean age of 55.7 (range 47 to 69 years). Twelve of the 16 were under 65. The mean follow-up time was 8 years. Table 1 demonstrates the baseline demographic information for these 16 cases and the comparison group of probable bvFTD patients and includes the mean ACE-R and the CBI scores on first assessment and length of follow-up for the phenocopy and the probable bvFTD group.

At presentation 10 of the 16 phenocopy patients scored above 88 on the ACE-R, and none of the remainder scored below 80/100. At last follow-up six of these patients still scored within the normal range. The profile of behavioural symptoms at presentation and last follow-up was typical of bvFTD with high endorsements for motivation (apathy), stereotyped and abnormal behaviours, changed appetite and eating and mood.

At presentation there was a significant difference in the ACE-R scores between the phenocopy cases and the probable bvFTD group ($p = 0.001$); the mean ACE-R score in the phenocopy group was 89/100, whereas the mean score for the probable bvFTD group was 73/100.

Table 1 Phenocopy cases – demographic details

Demographics at Presentation	Phenocopy bvFTD ($n = 16$)	Probable bvFTD ($n = 27$)	*P* value
Age at Onset, yrs	55.7 ± 6.3	59.7 ± 8.1	0.1
Sex (M:F)	15:1	22:5	0.4
Disease Duration, yrs.	3.9 ± 2.3	3.8 ± 2.4	0.1
Education, yrs.	11.4 ± 2.1	12.4 ± 3.4	0.3
ACE-R	89.2 ± 6.4	72.8 ± 14.6	0.001
CBI	91.3 ± 59	72.5 ± 21.5	0.3
Follow-up, yrs.	7.3 ± 4.2	3.2 ± 1.3	0.002

Demographic information (Mean ± standard deviation scores) for the phenocopy cases with blood available for *C9orf72* expansion testing, and probable bvFTD cases. *bvFTD* behavioural variant frontotemporal dementia, *ACE-R* Addenbrooke's Cognitive Examination-Revised, *CBI* Cambridge Behavioural Inventory

In contrast both groups had equivalently high scores on the CBI ($p = 0.3$).

The phenocopy group was then compared to a group of probable bvFTD cases using a mixed model analysis that took into account the variability of follow-up within and between the two groups. On a measure of global cognitive function, the ACE-R, the groups combined showed significant deterioration over time ($p < 0.001$) with a significant interaction between disease group and time ($p = 0.006$) indicating a faster rate of decline in probable bvFTD cases compared to phenocopy cases (Fig. 2). On a measure of behaviour, the CBI, the group as a whole showed significant deterioration over time ($p < 0.001$), however while the interaction between disease group and time was not significant there was a statistical trend ($p < 0.06$) suggesting a faster deterioration in behaviour in the probable bvFTD group compared to the phenocopy group.

The mean ACE-R and CBI scores with 95% confidence intervals, calculated according to the mixed model statistic, for standard times intervals, are demonstrated for the ACE-R and CBI in Table 2. Table 2 also shows the mean ACE-R and CBI scores at last follow-up for the phenocopy and probable bvFTD group; these are for illustrative purposes only as the follow-up times were variable within and between the groups and therefore statistical analysis based on these measures is not appropriate.

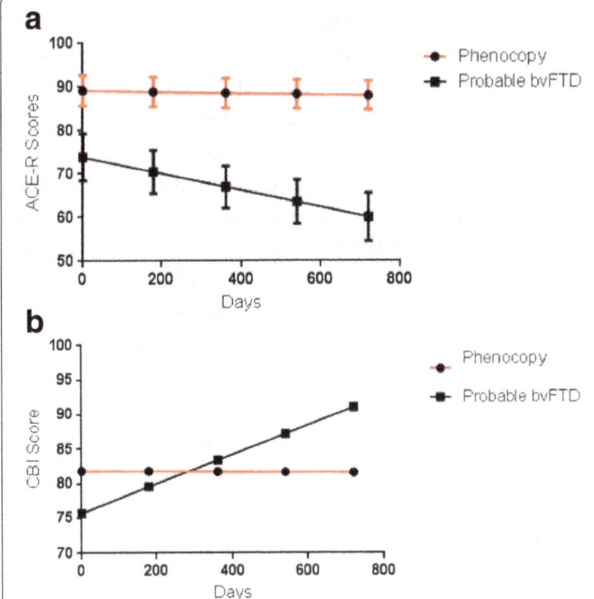

Fig. 2 Longitudinal changes in ACE-R and CBI – phenocopy and bvFTD cases. **a** demonstrates estimated marginal means based on the % change in ACE-R score across time for phenocopy and probable bvFTD cases. Time ($p < 0.001$). Time x Diagnosis ($p = 0.006$). **b** demonstrates estimated marginal means based on the change in CBI scores across time. Time ($p < 0.001$). Time x Diagnosis ($p = 0.06$)

Table 2 Phenocopy and bvFTD cases - Longitudinal changes in ACE-R and CBI

Time	Phenocopy bvFTD ($n = 16$)	Probable bvFTD ($n = 27$)
ACE-R – Scores (mean, 95% CI)		
Day 1	92 (84.1-99.9)	72 (65.7-78.3)
Day 180	91.6 (84.1-99.2)	69.5 (63.8-75.2)
Day 360	91.3 (84-98.6)	67 (61.5-72.5)
Day 540	91 (83.8-98.1)	64.5 (58.8-70.2)
Day 720	90.6 (83.7-97.5)	62 (55.7-68.2)
CBI Scores (mean, 95% CI)		
Day 1	81.8 (62.7-101)	75.7 (60.7-90.7)
Day 180	81.8 (63.4-100.1)	79.6 (66.1-93)
Day 360	81.7 (64.1-99.4)	83.4 (70.5-96.3)
Day 540	81.7 (64.6-98.8)	87.2 (73.9-100.6)
Day 720	81.6 (65-98.2)	91.1 (76.3-105.9)
Last Follow-up (mean, SD)		
ACE-R	85.1 ± 7.1	54.2 ± 23.6
CBI	77 ± 47.3	93.9 ± 33.7

Follow-up data according to the mixed model analysis with standard time intervals generated by the model, for phenocopy and probable bvFTD cases. Bottom rows show the mean ACE-R and CBI scores at last follow-up. *CI* confidence interval, *SD* standard deviation, *bvFTD* behavioural variant frontotemporal dementia, *ACE-R* addenbrooke's cognitive examination-Revised, *CBI* Cambridge behavioural inventory

MRI at baseline and follow-up

Grey matter density was judged as normal (0) or within normal range (1) in the orbitofrontal cortex, anterior temporal poles and insular cortex in each of the phenocopy cases at baseline and at follow-up.

Long-term clinical follow-up

In 2013 we attempted to contact the caregivers of the 15 living cases by post and to arrange a telephone interview. Three were still attending the clinic at regular intervals and we were successful in another three (total six), with lengths of follow-up ranging from 13 to 21 years from first visit to the clinic. All were living at home; 3 remained in the same relationship as at their presentation, and there had been no cases with progression to frank dementia.

Discussion

This study provides evidence for the validity of the bvFTD phenocopy syndrome. Only one of 16 phenocopy cases (6.25%) had the *C9orf72* expansion and it is interesting to note that this is the only patient in the cohort who is known to have died. This study had the benefit of very long-term follow-up information, between 13 and 21 years, in 6 cases. There was no evidence of progression to frank dementia in any of the phenocopy cases over many years of follow-up.

The underlying aetiology of the phenocopy syndrome is unknown. On a clinical level, these patients present with cognitive and behavioural changes, that are identical to the deficits seen in probable bvFTD cases, yet do not show significant brain atrophy [6, 16]. Furthermore, a previous clinicopathological study found that 2 phenocopy cases did not have FTLD pathology at autopsy [17]. While it is possible that the phenocopy syndrome represents a late onset decompensated developmental disorder in the Asperger-Autism spectrum, it remains to be proven. In keeping with this hypothesis, such patients, although scoring normally on tests such as the ACE-R and measures of memory, may show mild deficits on tests of inhibitory control and emotion processing [18] as do patients on the Asperger-Autism spectrum [19, 20]. A recent study comparing phenocopy and probable bvFTD cases showed a high rate of adverse life events, relationship problems and cluster C personality traits comprising the avoidant, dependent, and obsessive-compulsive personality traits [21]. Putting these findings together it seems highly likely that the phenocopy syndrome is a final common pathway for a complex interaction of a number of personality and psychiatric factors.

Interestingly long-term assessments show that, although some patients continue to exhibit behavioural symptoms, these symptoms are rated as less marked by caregivers over time. This could, of course, simply reflect the fact that family members adjust to and are less troubled by the symptoms. A study of possible bvFTD patients followed over several years showed that a subgroup, many of whom had the *C9orf72* expansion, progressed on cognitive and functional measures while others, who lacked the expansion, demonstrated no change and conformed, therefore, to the phenocopy syndrome [3]. Although the former work did not have the benefit of such long-term follow-up, it mirrors the results from this study, which showed that the phenocopy cases did not progress on the CBI, and together these findings point towards a non-progressive non-neurodegenerative aetiology in phenocopy cases. The probable bvFTD patients were also significantly more impaired on the ACE-R at presentation, and the mixed model analysis revealed a significant deterioration in ACE-R scores over time in the probable bvFTD group compared to the phenocopy group further demonstrating the relative cognitive stability of phenocopy cases.

Studies of FTD have established that the *C9orf72* expansion, whilst variable in prevalence around the world, is a common Mendelian genetic cause of familial disease, and is also present in a proportion of sporadic cases [22]. The full clinical spectrum associated with the expansion is not yet clear but it has been shown that such patients have a high rate of psychotic symptoms and that there is considerable variability in the rate of progression. While some patients present with a long insidious history of gradual decline others have a more fulminating illness [8, 9]. Studies have also linked *C9orf72* to other clinical phenotypes outside of FTD and MND, including Parkinson's disease, multiple system atrophy (MSA) and Alzheimer's disease (AD), although many lacked neuropathological confirmation [22]. Nonetheless, there does appear to be partial penetrance as *C9orf72* carriers may remain asymptomatic into their 80's [23]. We have confirmed that patients with the phenocopy syndrome may also harbor the expansion but in a well-characterized cohort with long term follow up this appears to be the exception. Interestingly, the only *C9orf72* carrier in our phenocopy cohort did not show any abnormalities on MRI or FDG-PET, in keeping with reports from prior studies [8, 9]. Our work provides data to support the informed genetic counseling of this clinical group. A lack of understanding of the phenocopy syndrome and support for the patients and their families can make recruitment into a research programme difficult. Nonetheless further work is necessary to confirm the proportion of the FTD phenocopy syndrome that has a genetic aetiology and also to confirm the underlying pathology in these cases. Moreover, study of the phenocopy syndrome may help clarify the link between psychiatric illness and frontotemporal dementia. As in this project, cases that have a psychiatric history are usually excluded from studies however this design may need to be reconsidered in the future in light of this apparent link and co-existence of psychiatric and neurodegenerative disorders.

Conclusion

We propose that the phenocopy syndrome is a valid entity. These patients are almost always male and experience symptom onset between the ages of 45 and 65. Despite reported behavioural changes, they perform relatively normally on general cognitive tests such as the ACE-R or ACE-III, have preserved basic activities of daily living, lack atrophy on MRI and critically show no decline after 3 years of follow-up. Within the first two to 3 years of evaluation of possible bvFTD cases physicians should exhibit caution in diagnosing the phenocopy syndrome, since the majority will progress to probable disease over time and almost one half will progress within the first 3 years. It should be also stressed that although phenocopy cases may not harbour underlying neurodegenerative pathology, this is not a benign condition and caregiver burden can be high.

Abbreviations

ACE-R: Addenbrookes cognitive examination – Revised; bvFTD: behavioural variant frontotemporal dementia; CBI: Cambridge behavioural inventory; FDG-PET: Fludeoxyglucose (18F)-Positron emission tomography

Acknowledgements

We are grateful to the research participants involved with the research studies. Work at University College London Institute of Neurology was supported by the Medical Research Council (UK) and the National Institute of Health Research's Biomedical Research Centre at University College London Hospital.

Funding
This work was supported by funding to Forefront, a collaborative research group dedicated to the study of frontotemporal dementia and motor neurone disease, from the National Health and Medical research Council of Australia program grant (#1037746) and the Australian Research Council Centre of Excellence in Cognition and its Disorders Memory Node (#CE110001021). The funding body did not have a role in the design of the study and collection, analysis, and interpretation of data and in writing the manuscript.
Dr. Devenney is supported by the Motor Neurone Disease Research Institute Australia. Professor Eneida Mioshi is supported by the Alzheimer's Association (USA) and the Alzheimer's Society (UK). Professor Michael Hornberger is supported by Alzheimer's Research UK, Medical Research Council and the Wellcome Trust. Professor James Rowe is supported by the Wellcome Trust (#103838) and the National Institute for Health Research Cambridge Biomedical Research Centre.

Authors' contributions
ED contributed to the study design, data analysis, manuscript preparation, writing and review. TS contributed to study design, data collection, and review. EM, MH, SM, JRH contributed to study design, data collection, manuscript preparation and review. KED contributed to study design, data collection and review. JBR contributed to study design, data collection, data analysis, manuscript preparation and review. All authors read and approved the final manuscript.

Competing interests
Professor E Mioshi was previously a member of the editorial board for BMC Neurology. On behalf of all the other authors, the corresponding author states that there is no competing interest.

Author details
[1]Brain and Mind Centre, University of Sydney, Sydney, NSW 2050, Australia. [2]ARC Centre of Excellence in Cognition and its Disorders, Sydney, Australia. [3]Medical Research Council Cognition and Brain Sciences Unit, Cambridge, UK. [4]Faculty of Medicine and Health Sciences, University of East Anglia, Norwich, UK. [5]Department of Clinical Neurosciences, University of Cambridge, Cambridge, UK. [6]MRC Prion Unit, Department of Neurodegenerative Disease, UCL Institute of Neurology, Queen Square, London, UK.

References
1. Rascovsky K, Hodges JR, Knopman D, Mendez MF, Kramer JH, Neuhaus J, van Swieten JC, Seelaar H, Dopper EG, Onyike CU, et al. Sensitivity of revised diagnostic criteria for the behavioural variant of frontotemporal dementia. Brain. 2011;134(Pt 9):2456–77.
2. Chare L, Hodges JR, Leyton CE, McGinley C, Tan RH, Kril JJ, Halliday GM. New criteria for frontotemporal dementia syndromes: clinical and pathological diagnostic implications. J Neurol Neurosurg Psychiatry. 2014; 85(8):865–70.
3. Devenney E, Bartley L, Hoon C, O'Callaghan C, Kumfor F, Hornberger M, Kwok JB, Halliday GM, Kiernan MC, Piguet O, et al. Progression in Behavioural variant frontotemporal dementia: a longitudinal study. JAMA Neurol. 2015:72(12):1501–9.
4. Hornberger M, Shelley BP, Kipps CM, Piguet O, Hodges JR. Can progressive and non-progressive behavioural variant frontotemporal dementia be distinguished at presentation? J Neurol Neurosurg Psychiatry. 2009;80(6):591–3.
5. Hornberger M, Piguet O, Kipps C, Hodges JR. Executive function in progressive and nonprogressive behavioural variant frontotemporal dementia. Neurology. 2008;71(19):1481–8.
6. Kipps CM, Hodges JR, Fryer TD, Nestor PJ. Combined magnetic resonance imaging and positron emission tomography brain imaging in behavioural variant frontotemporal degeneration: refining the clinical phenotype. Brain. 2009;132(Pt 9):2566–78.
7. Mioshi E, Hsieh S, Savage S, Hornberger M, Hodges JR. Clinical staging and disease progression in frontotemporal dementia. Neurology. 2010;74(20):1591–7.
8. Khan BK, Yokoyama JS, Takada LT, Sharon JS, Rutherford NJ, Fong JC, Karydas AM, Wu T, Ketelle RS, Baker MC. Atypical, slowly progressive behavioural variant frontotemporal dementia associated with C9ORF72 hexanucleotide expansion. J Neurol Neurosurg Psychiatry. 2012;83(4):358–64.
9. Devenney E, Foxe D, Dobson-Stone C, Kwok JB, Kiernan MC, Hodges JR: Clinical heterogeneity of the C9orf72 genetic mutation in frontotemporal dementia.Neurocase 2014(ahead-of-print):1-7.
10. Kipps CM, Davies RR, Mitchell J, Kril JJ, Halliday GM, Hodges JR. Clinical significance of lobar atrophy in frontotemporal dementia: application of an MRI visual rating scale. Dement Geriatr Cogn Disord. 2007;23(5):334–42.
11. Ambikairajah A, Devenney E, Flanagan E, Yew B, Mioshi E, Kiernan MC, Hodges JR, Hornberger M. A visual MRI atrophy rating scale for the amyotrophic lateral sclerosis-frontotemporal dementia continuum. Amyotroph Lateral Scler Frontotemporal Degener. 2014;0:1–9.
12. Wedderburn C, Wear H, Brown J, Mason SJ, Barker RA, Hodges J, Williams-Gray C. The utility of the Cambridge Behavioural inventory in neurodegenerative disease. J Neurol Neurosurg Psychiatry. 2008;79(5):500–3.
13. Mioshi E, Dawson K, Mitchell J, Arnold R, Hodges JR. The Addenbrooke's cognitive examination revised (ACE-R): a brief cognitive test battery for dementia screening. Int J Geriatr Psychiatry. 2006;21(11):1078–85.
14. Renton AE, Majounie E, Waite A, Simón-Sánchez J, Rollinson S, Gibbs JR, Schymick JC, Laaksovirta H, Van Swieten JC, Myllykangas L. A Hexanucleotide repeat expansion in< i> C9ORF72</i> is the cause of chromosome 9p21-linked ALS-FTD. Neuron. 2011;72(2):257–68.
15. Laird NM, Ware JH. Random-effects models for longitudinal data. Biometrics. 1982;38(4):963–74.
16. Kipps CM, Hodges JR, Hornberger M. Nonprogressive behavioural frontotemporal dementia: recent developments and clinical implications of the 'bvFTD phenocopy syndrome'. Curr Opin Neurol. 2010;23(6):628–32.
17. Devenney E, Forrest SL, Xuereb J, Kril JJ, Hodges JR. The bvFTD phenocopy syndrome: a clinicopathological report. J Neurol Neurosurg Psychiatry. 2016; 87(10):1155–6.
18. Kumfor F, Irish M, Leyton C, Miller L, Lah S, Devenney E, Hodges JR, Piguet O. Tracking the progression of social cognition in neurodegenerative disorders. J Neurol Neurosurg Psychiatry. 2014;85(10):1076–83.
19. Happé F, Booth R, Charlton R, Hughes C. Executive function deficits in autism spectrum disorders and attention-deficit/hyperactivity disorder: examining profiles across domains and ages. Brain Cogn. 2006;61(1):25–39.
20. Ashwin C, Chapman E, Colle L, Baron-Cohen S. Impaired recognition of negative basic emotions in autism: a test of the amygdala theory. Soc Neurosci. 2006;1(3-4):349–63.
21. Gossink FT, Dols A, Kerssens CJ, Krudop WA, Kerklaan BJ, Scheltens P, Stek ML, Pijnenburg YA. Psychiatric diagnoses underlying the phenocopy syndrome of behavioural variant frontotemporal dementia. J Neurol Neurosurg Psychiatry. 2016;87(1):64–8.
22. Beck J, Poulter M, Hensman D, Rohrer JD, Mahoney CJ, Adamson G, Campbell T, Uphill J, Borg A, Fratta P. Large C9orf72 hexanucleotide repeat expansions are seen in multiple neurodegenerative syndromes and are more frequent than expected in the UK population. Am J Hum Genet. 2013; 92(3):345–53.
23. Galimberti D, Arosio B, Fenoglio C, Serpente M, Cioffi SM, Bonsi R, Rossi P, Abbate C, Mari D, Scarpini E. Incomplete penetrance of the C9ORF72 hexanucleotide repeat expansions: frequency in a cohort of geriatric non-demented subjects. J Alzheimers Dis. 2014;39(1):19–22.

Cases of visual impairment caused by cerebral venous sinus occlusion-induced intracranial hypertension in the absence of headache

Tongtao Zhao[1], Gang Wang[1], Jiaman Dai[1], Yong Liu[1], Yi Wang[1,2] and Shiying Li[1*]

Abstract

Background: Cerebral venous sinus thrombosis or stenosis (here collectively referred to as cerebral venous sinus occlusion, CVSO) can cause chronically-elevated intracranial pressure (ICP). Patients may have no neurological symptoms other than visual impairment, secondary to bilateral papilledema. Correctly recognizing these conditions, through proper ophthalmological examination and brain imaging, is very important to avoid delayed diagnosis and treatment.

Case presentation: We report a case series of 3 patients with chronic CVSO, who were admitted to an ophthalmological department in Chongqing, China, from 2015 March to 2017 February. All patients presented with decreased vision and bilateral papilledema, but had no headache or other neurological symptoms. The visual fields of all patients were impaired. Flash visual evoked potentials (VEPs) in two patients showed essentially normal peak time of P2 wave, and pattern VEPs in one patient displayed decreased P100 amplitude in one eye, while a normal P100 wave in the other eye. In all patients, lumbar puncture (LP) revealed significantly elevated ICP. And magnetic resonance venography (MRV) demonstrated cerebral venous sinus abnormalities in every patient: one right sigmoid sinus thrombosis, one superior sagittal sinus thrombosis, and one right transverse sinus stenosis.

Conclusions: CVSO can cause chronically-elevated ICP, leading to bilateral papilledema and visual impairment. A considerable amount of patients have no apparent neurological symptoms other than visual loss. Unlike other optic nerve lesions, such as neuritis or ischemic optic neuropathy, the optic disc edema in CVSO is usually bilateral, the flash or pattern VEP is often normal or only mildly affected, and patients are often not sensitive to steroid therapy. CVSO should be suspected in such patients when unenhanced brain imaging is normal. Further investigations, such as LP and contrast-enhanced imaging (MRV and digital subtraction angiography), should be performed to diagnose or exclude CVSO.

Keywords: Cerebral venous sinus occlusion, Intracranial hypertension, Papilledema

* Correspondence: shiying.li@tmmu.edu.cn
[1]Department of Ophthalmology, Southwest Hospital, The Third Military Medical University (Army Medical University), Chongqing, China
Full list of author information is available at the end of the article

Background

Cerebral venous sinus diseases, such as cerebral venous sinus thrombosis (CVST) and cerebral venous sinus stenosis (CVSS), are conditions affecting the intracranial venous drainage, causing either complete or partial cerebral venous sinus occlusion (CVSO) [1, 2]. This typically leads to elevated intracranial pressure (ICP), which can cause papilledema (usually bilateral) and visual impairment. When CVSO is acute (e.g., secondary to acute CVST), it typically causes severe headache and stroke-like neurological signs. However, when the onset is chronic, the symptoms of elevated ICP, like headache, are often absent, and the diagnosis may be delayed [3]. Here we report a case series of 3 patients with CVSO and elevated ICP, who had no apparent symptoms other than visual impairment, and firstly were admitted to ophthalmologists clinics.

Case presentation

Case 1

A 20 year-old man presented with a 1-month history of impaired vision, binocular horizontal diplopia and metamorphopsia. There was no history of headache, vomiting, fever, or trauma. He denied any history of hematological or neurological diseases, and was not on any medication. Notable in his past medical history was that he had undergone surgery for mastoiditis 8 years previously.

On presentation, the patient appeared in clear consciousness. Vital signs were stable, with blood pressure 121/82 mmHg, pulse 88 bpm and a body temperature of 37 °C. Best corrected visual acuity was 0.15 (Decimal Fraction) in both eyes. Ocular motilities of both eye were normal. Ophthalmoscopy revealed significant bilateral optic disc swelling with peri-papillary hemorrhages (Fig. 1a, b), but the eyes were otherwise normal. Fundus fluorescein angiography (FFA) showed hyperfluorescent leaking defects at the optic discs (Fig. 1c, d). Humphrey automated perimetry (HAP) revealed bilateral inferior arcuate scotomas (Fig. 4). Optical coherence tomography (OCT) showed bilateral papilledema, but the macular morphology was normal (Fig. 1e, f). Flash visual evoked potentials (FVEPs) showed normal peak time of the P2 wave (Fig. 4). The electroretinogram (ERG) also showed normal retinal function. Routine hematological and biochemical tests showed no significant abnormalities. Unenhanced brain and orbital magnetic resonance imaging (MRI) showed neither abnormal signals nor any signs of increased intracranial pressure, such as enlarged ventricles or mid-line shift, partially empty sella, flattening of the globe, or enlarged optic nerve sheaths (Fig. 1g, h). The patient was examined by neurologist, and no positive neurological signs were found. Considering the poor vision of both eyes, he was administrated with systemic steroids, but the visual acuity did not improve afterwards.

Given the patient's manifestation and ophthalmological and systemic investigations, primary optic neuropathies, including optic neuritis and ischemic optic neuropathy, were basically ruled out. Specialized investigations for intracranial pathology were therefore performed. Magnetic resonance

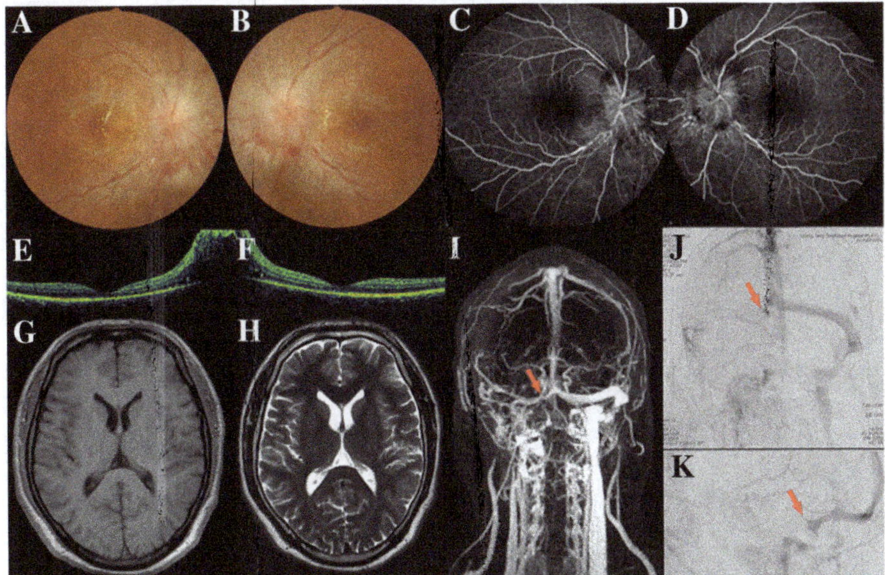

Fig. 1 *Case 1, 20-year-old male patient with severe bilateral papilledema* **a, b,** Ophthalmoscopy images of right and left eye, respectively. **c, d,** FFA images, showing hyperfluorescence of optic discs bilaterally, without other abnormal leakage. **e f,** OCT images, showing relatively normal macular morphology in both eyes. **g, h,** Unenhanced T1- and T2-weighted MRI images, respectively, showing no abnormalities. **i,** MRV image, showing a poorly-visualized right sigmoid and transverse sinuses (*red arrow*). **j, k,** DSA images, showing a filling-defect (*red arrows*) in the right sigmoid and transverse sinuses

venography (MRV) showed a loss-of-signal void in the right sigmoid sinus (Fig. 1i). LP at the time showed an elevated cerebrospinal fluid (CSF) opening-pressure of over 40 cm H_2O (normal, 18–20 cm H_2O). CSF protein, glucose, and cell counts were all within normal limits. After neurological consultation, a digital subtraction angiography (DSA) was performed, which showed a filling-defect in the right sigmoid sinus (Fig. 1j, k). The patient was diagnosed with right sigmoid sinus thrombosis, and was referred to the neurology department for conservative treatment. At 6 months follow up, the visual acuities improved to 0.2 in right eye and 0.3 in left eye.

Case 2

A 72 year-old man presented with visual loss in his left eye for 7 months and decreased vision in his right eye for 8 months. He had been diagnosed with multiple lacunar cerebral infarctions and non-arteritic anterior ischemic optic neuropathy (NAAION) in the neurology department, but no positive neurological signs were found. He was given oral steroid therapy for several months, but with no improvement in vision. The patient had no history of hypertension or diabetes and no history of systemic or local infection.

The patient came to the ophthalmology outpatient department for further investigation. On presentation, he was in clear consciousness. Best corrected visual acuity was 0.3 (right) and no light perception (left). Relative afferent pupillary defect was present in the left eye. Mild lens opacity was observed in both eyes. In the right eye, the optic disc was slightly edematous (Fig. 2a). In the left eye, the optic disc was slightly pale in color (Fig. 2b). Signs as gliosis of peripapillary retinal nerve fiber layers, optociliary shunt vessels, or refractile bodies were not found. FFA showed hyperfluorescence of the right optic disc, and hypofluorescence in the left optic disc (Fig. 2c, d). HAP revealed superior and nasal scotomas (Fig. 4). OCT revealed that both macula had normal morphology (Fig. 2e, f). FVEP showed a mild decrease in amplitude of the P2 wave in the right eye, and a severe decrease in the left eye (Fig. 4). The ERG was relatively normal bilaterally. In the neurology department, he had previously undergone a contrast-enhanced CT-head (Fig. 2g) and CTA (computed tomographic angiography), which showed no abnormalities (Fig. 2h). An unenhanced MRI brain showed multiple lacunar cerebral infarctions and mild cerebral atrophy. Laboratory tests ruled out any blood disorders or infections. To further investigate for intracranial conditions, an MRV was performed, which demonstrated superior sagittal sinus thrombosis (Fig. 2i, j). LP showed an elevated cerebrospinal fluid (CSF) opening-pressure of 30 cm H_2O. CSF protein, glucose, and cell counts were all within normal limits. The patient was referred back to the neurology department for endovascular intervention and stent placement. The best corrected visual acuity of right eye improved to 0.4 at six months following treatment.

Case 3

A 20 year-old woman presented with a 1-month history of deteriorating vision. There was no history of eye pain, headache, vomiting, fever, or trauma. She denied any

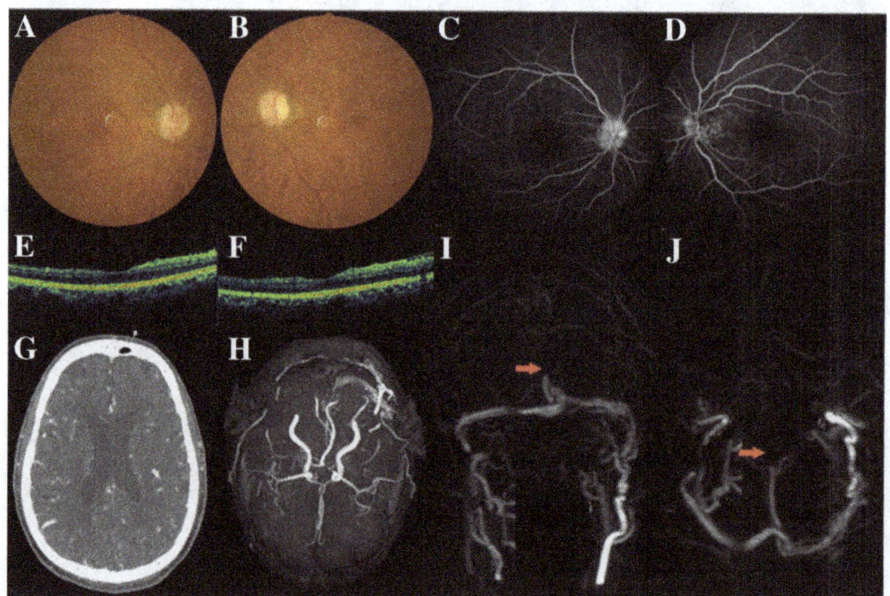

Fig. 2 *Case 2, 72-year-old male patient with mild bilateral papilledema.* **a, b,** Ophthalmoscopy images. **c, d,** FFA images, showing hyperfluorescence of the right optic disc, and hypofluorescence in the left optic disc, without other abnormal leakage. **e, f,** OCT images, showing relatively normal macular morphology in both eyes. **g,** Contrast-enhanced CT image, showing no signs of elevated ICP. **h,** CTA image, showing a normal cerebral arterial system. **i, j,** MRV image, consistent with thrombosis (*red arrows*) of the superior sagittal sinus

history of infection or surgery, and was not taking oral contraceptives, or any other medication. There was no notable past medical history.

On presentation, the patient's best corrected visual acuity was 0.9 (right) and 0.5 (left), and she had normal pupil diameter and pupillary reflexes. Ophthalmoscopy revealed significant bilateral optic disc swelling and peri-papillary hemorrhages, but no other abnormalities (Fig. 3a, b). The papilledema was surprisingly severe given her moderate visual impairment. The intra-ocular pressure (IOP) of both eyes was normal. Examined by neurologist, the patient showed no positive neurological signs. FFA showed hyperfluorescence of both optic discs and dilated peri-papillary capillaries (Fig. 3c, d). There was no other abnormal fluorescence observed. OCT showed bilateral papilledema but normal macular morphology (Fig. 3e, f). HAP showed non-specific bilateral inferior nasal scotomas (Fig. 4). Pattern VEPs (PVEPs) indicated a nearly normal amplitude of the P100 wave in the right eye (visual acuity of 0.9) and a decreased amplitude with normal peak time of the P100 wave in the left eye (Fig. 4).

Blood tests showed no evidence of systemic infection or biochemical abnormalities. No abnormalities were seen on an unenhanced MRI of the brain (Fig. 3g, h). An LP demonstrated an elevated CSF opening pressure of 29 cm H_2O. To further investigate for intracranial conditions, an MRV was performed, which showed a narrowed right transverse sinus, but no other abnormalities (Fig. 3i–k). From this imaging, the patient was diagnosed with right transverse sinus stenosis and referred to the neurosurgery department for further investigation of venous anatomy, prior to treatment. At 6 months follow up, the visual acuity kept unchanged. Due to personal reasons, the patient refused the ventriculoperitoneal shunt suggested by neurologists.

Discussion and conclusions

Papilledema is swelling of the optic nerve head (optic disc), secondary to elevated intracranial pressure (ICP) [4]. It is usually bilateral. Optic disc edema in the absence of elevated ICP is commonly referred to as "disc swelling", which is usually associated with ocular diseases like optic neuritis and ischemic optic neuropathy. However, patients with bilateral optic disc swelling should be suspected of having an elevated ICP, whether or not they have neurological manifestations. Causes of elevated ICP include obstruction of the ventricular system by congenital or acquired lesions, space-occupying intracranial lesions, subarachnoid hemorrhage, cerebral trauma, cerebral venous sinus thrombosis/stenosis, and idiopathic intracranial hypertension.

Elevated ICP usually causes dramatic neurological symptoms, including headaches, nausea, vomiting and deterioration of consciousness, as well as visual impairment. Such patients are most commonly diagnosed in the neurology department. However, chronic cerebral venous sinus occlusion (CVSO), either complete or partial, can cause chronically elevated ICP, and can produce visual impairment as the only clinical symptom. Thus

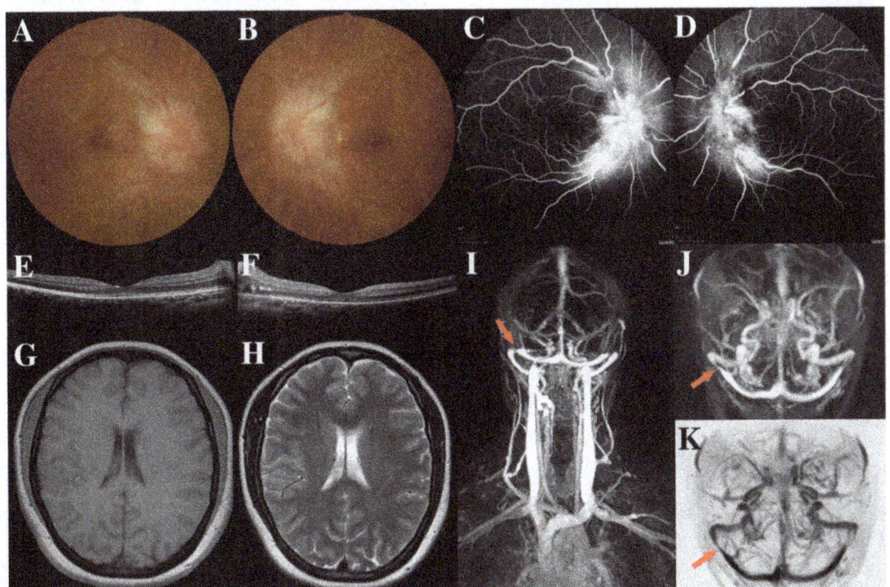

Fig. 3 *Case 3, 20-year-old female patient with mild bilateral papilledema.* **a, b,** Ophthalmoscopy images. **c, d,** FFA images, showing hyperfluorescence of optic discs bilaterally, without other abnormal leakage. **e, f,** OCT images, showing normal macular morphology in both eyes. **g, h,** Unenhanced T1- and T2-weighted MRI images, respectively, showing no abnormalities. **i–k,** MRV images, showing a narrowed right transverse sinus (*red arrows*)

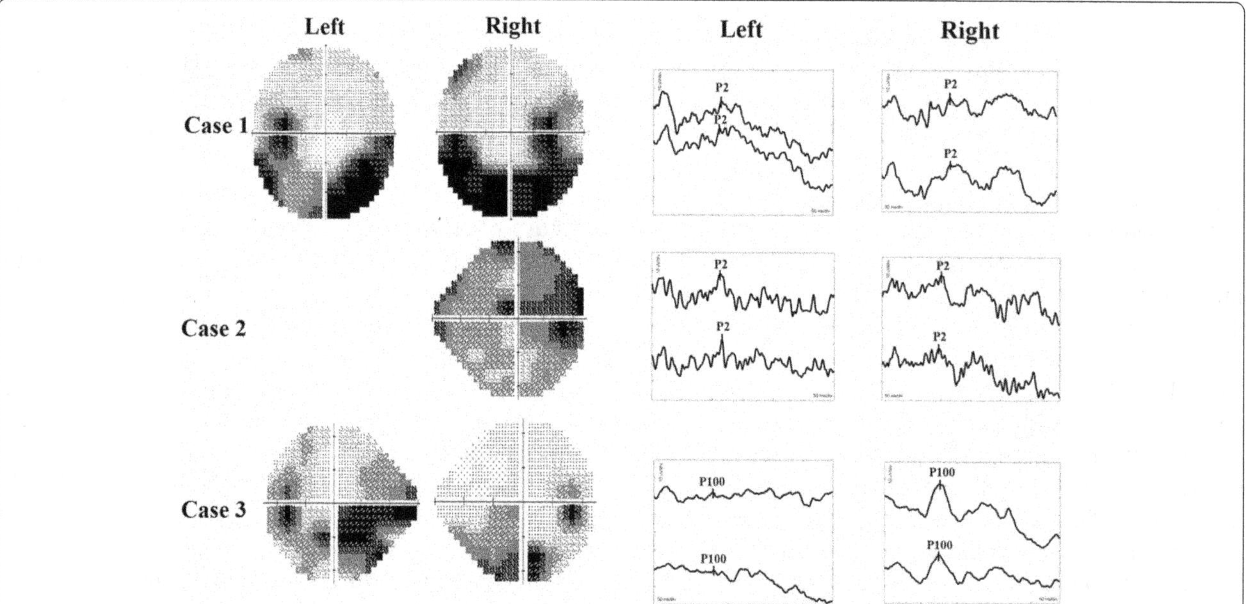

Fig. 4 *Visual fields and FVEP/PVEP of the 3 cases.* Left, Humphrey visual field plots of both eyes. All patients had impairment of visual fields, secondary to papilledema. With case 2, the visual field of the left eye couldn't be tested due to the poor vison. Right, FVEP plots for cases 1 and 2, showing only mild abnormalities (normal peak time, in contrast to delayed peak time in optic neuritis). PVEP plots for case 3, showing a nearly normal amplitude of the P100 wave in the right eye (visual acuity of 0.9) and a decreased amplitude with normal peak time of the P100 wave in the left eye (visual acuity of 0.5)

such patients often present to the optometrist or ophthalmologist. As well as producing decreased visual acuity, chronic papilledema induced by elevated ICP can produce visual field defects if the optic disc edema persists. However, unlike primary optic nerve diseases like optic neuritis, the flash VEP in patients with papilledema secondary to elevated ICP is often normal or only mildly affected [5, 6].

In case 1, the symptoms, other than blurred vison, were relatively occult. Although the bilateral optic disc swelling strongly indicated elevated ICP, there were no positive findings on CT or MRI. However, vision was not improved following treatment with systemic steroids. Therefore, further investigation was performed, which demonstrated elevated ICP secondary to right sigmoid sinus thrombosis. In retrospect, the patient's history of mastoiditis and surgery eight years prior was highly significant. Mastoiditis is an important cause of sigmoid sinus thrombosis, especially in younger patients.

In case 2, the patient was a septuagenarian male with a long history of impaired vision, but no neurological symptoms. Due to the likely chronicity of the elevated ICP at presentation, the optic disc swelling in the right eye was not prominent, and the optic nerve in the left eye was already slightly atrophied, and the eye was blind. Prior to ophthalmology consultation, his visual impairment may be partially attributed to his multiple lacunar cerebral infarctions. But this multiple lacunar cerebral infarction as Fig. 3 showed can't explain the severity of his visual impairment of both eyes, which indicated that the cerebral infarctions did not distinctly affect his visual pathway. Given his age, a diagnosis of non-arteritic anterior ischemic optic neuropathy was also made. However, the severity of visual impairment and lack of response to steroid therapy indicated the need for further investigation. Following MRV imaging, a diagnosis of superior sagittal sinus thrombosis was made. The patient's visual impairment improved following endovascular stenting of the venous sinus.

Case 3 was that of a young adult female with blurred vision and bilateral papilledema, but no other neurological symptoms, and no history of systemic disease or infection. Her elevated ICP was confirmed by lumbar puncture, but unlike the other two cases, her radiological findings were less prominent. There were no definite signs of sinus thrombosis observed from the MRV, but a narrowed section was noted at the junction between the right transverse and sigmoid sinus. With no evidence of any intracranial mass, the patient was diagnosed with right transverse sinus stenosis. However, the etiology of this stenosis is currently still unknown, and the patient is under continued management by the neurosurgical team.

CVSO (partial or complete) affects the dural venous sinuses that drain blood from the brain, and is usually caused by either venous thrombosis or stenosis. Cerebral venous sinus thrombosis (CVST) most commonly affects the transverse sinus (86% of cases), followed by the superior sagittal sinus (62%), straight sinus (18%), then least commonly, the cortical veins (17%) [1]. Risk factors for CVST include thrombophilia, chronic inflammatory diseases, use of hormonal contraception, infections such as meningitis, mastoiditis and sinusitis, and invasive procedures in the head and neck area [7, 8]. Symptoms of CVST include headache, visual impairment, symptoms of stroke (such as unilateral limb and facial weakness), and seizures. However, neurological symptoms are absent in a notable proportion of patients, and these patients may present later with impaired visual acuity due to chronic, advancing papilledema [9, 10].

Cerebral venous sinus stenosis (CVSS) is a rare intracranial abnormality. Stenosis may be caused by abnormal intrinsic dural sinus anatomy or by extrinsic compression; for example, due to an intracranial tumor or enlarged arachnoid granulation. In many cases the cause of stenosis is unknown. The stenosis is most often found at the junction of the transverse and sigmoid sinuses, and is typically diagnosed by venography [11, 12]. Regardless of the underlying cause, stenting has proved (in multiple retrospective, non-controlled studies) to be an effective method for improving the symptoms of elevated ICP and papilledema [13, 14].

Imaging of patients with CVSO, using unenhanced CT or MRI, may demonstrate gross abnormalities, such as cerebral edema, venous infarction and dilated ventricles. However in some cases, unenhanced imaging may be totally normal, especially in patients with a chronic disease course. Therefore, when elevated ICP is suspected, contrast-enhanced MR venography is required to image the cerebral veins for thrombus or stenosis, and lumbar puncture (LP) may be needed, to measure the opening pressure and test for constituent changes in the CSF.

In summary, CVST and CVSS (here collectively referred to as CVSO) are severe conditions which can cause elevated ICP, leading to visual impairment. A considerable amount of patients with CVSO have no apparent neurological symptoms other than visual loss. VEP could be normal or abnormal. When encountering patients with bilateral papilledema, especially those with normal unenhanced brain imaging, CVSO should always be considered. Further investigations such as LP, MRV or DSA are necessary to diagnose or rule-out CVST or CVSS.

Abbreviations

CSF: Cerebrospinal fluid; CTA: Computed tomographic angiography; CVSO: Cerebral venous sinus occlusion; CVSS: Cerebral venous sinus stenosis; CVST: Cerebral venous sinus thrombosis; DSA: Digital subtraction angiography; ERG: Electroretinogram; FFA: Fundus fluorescein angiography; HAP: Humphrey automated perimetry; ICP: Intracranial pressure; IOP: Intraocular pressure; LP: Lumbar puncture; MRI: Magnetic resonance imaging; MRV: Magnetic resonance venography; NAAION: Non-arteritic anterior ischemic optic neuropathy; OCT: Optical coherence tomography; VEPs: Visual evoked potentials

Acknowledgements

The authors thank Prof. Xiaohong Meng for data collecting.

Author contributions

TTZ, YW, and SYL designed the study. YL, GW and JMD helped to collect and analyze data. TTZ wrote the manuscript. TTZ and SYL critical revised the manuscript. All authors read and approved the final manuscript.

Funding

This study was supported by the Translational Grant (SWH2016LHZH-02) of Southwest Hospital, Third Military Medical University(Army Medical University), Translational Grant (2016xzh07) of Third Military Medical University(Army Medical University) and Southwest Hospital Innovation Grant(SWH2015LC15).

Competing interests

The authors declare that they have no competing interests.

Author details

[1]Department of Ophthalmology, Southwest Hospital, The Third Military Medical University (Army Medical University), Chongqing, China. [2]Aier Eye Hospital, Chongqing, China.

References

1. Stam J. Thrombosis of the cerebral veins and sinuses. N Engl J Med. 2005; 352(17):1791–8.
2. Ridh MA, Saindane AM, Bruce BB, et al. Magnetic resonance imaging findings of elevated intracranial pressure in cerebral venous thrombosis versus idiopathic intracranial hypertension with transverse sinus stenosis. Neuro-Ophthalmology. 2013;37(1):1–6.
3. Coutinho JM, Stam J, Canhão P, et al. Cerebral venous thrombosis in the absence of headache. Stroke. 2015;46:245–7.
4. Trobe JD. Papilledema: the vexing issues. J Neuroophthalmol. 2011;31(2): 175–86.
5. Eliseeva N, Serova N, Yakovlev S, et al. Neuro-ophthalmological features of cerebral venous sinus thrombosis. Neuro-Ophthalmology. 2015;39(2):69–76.
6. O'Rourke TL, Slagle WS, Elkins M, et al. Papilloedema associated with dural venous sinus thrombosis. Clin Exp Optom. 2014;97:133–9.
7. Ferro JM, Canhão P, Stam J, et al. Prognosis of cerebral vein and dural sinus thrombosis: results of the international study on cerebral vein and Dural sinus thrombosis (ISCVT). Stroke. 2004;35(3):664–70.
8. Micieli JA, Margolin E. A 55-year-old man with severe papilledema. JAMA. 2015;313(9):963–4.
9. Pakter GJ. Bilateral optic disc swelling as a presenting sign of superior sagittal sinus thrombosis. BMJ Case Reports 2012;10.1136/bcr-2012-006814.
10. Shah S, Saxena D. Bilateral papilledema: a case of cerebral venous sinus thrombosis. Oman J Ophthalmol. 2014;7:33–4.
11. Woodall MN, Nguyen KD, Alleyne CH, et al. Bilateral transverse sinus stenosis causing intracranial hypertension. BMJ Case Reports 2013;2013: bcr2013010513.
12. Honarmand AR, Hurley MC, Ansari SA, et al. Focal stenosis of the sigmoid sinus causing intracranial venous hypertension: case report, endovascular management, and review of the literature. Interv Neuroradiol. 2016;22(2): 240–5.
13. Shazly TA, Jadhav AP, Aghaebrahim A, et al. Venous sinus stenting shortens the duration of medical therapy for increased intracranial pressure secondary to venous sinus stenosis. J Neurointerv Surg 2017 May 9. pii: neurintsurg-2017-013103.
14. Dinkin MJ, Patsalides A. Venous sinus stenting for idiopathic intracranial hypertension: where are we now? Neurol Clin. 2017 Feb;35(1):59–81.

19

Biochemical markers in vascular cognitive impairment associated with subcortical small vessel disease - A consensus report

A. Wallin[1,18*], E. Kapaki[2], M. Boban[3], S. Engelborghs[4,5], D. M. Hermann[6], B. Huisa[7], M. Jonsson[1], M. G. Kramberger[8], L. Lossi[9], B. Malojcic[3], S. Mehrabian[10], A. Merighi[9], E. B. Mukaetova-Ladinska[11], G. P. Paraskevas[2], B. O. Popescu[12], R. Ravid[13], L. Traykov[10], G. Tsivgoulis[14], G. Weinstein[15], A. Korczyn[16], M. Bjerke[5] and G. Rosenberg[17]

Abstract

Background: Vascular cognitive impairment (VCI) is a heterogeneous entity with multiple aetiologies, all linked to underlying vascular disease. Among these, VCI related to subcortical small vessel disease (SSVD) is emerging as a major homogeneous subtype. Its progressive course raises the need for biomarker identification and/or development for adequate therapeutic interventions to be tested. In order to shed light in the current status on biochemical markers for VCI-SSVD, experts in field reviewed the recent evidence and literature data.

Method: The group conducted a comprehensive search on Medline, PubMed and Embase databases for studies published until 15.01.2017. The proposal on current status of biochemical markers in VCI-SSVD was reviewed by all co-authors and the draft was repeatedly circulated and discussed before it was finalized.

Results: This review identifies a large number of biochemical markers derived from CSF and blood. There is a considerable overlap of VCI-SSVD clinical symptoms with those of Alzheimer's disease (AD). Although most of the published studies are small and their findings remain to be replicated in larger cohorts, several biomarkers have shown promise in separating VCI-SSVD from AD. These promising biomarkers are closely linked to underlying SSVD pathophysiology, namely disruption of blood-CSF and blood–brain barriers (BCB-BBB) and breakdown of white matter myelinated fibres and extracellular matrix, as well as blood and brain inflammation. The leading biomarker candidates are: elevated CSF/blood albumin ratio, which reflects BCB/BBB disruption; altered CSF matrix metalloproteinases, reflecting extracellular matrix breakdown; CSF neurofilment as a marker of axonal damage, and possibly blood inflammatory cytokines and adhesion molecules. The suggested SSVD biomarker deviations contrasts the characteristic CSF profile in AD, i.e. depletion of amyloid beta peptide and increased phosphorylated and total tau.

Conclusions: Combining SSVD and AD biomarkers may provide a powerful tool to identify with greater precision appropriate patients for clinical trials of more homogeneous dementia populations. Thereby, biomarkers might promote therapeutic progress not only in VCI-SSVD, but also in AD.

Keywords: Vascular cognitive impairment, Subcortical small vessel disease, Biomarkers, Blood, CSF, Alzheimer's disease, Mixed type dementia, Dementia

* Correspondence: anders.wallin@neuro.gu.se
[1]Department of Psychiatry and Neurochemistry, Institute of Neuroscience and Physiology, Sahlgrenska Academy at the University of Gothenburg, Mölndal, Sweden
[18]Memory Clinic at Department of Neuropsychiatry, Sahlgrenska University Hospital, Institute of Neuroscience and Physiology at Sahlgrenska Academy, University of Gothenburg, Wallinsgatan 6, SE-431 41 Mölndal, Sweden
Full list of author information is available at the end of the article

Background

There are not yet efficient ways of treating or preventing dementia disorders of which Alzheimer's disease (AD) remains the most common target for therapeutic interventions. In contrast, only few clinical pharmacological trials have been conducted in subjects with vascular cognitive impairment (VCI). The lack of treatment success in VCI may be largely due to the heterogeneity of cerebrovascular diseases, with the majority of VCI clinical trials being performed in stroke patients. Only few clinical trials have been performed in patients with subcortical small vessel disease (SSVD), a common, fairly homogeneous, but often under-recognized type of VCI (VCI-SSVD) [1–4]. The clinical phenotype of combined AD and vascular pathologies is often referred to as mixed type dementia (MD). The overlap of SSVD, AD and normal aging makes the underlying clinical diagnosis challenging, and it may lead to misclassification of patients in treatment trials. One way of moving the field forward is to be more specific about disease definitions along the AD – SSVD axis. This, in turn, will allow for refinements of diagnostic criteria with more sharply defined patient cohorts.

Method

A focused meeting on VCI-SSVD biochemical markers was held as a part of the 9th International Congress on Vascular Dementia in Ljubljana, Slovenia, on 18 October, 2015. Experts in this field reviewed the current evidence and literature data. For the purpose of this narrative review, we conducted a comprehensive search on Medline, PubMed and Embase databases for studies published until 15.01.2017. The key words used in the current search were: subcortical small vessel disease, vascular dementia, vascular cognitive impairment, Alzheimer's disease, Binswanger's disease, biomarker(s), cerebrospinal fluid, blood, serum, plasma, blood brain barrier, white matter, genetics, tau protein(s), amyloid, inflammation. We critically reviewed all abstracts and obtained the full text of relevant papers. We grouped the identified relevant subcortical small vessel disease biomarkers into themes and report the major relevant findings. The proposal on current status of biochemical markers in VCI-SSVD was reviewed by the group, including additional experts who did not attend the meeting. The draft was repeatedly circulated and discussed before it was finalized.

Types of cerebral small vessel diseases, other vascular lesions and Alzheimer pathology

Cerebral SSVD refers to pathological processes affecting a spectrum of subcortical vascular changes visible on Computed Tomography/Magnetic Resonance Imaging (CT/MRI) as white matter lesions (WML), lacunes and cerebral microbleeds. Underlying vascular pathologies are arteriolosclerosis, lipohyalinosis, fibroid necrosis, oedema and damage to the blood-cerebrospinal fluid and blood–brain barriers (BCB/BBB), the latter resulting in chronic leakage of fluid and macromolecules in the white matter and inflammation (reviewed by Kalaria, 2016) [5]. Although SSVD pathogenesis remains poorly understood, it is an age-related condition, associated with a number of risk factors including systemic hypertension [6–9], chronic kidney disease [10, 11], smoking [12], metabolic syndrome [8, 13, 14], osteoporosis [15], chronic obstructive pulmonary disease [16] and sleep-apnoea syndrome [17]. The SSVD clinical manifestations are largely due to complete (lacunes) or incomplete (WML) infarction(s) and microbleeds resulting in cognitive, motor and mood disturbances and eventually functional disability [2], although same lesions might appear in cognitively intact persons during normal ageing. In patients with hypertension and WML, cerebral blood flow autoregulation is restricted, resulting in lack of physiological vasodilation during times of increased oxygen and nutrient needs. This renders the brain vulnerable to ischemic hypoperfusion, particularly in the watershed regions of the white matter [18].

Clinico-pathological studies have associated the characteristic clinical symptoms of VCI-SSVD (i.e. presence of motor and executive slowing, forgetfulness and dysarthria) with the bidirectional disruption of pathways connecting the prefrontal cortex with the basal ganglia and thalamus [2]. As opposed to other vascular subtypes, VCI-SSVD patients presents with a slow progressive course, which may mimic AD. On the other hand, late-onset AD patients frequently have significant SSVD burden, not necessarily related to their amyloid load [19]. The disruption of white matter network may be mediated via the effect of the small vessel pathology, rather than amyloid deposits [20]. A recent study showed age at onset as a crucial factor that determines distinct features in subcortical VCI patients, such as pathologic burden, structural changes and cognitive function. Early onset subcortical vascular cognitive impairment was reported to be associated with more lacunes, more severe frontal structural network disruption and more affected frontal executive functions. In contrast, later onset VCI-SSVD shows more pronounced amyloid burden, cortical and hippocampal atrophy [21]. The genetic component of VCI-SSVD is supported by the presence of monogenic forms representing a small portion of VCI-SSVD cases [22].

Biochemical markers

Although several studies using biochemical markers have been completed and reviewed in AD, such information is still lacking for VCI-SSVD. Here we review studies using a broad range of biochemical markers from cerebrospinal fluid (CSF), plasma or serum in VCI-SSVD.

Our primary question is whether they are useful to identify VCI-SSVD. We also review whether there are overlapping and differentiating findings between VCI-SSVD and AD.

Blood-CSF/blood–brain barriers (BCB/BBB)

The BCB/BBB are highly selective permeability barriers that separate the circulating blood from the brain. The function and structure of BCB/BBB alter with aging. Disruption of BCB/BBB function, followed by blood-to-brain extravasation of circulating neuroinflammatory molecules, may increase the risk of brain injury. This may be an important factor for disease progression in both VCI and AD [23], and increasing evidence, also from pre-clinical translational studies, indicates that dysfunction of the BCB/BBB may play a significant role in the pathogenesis of vascular dementia [24–26]. The CSF/serum albumin quotient (QA) is the gold-standard measure of BCB/BBB integrity, with increases in this ratio indicating increased permeability. QA requires the measurement of albumin in CSF and serum collected concurrently [27, 28]. Advancing age is associated with increased BCB/BBB permeability, which is further increased in patients with VCI (as compared to AD) and with worsening of WML [29]. Altered BCB/BBB has consistently been reported in VCI-SSVD patients, and it is thought to contribute to the pathogenic process in AD [30–34].

Several lines of evidence suggested that the astrocytic protein S100β is a potentially useful peripheral marker of BCB/BBB permeability [35]. S100β can be released from injured astrocytes and enter the extracellular space and hence the bloodstream. This protein is elevated in radiologically defined SSVD [36, 37]. A positive correlation of S100β levels with the severity of depression, a common symptom in SSVD, has also been reported [38]. Changes in BCB/BBB function correlate strongly with an increase of two other proteins, namely glial fibrillary acidic protein (GFAP) and neuron specific enolase (NSE) in serum, indicating BCB/BBB leakage [39]. However, they are both unspecific biological markers in dementia disorders [40–42].

Inflammatory and glial activation markers

Both the innate immune system and systematic inflammation have central roles in the pathophysiology of cognitive impairment [43, 44]. While many molecules within the inflammatory pathway are likely to be involved, only few of them have been investigated in the context of VCI-SSVD.

C reactive protein (CRP), a biomarker of systemic inflammation, is perhaps the most extensively studied circulatory biomarker of cerebral SSVD pathology. Although its association with SSVD (particularly in the presence of WML) is inconclusive [45–48], several studies have suggested that elevated peripheral CRP level increases the risk of VCI, but not AD [49, 50]. In addition, elevated serum CRP appears to be consistently associated with measures of white matter integrity [51, 52], whereas a rapid decline in CRP levels predicts a healthier white matter microstructure [53].

Interleukins (ILs) are a group of cytokines participating in the regulation of the immune response. A classification that proves useful in clinical practice (outside of structural biology) divides immunological cytokines into type 1 (IFN-γ, TNFα, TNFβ, IL-2, and IL-12-b), that enhances cellular immune responses and type 2 (TGF-β, IL-4, IL-5, IL-6, IL-10 and IL-13), which controls antibody responses. In the vasculature, interleukin-6 (IL-6) is secreted as a pro-inflammatory cytokine by *tunica muscularis* cells of the blood vessels. As a response to IL-6, the liver synthesizes the CRP. Although the majority of studies reported a positive association [54], the usefulness of IL-6 and CRP as biomarkers of SSVD, particularly in the presence of WML, remains to be fully established [48]. In contrast, CSF TNF-α, TGF-β and vascular endothelial growth factor (VEGF) levels are all elevated in VCI-SSVD patients [55, 56].

CSF *α1-antichymotrypsin*, an acute phase inflammatory protein, was also increased in individuals with VCI-SSVD compared to healthy controls as well as in prodromal VCI-SSVD patients who later progressed to dementia, whereas in AD it was elevated only in manifest dementia [57]. Interestingly, higher levels of serum α1-antichymotrypsin in individuals with VCI, but not AD, compared to controls have also been reported [58].

YKL-40, a marker of glial activation, was elevated in CSF of patients with prodromal VCI but not prodromal AD [59].

Markers of extracellular matrix breakdown

Matrix metalloproteinases (MMPs) are a large family of enzymes active in the extracellular matrix, at the cell surface and intracellularly. Although there are 26 family members, MMP-2, −3, −7, −9, −10 and −12 are mainly active in the brain. Some MMPs, i.e. MMP-2, are constitutively produced and are normally present in the CSF. Others (mainly MMP-3 and MMP-9) are inducible with very low levels in the CSF until an inflammatory response is elicited [60, 61]. Changes in several MMPs have been found in SSVD [33]. Measurement of MMPs and tissue inhibitor of metalloproteinases-1 (TIMP-1) are promising SSVD biomarkers, and have high validity in discriminating VCI-SSVD from cognitive impairment of primarily neurodegenerative etiology [33, 34, 57, 62, 63].

Markers of subcortical neuronal degeneration and myelin damage

Neurofilaments

Neurofilaments (NFs) are major structural proteins of neurons. They consist of three subunits of low (NF-L), medium (NF-M), or high (NF-H) molecular weight with varying degrees of phosphorylation [64]. NFs may be sensitive surrogate markers for neuronal death and axonal loss [65]. Several early studies detected NF peptides in the CSF of several neurological/neurodegenerative disorders [66–69]. NF-L subunit is a protein expressed in large-caliber myelinated axons [70]. Slightly increased CSF NF-L levels occur in healthy older individuals and correlate with increasing age [66]. However, a more significant increase in CSF NF-L levels is also present in individuals with WML [32, 33, 71, 72]. A positive association of CSF-NF-L levels with increasing severity of WML in non-demented subjects has also been reported [73].

In acute cerebral infarction, very high NF-L levels were reported [66]. The CSF levels of NF-L were higher in dementia disorders engaging subcortical brain regions, such as VCI and MD, but also in fronto-temporal dementia (FTD) [74, 75]. In VCI-SSVD the CSF NF-L concentrations were consistently higher than in controls, however with considerable overlap among other dementia disorders [32, 72]. In a recent meta-analysis comparing 106 VCI-SSVD patients with 283 healthy age-matched controls, the patient group had increased CSF NF-L levels. However, the overall elevation was smaller than that for either AD or FTD patients versus controls [76].

Increased WML load and ventricular dilation were related to increased CSF levels of TIMP-1 and NF-L and to decreased sAPPβ (a marker of amyloid pathology), suggesting that these molecules may function as biological markers of white matter damage [77].

Far less is known about CSF levels of the other NF isoforms. One study reported increased CSF levels of phosphorylated NF-H/M in AD compared with VCI and controls [67]. Others have found elevated CSF NF-H levels in AD and VCI in comparison with controls, but no differences between FTD and controls, or between AD, VCI and FTD patients [78].

Myelin basic protein

Myelin basic protein (MBP) is a major structural constituent of the myelin sheath [79]. Its function is to maintain the structure of the myelin and together with myelin-associated glycoprotein (MAG) to modulate the caliber of myelinated axons [80]. One of the hallmarks of VCI-SSVD is the rarefaction of white matter, due to nerve fiber degeneration, gliosis, demyelination or a combination of all three [81, 82]. Significantly elevated MBP CSF levels have been reported in stroke with subcortical infarcts affecting the white matter, as opposed to stroke with cortical infarcts [83], indicating its potential as a regional marker of infarction, as well as a marker of WML. Increased CSF levels of MBP and NF-L were found in acute ischemic stroke patients. In mild stroke {NIHSS <5 (National Institute of Health Stroke Scale)}, the concentration of MBP was significantly lower compared to more severe stroke (NIHSS >5), while NF-L was a stronger marker for stroke in general, independent of severity [84]. Increased CSF levels of MBP and NF-L were also described in patients with WML as compared to controls. However, compared to controls, MBP and NF-L were increased in both VCI-SSVD and AD patients, with considerable overlap between patient groups [33].

CSF sulfatide

CSF sulfatide is an acidic glycophospholipid of oligodendrocyte-produced myelin sheaths considered as a marker of white matter degradation. It was found to be 200% higher in patients with VCI-SSVD compared to controls and patients with AD [85], while CSF sulfatide levels distinguished between patients with subcortical arteriosclerotic encephalopathy and those with normal pressure hydrocephalus with a sensitivity and specificity of 74 and 94% respectively [86]. CSF sulfatide has also been shown to predict WML progression in nondisabled patients with WML [87].

Furthermore, this marker was lower in mild cognitive impairment and mild AD compared to control subjects [88]. In another study TNF-α levels were significantly correlated with sulfatide levels [89], suggesting that this apoptosis-inducing cytokine may lead to oligodendrocytes death, thus contributing to white matter degeneration, a hallmark of SSVD.

Markers of cortical neuronal degeneration

Tau proteins

Tau protein is the major component of intracellularly located neurofibrillary tangles and, in the neurofibrillary pathology, it is present in a hyperphosphorylated form. Both total and hyperphosphorylated tau have been found to be increased in the CSF of patients with AD [90]. Total tau (T-tau) is viewed as a marker of neuronal and/or axonal degeneration, while hyperphosphorylated tau (P-tau) is a more specific marker of tangle formation in AD [91]. Although their diagnostic accuracy may be reduced to variable degree when attempting differentiating AD from other types of dementia, the above biomarkers, especially when combined with Aβ42, achieve sensitivities and specificities >90% for the discrimination of AD at least from normal ageing. They have now been incorporated in *research* guidelines for diagnosing incipient and manifest AD [92, 93].

In VCI, CSF T-tau levels have been reported to be either normal [94–96], increased [97–101], or intermediate between those found in controls and AD, but much lower as compared to those of AD [102, 103]. Even then, some patients with VCI do present with high or, sometimes, very high T-tau levels [96, 103–106]. When patients with VCI, MD or AD with WML were clinically separated, the results were again conflicting: T-tau in VCI was reported as comparable to controls [96], increased [101] or intermediate but much lower in comparison to those of AD [103], while patients with MD presented with increased T-tau in all studies. However, patients with lacunar infarcts [94], progressive WML [99] or VCI-SSVD (pure and/or combined with AD) [32, 33, 107, 108] had normal T-tau levels. The CSF levels of P-tau have been described as normal in VCI or VCI-SSVD [33, 100, 101, 103, 107, 108], while in MD, levels were increased to the level of AD [103] or intermediate between controls and AD [107].

Markers of amyloid pathology

β-amyloid

Beta-amyloid peptides with 40 (Aβ40) and, especially, with 42 amino acids (Aβ42) are the major components of extracellular AD amyloid plaques. Aβ42 is considered to inversely reflect amyloid pathology, having high sensitivity and specificity (>85%) as compared to cognitively intact old subjects and is now recognized as one of the three clinically useful CSF biomarkers (the other two being T-tau and P-tau) for AD [28, 91]. Reduction of CSF Aβ42 in VCI of any type [106] and VCI-SSVD with or without signs of AD [33, 72, 108, 109], at levels similar to AD or intermediate between controls and AD have been reported. In other studies, the levels of Aβ42 in VCI were described as comparable to those of controls and higher than in AD [95, 98, 100, 101, 103], although overlap exists, with some VCI patients presenting with low levels [103]. Most of the above studies agreed that in MD, Aβ42 levels were reduced in a degree comparable to AD. However, the ratio of Aβ42/40, which is reduced in AD, has been found to be comparable to controls in "pure" VCI [110].

Amyloid precursor protein β

Soluble amyloid precursor protein β peptide (sAPPβ) is a product of APP cleavage with potential neurotrophic properties on axons [111]. CSF sAPPβ has been shown to correlate with white matter lesion load in CSF [77] and seems to be unaltered in the CSF in AD patients [112].

Markers of hypercoagulable state

Several plasma markers of coagulation/fibrinolysis have been associated with VCI-SSVD [54]. The clotting cascade is regulated by balance of activators and inhibitors. Activators may be raised in hypercoagulable state either independently or in parallel with the lowering of inhibitors. The validation of candidate biomarkers is complicated by the existence of heterogeneity among cerebral vessels in different brain regions in response to coagulation dysfunction [113]. In addition, a tenable association with VCI-SSVD has often been difficult to demonstrate with certainty for most proposed markers [114]. Clinical observations have been strengthened, at least in part, by a recent demonstration of a number of downregulated coagulation-related genes in SSVD, after postmortem gene-expression microarray analysis [115].

Markers of coagulation cascade

Fibrinogen is the endpoint plasma protein of the clotting cascade. Conflicting results have been published regarding its possible significance as a biomarker in VCI-SSVD [116–122].

Factor VII (also known as serum prothrombin conversion accelerator) has been found increased [123], whereas *antithrombin III*, a plasma protein that inactivates thrombin, and *D-dimer*, a fibrin degradation product, were found to be reduced in VCI-SSVD [113, 114, 124].

Markers derived from the endothelial cells, nearby tissue, or platelets

Many studies report that numerous proteins expressed by the endothelial cells are positively associated with lacunar infarcts or WML and thus increased in VCI-SSVD because of endothelial damage [113, 123, 125–128]. There is a still growing list of these molecules, which includes: *von Willebrand factor* (vWF) [123]; *thrombomodulin* (CD141 or BDCA-3); *the monokine induced by γ-interferon* (MIG) or *chemokine (C-X-C motif) ligand 9* (CXCL-9) [129]; *soluble intercellular adhesion molecule-1* (sICAM-1 also known as CD54); *soluble vascular cell adhesion molecule-1* (sVCAM-1); and *soluble E-selectin* (sE-selectin), the two latter mediating the adhesion of white cells (except neutrophils) to the vascular endothelium [130–133]. However, other neuropathology studies did not confirm a local endothelial activation, and showed that the endothelial layer remains intact in VCI-SSVD [134, 135]. Specifically, the local expression of ICAM-1 and thrombomodulin in the vascular endothelium of small arteries was not confirmative of an association with VCI-SSVD [136]. Thus, the usefulness of these markers for diagnostic purposes remains to be established, as recently reviewed [137].

Other neurotoxic/metabolic biomarkers

Homocysteine (Hcy) is the metabolic product of dietary methionine. Hcy is also synthesized in the liver and kidney. Increased total Hcy plasma levels is associated with risk, clinical deterioration and severity of WML in symptomatic patients with SSVD [138, 139]. Still, the links between hyperhomocysteinemia and SSVD (including a possible endothelial mechanism) are poorly understood [138]. As recently reviewed, when Hcy plasma levels are below 100 μM vascular effects are primarily seen, whereas adverse effects on the nerve cells appear, only when concentrations exceed 100 μM (above clinically-relevant range) [140]. Still we are far from a full identification and characterization of the key molecular pathways linking Hcy to VCI-SSVD. However, preclinical and clinical data support the notion that Hcy is an important mediator of VCI-SSVD.

B-type natriuretic peptide (BNP, also referred to as ventricular natriuretic peptide) is a polypeptide secreted by heart ventricles in response to excessive stretching of cardiomyocytes. Similarly, cardiac troponin T is a very sensitive and specific indicator of myocardial damage. A few studies report that serum levels of BNP [141, 142] or cardiac troponin T [143] are elevated in VCI-SSVD. These results need to be substantiated by other investigations to propose these molecules as relevant biomarkers for VCI-SSVD.

Oxidative stress markers

Clinical studies on markers of oxidative stress in patients with VCI-SSVD and cognitive impairment are scarce. The Framingham study reported lower plasma levels of *myeloperoxidase* in participants with greater WML volumes and silent brain infarcts [47]. *Asymmetric dimethylarginine* (ADMA) is a key chemical involved in normal endothelial function and thus cardiovascular health. Higher plasma ADMA levels were associated with an increased prevalence of silent brain infarcts after adjustment for traditional stroke risk factors, indicating its potential usefulness as a new biomarker of subclinical vascular brain injury [144]. Patients with large-vessel disease had higher oxidative stress (as measured by the serum levels of thiobarbituric acid-reactive substances), but lower antioxidant defense (as measured by serum levels of free thiol) compared to those with SSVD after an acute ischemic stroke [145].

Results and discussion

Overlapping and differentiating biomarker findings in VCI-SSVD and AD

Hitherto, there are no yet established biochemical markers for VCI-SSVD, although there are potential candidates. For AD, CSF T-tau, P-tau and Aβ42 have been included in the diagnostic criteria by the National Institute on Aging and the Alzheimer's Association workgroup for all phases of AD, published in 2011 [92]. By analogy, in VCI-SSVD a major step forward will be to stratify biochemically homogenous patient groups. From the evidence presented in the current work, a significantly elevated albumin ratio reflecting BCB/BBB dysfunction, a hallmark of VCI-SSVD, is a consistent finding in studies with VCI-SSVD and MD [32, 33, 146, 147]. In AD, the albumin ratio is not different from that of controls [33, 72, 147, 148].

Other promising biomarkers are those reflecting damage to the white matter, such as CSF NF-L and MBP. Both markers correlate with SSVD, but they have also been found to be elevated in AD. This overlap possibly reflects concomitant AD and SSVD pathology. However, both CSF NF-L and MBP can be of value in detecting damage to white matter in patients with VCI-SSVD or MD regardless of the white matter etiology. Markers, such as sulfatide, sAPPβ, MMP-2, MMP-3, MMP-9 and TIMP-1, also hold potential for VCI-SSVD biomarkers, though some of them (MMP-2, MMP-3 and MMP-9) have also been described to be altered in AD [33, 57, 62, 63, 77, 85–87, 149, 150]. Other glial and neuronal markers, such as YKL-40, GFAP, S100B and NSE, are also related to AD and are thus not specific [41, 42, 151–153]. Markers of inflammation (i.e. IL-6, TNF-α, TGF-β, VEGF, sICAM-1, sVCAM and sE-selectin) have all been found to be increased in both diseases [56, 154, 155]. Other markers of questionable specificity for SSVD, as compared to AD, are CRP, ADMA and Hcy, since they have also been found to be elevated in AD [57, 155]. Biomarkers closely related to alterations of the vessel wall (vWF, thrombomodulin) and partakers in the coagulation/fibrinolysis system (D-dimer, Factor VII, antithrombin III), rather than inflammation in general, may prove to be more specific for VCI-SSVD and need to be investigated in the context of AD differential diagnosis. It should be noted that the overlap among the above-mentioned biomarkers might be a result of heterogeneous AD populations containing MD patients emphasizing the need for further investigations of "pure" VCI-SSVD and AD cases.

At present, combination of markers reflecting SSVD with markers that seem to be more specific for AD pathology such as Aβ42, T-tau and especially P-tau, appears promising for the exclusion of pure AD or favoring the diagnosis of MD [33].

Are biomarkers useful for detection of VCI –SSVD in clinical practice?

Thus far, biochemical markers with potential benefit for the diagnosis of VCI-SSVD have limited use in every day clinical practice (see Table 1). Since combination of biomarkers increases accuracy of the AD diagnosis, it seems feasible that a multimodal biomarker approach may be beneficial for the diagnosis of VCI-SSVD as well. In the Ten Point Scale of Binswanger's disease (which is synonymous with VCI-SSVD), three axes of biomarkers are included: biochemical, imaging and clinical [34, 156]. Increased albumin ratio, reduced MMP-2, elevated NF-L in the absence of a characteristic AD CSF profile are emphasized as the most significant among biochemical markers [34, 156]. Individuals with the highest scores, i.e. presence of the most of the aforementioned biomarkers, are most likely to have VCI-SSVD. Of course, this scoring system requires

Table 1 Summary of studies on candidate CSF biomarkers for VaD, VCI and SSVD according to their discrimination power (vs. Controls and/or AD)

Candidate biomarker	Study [Ref]	Date	Change	HC *n*	NC *n*	VaD *n*	VCI *n*	SSVD *n*	AD *n*	Difference vs. Controls	Difference vs. AD	Sn/Sp vs. Controls	Sn/Sp vs. AD
Albumin ratio (CSF/serum)	Wallin et al. [30]	1990	↑	30	-	53	-	-	-	$P < 0.001$	-	-	-
	Bjerke et al [72]	2009	→	52	-	-	-	9	20	NS	NS	-	-
	Bjerke et al. [33]	2011	↑	30	-	-	-	26	30	$P < 0.005$	$P < 0.01$	-	-
	Wallin et al. [32]	2001	↑	18	-	-	-	25	-	$P < 0.001$	-	-	-
NSE	Blennow et al. [41]	1994	↑	33	-	19	-	-	45	$P < 0.0001$	NS	-	-
TNF-α	Tarkowski et al. [55]	1999	↑	25	-	33	-	-	34	$P < 0.001$	-	-	-
VEGF	Tarkowski et al. [56]	2002	↑	27	-	26	-	-	20	$P = 0.03$	NS	-	-
TGF-beta	Tarkowski et al. [56]	2002	↑	27	-	26	-	-	20	$P < 0.0004$	NS	-	-
YKL-40	Olsson et al. [59]	2013	↑	-	65	19	-	-	-	$P < 0.05$	-	-	-
MMP-9	Adair et al. [62]	2004	↑	8	-	15	-	-	30	$P < 0.003$	$P < 0.0001$	-	-
	Bjerke et al. [33]	2011	↑	30	-	-	-	26	30	$P < 0.05$	$P < 0.05$	-	-
MMP-10	Bjerke et al. [33]	2011	↑	30	-	-	-	26	30	$P < 0.005$	NS	-	-
MMP-2	Bjerke et al. [33]	2011	→	30	-	-	-	26	30	NS	NS	-	-
MMP-3	Bjerke et al. [33]	2011	→	30	-	-	-	26	30	NS	NS	-	-
TIMP-1	Ohrfelt et al. [57]	2011	↑	52	-	-	-	7	15	$P = 0.01$	-	-	-
	Ohrfelt et al. [57]	2011	↑	52	-	-	-	8	24	$P = 0.03$	-	-	-
	Bjerke et al. [33]	2011	↑	30	-	-	-	26	30	$P < 0.05$	$P < 0.005$	-	-
TIMP-2	Bjerke et al. [33]	2011	→	30	-	-	-	26	30	NS	NS	-	-
NF-L	Wallin et al. [32]	2001	↑	18	-	-	-	25	-	$P < 0.001$	-	Sn 68% Sp 85%	-
	Bjerke et al. [72]	2009	↑	52	-	-	-	9	20	$P < 0.001$	NS	-	-
	Bjerke et al. [33]	2011	↑	30	-	-	-	26	30	$P < 0.0001$	$P < 0.05$	-	-
MBP	Bjerke et al. [33]	2011	↑	30	-	-	-	26	30	$P < 0.0001$	$P < 0.005$	-	-
Sulfatide	Fredman et al. [85]	1992	↑	19	-	20	-	-	43	$P < 0.0001$	$P < 0.0001$	-	-
Total tau (τ_T)	Wallin et al. [32]	2001	→	18	-	-	-	25	-	NS	-	Sn 85% Sp 36%	-
	Paraskevas et al. [103]	2009	↑	68	-	23	-	-	92	$P < 0.05$	$P < 0.05$	-	Sn 80% Sp 86%
	Bjerke et al. [72]	2009	→	52	-	-	-	9	20	NS	$P < 0.005$	-	-
	Bjerke et al. [33]	2011	↑	30	-	-	-	26	30	$P < 0.005$	NS	-	-
Phospho-tau ($\tau_{p\text{-}181}$)	Paraskevas et al. [103]	2009	→	68	-	23	-	-	92	NS	$P < 0.01$	-	Sn 84% Sp79%
	Bjerke et al. [72]	2009	→	52	-	-	-	9	20	NS	$P < 0.005$	-	-
	Bjerke et al. [33]	2011	→	30	-	-	-	26	30	NS	$P < 0.05$	-	-
$A\beta_{42}$	Paraskevas et al. [103]	2009	→	68	-	23	-	-	92	NS	NS	-	Sn 73% Sp 70%
	Bjerke et al. [72]	2009	↓	52	-	-	-	9	20	$P < 0.05$	$P < 0.005$	-	-
	Bjerke et al. [33]	2011	↓	30	-	-	-	26	30	$P < 0.001$	NS	-	-
$A\beta_{42}$, τ_T, $\tau_{p\text{-}181}$ (combination)	Paraskevas et al. [103]	2009	↑	68	-	23	-	-	92	NS	$P < 0.01$	-	Sn 87% Sp 89%
$sAPP_\beta$	Bjerke et al. [77]	2014								Correlation with WML	-	-	-

VaD Vascular Dementia, *VCI* Vascular Cognitive Impairment, *SSVD* Subcortical Small Vessel Disease, *AD* Alzheimer's disease, *HC* Healthy Controls, *NC* Neurological Controls, *Sn/Sp* Sensitivity/Specificity, *n* number of controls/patients, ↓ reduced levels, ↑ increased levels, → no difference vs. controls, – not included, *NS* Not Significant validation and standardization in large multi-centers longitudinal studies.

Conclusion and future directions

VCI-SSVD is a common neurocognitive disorder with similar clinical manifestations similar to other disorders, such as AD. Underestimation of the impact of SSVD on cognition and insufficient knowledge of SSVD in AD may explain why VCI-SSVD is under-recognized in clinical practice and not often studied in research contexts. Biochemical markers may be of help for the (differential) diagnosis of VCI-SSVD. They can also be used for identifying patients with preclinical SSVD from apparently healthy controls. Furthermore, they have a potential to define a spectrum disorder with pure subcortical vascular disease (i.e. Binswanger's disease) at one end of the spectrum and pure AD at the other. In between will be the large group of MD patients that will remain a major diagnostic challenge.

This review of all biological markers studied in patients with VCI-SSVD identified several fluid biomarkers with evidence for use in diagnostic settings, while others are too early to be considered as potential SSVD biomarkers. There is little value of blood tests at this time since none of the above biomarkers have been adequately studied, whereas CSF helps to separate vascular and neurodegenerative causes based on the presence of BCB/BBB disruption and extracellular matrix breakdown. Obviously, many of the CSF reports cited in this review are based on small series of cases. Replication studies should be done to ensure the reproducibility of the results and calculation of positive and negative predictive values should be provided. At present, it is unlikely that single markers may be sufficient for diagnostic and differentiating purposes. Instead, a combination of biochemical and imaging markers as well as psychometrics will be necessary to improve the diagnostic accuracy.

A third potential use of fluid biomarkers is their application as surrogates for disease progression e.g. in clinical pharmacological trials. For that purpose, such biomarkers could be used if different levels of the biomarkers can reflect patients' clinical severity or extent of WML. If a biomarker fulfills this definition, it could be very valuable in clinical trials obviating the need for repeated expensive MRI examinations.

A fourth potential use of fluid biomarkers is to clarify the pathogenesis of the disorder, for example to verify an inflammatory underlying process, perhaps in a subgroup of patients, thus suggesting a (novel) target for therapy. Clearly, much further work needs to be done along these lines.

The search for an optimal panel of biomarkers with high sensitivity and specificity through a collaborative international network of biobanks, multi-center collections based on large patient cohorts, combined with population genetics, clinical trials and harmonized protocols and procedures will provide the crucial tools needed to enhance the likelihood of success in identifying valid biomarkers in VCI-SSVD [157]. In addition, research will benefit from innovative statistical approaches that allow handling large datasets, e.g. strategies used in the field of artificial intelligence. With combined efforts, the development of biomarkers in the VCI-SSVD field may not only foster therapeutic progress in VCI-SSVD but also in AD.

Abbreviations

AD: Alzheimer's disease; ADMA: Asymmetric dimethylarginine; Aβ40: Beta-amyloid peptide with 40 amino acids; Aβ42: Beta-amyloid peptide with 42 amino acids; BBB: Blood–brain barrier; BCB: Blood-cerebrospinal fluid barrier; BNP: B-type natriuretic peptide; CRP: C reactive protein; CSF: Cerebrospinal fluid; CT: Computed tomography; CXCL-9: Chemokine (C-X-C motif) ligand 9; FTD: Fronto-temporal dementia; GFAP: Glial fibrillary acidic protein; Hcy: Homocysteine; IL-6: Interleukin-6; ILs: Interleukins; MAG: Myelin-associated glycoprotein; MBP: Myelin basic protein; MD: Mixed type dementia; MIG: Monokine induced by γ-interferon; MMPs: Matrix metalloproteinases; MRI: Magnetic resonance imaging; NF-H: Neurofilament heavy subunit; NF-L: Neurolfilament light subunit; NF-M: Neurofilament medium subunit; NFs: Neurofilaments; NIHSS: National institute of health stroke scale; NSE: Neuron specific enolase; P-tau: Hyperphosphorylated tau; QA: Cerebrospinal fluid/serum albumin quotient; sAPPβ: soluble amyloid precursor protein β peptide; sE-selectin: soluble E-selectin; sICAM-1: soluble intercellular adhesion molecule-1; SSVD: Subcortical small vessel disease; sVCAM-1: soluble vascular cell adhesion molecule-1; TIMP-1: Tissue inhibitor of metalloproteinases-1; T-tau: Total tau; VCI: Vascular cognitive impairment; VCI-SSVD: Vascular cognitive impairment of the subcortical small vessel disease type; WML: White matter lesions

Acknowledgements

We would like to thank Dr. Vasilios Constandinides for his contribution in the preparation of the final version of the manuscript.

Funding

No funding was obtained for the preparation of the present manuscript.

Author's contributions

AW and EK contributed substantially and equally to the conception and design of the consensus report. Drafting and revising the manuscript critically for intellectual content was jointly performed by AW, EK, MB, SE, DH, BH, MJ, MK, LL, BM, SM, AM, EM-L, GP, BP, RR, LT, GT, GW, AK, MB and GR. All authors approved the final version of the manuscript.

Competing interests

EBM-L - none, EK - none, GP – none, MGK – none, ADK – none, MB - none. AW was consultant/speaker for Esai, Nutricia and received research funding from Roche diagnostics. SE was/is consultant for and/or received research funding from Janssen, ADxNeuroSciences, Innogenetics/Fujirebio Europe, Lundbeck, Pfizer, Novartis, UCB, Roche diagnostics, Nutricia/Danone.

Author details
[1]Department of Psychiatry and Neurochemistry, Institute of Neuroscience and Physiology, Sahlgrenska Academy at the University of Gothenburg, Mölndal, Sweden. [2]1st Department of Neurology, Eginition Hospital, Medical School, National and Kapodistrian University of Athens, Athens, Greece. [3]Department of Neurology, University Hospital Centre Zagreb, Medical School, University of Zagreb, Zagreb, Croatia. [4]Memory Clinic and Department of Neurology, Hospital Network Antwerp (ZNA) Middelheim and HogeBeuken, Antwerp, Belgium. [5]Reference Center for Biological Markers of Dementia, Department of Biomedical Sciences, Institute Born-Bunge, University of Antwerp, Antwerp, Belgium. [6]Department of Neurology, University Hospital Essen, Essen, Germany. [7]Department of Neurology, University of California, Irvine, California, USA. [8]Department of Neurology, University Medical Center Ljubljana, Ljubljana, Slovenia. [9]Department of Veterinary Sciences, University of Turin, Turin, Italy. [10]Department of Neurology, University Hospital "Alexandrovska", Medical University, Sofia, Bulgaria. [11]Institute of Neuroscience, Campus for Ageing and Vitality, Newcastle University, Newcastle upon Tyne NE4 5PL, UK. [12]Department of Neurology, Colentina Clinical Hospital, School of Medicine, 'Carol Davila' University of Medicine and Pharmacy, Bucharest, Romania. [13]Brain Bank Consultants, Amsterdam, The Netherlands. [14]2nd Department of Neurology, Attikon Hospital, Medical School, National and Kapodistrian University of Athens, Athens, Greece. [15]School of Public Health, University of Haifa, Haifa, Israel. [16]Department of Neurology, Sackler School of Medicine, Tel Aviv University, Tel Aviv, Israel. [17]University of New Mexico Health Sciences Center, Albuquerque, NM 87131, USA. [18]Memory Clinic at Department of Neuropsychiatry, Sahlgrenska University Hospital, Institute of Neuroscience and Physiology at Sahlgrenska Academy, University of Gothenburg, Wallinsgatan 6, SE-431 41 Mölndal, Sweden.

References

1. Erkinjuntti T. Diagnosis and management of vascular cognitive impairment and dementia. J Neural Transm Suppl. 2002;63:91–109.
2. Roman GC, Erkinjuntti T, Wallin A, Pantoni L, Chui HC. Subcortical ischaemic vascular dementia. Lancet Neurol. 2002;1(7):426–36.
3. Salvadori E, Poggesi A, Valenti R, Della Rocca E, Diciotti S, Mascalchi M, et al. The rehabilitation of attention in patients with mild cognitive impairment and brain subcortical vascular changes using the attention process training-II. The RehAtt study: rationale, design and methodology. Neurol Sci. 2016; 37(10):1653–62.
4. Jia J, Wei C, Liang J, Zhou A, Zuo X, Song H, et al. The effects of DL-3-n-butylphthalide in patients with vascular cognitive impairment without dementia caused by subcortical ischemic small vessel disease: a multicentre, randomized, double-blind, placebo-controlled trial. Alzheimers Dement. 2016;12(2):89–99.
5. Kalaria RN. Neuropathological diagnosis of vascular cognitive impairment and vascular dementia with implications for Alzheimer's disease. Acta Neuropathol. 2016;131(5):659–85.
6. de Leeuw FE, de Groot JC, Oudkerk M, Witteman JC, Hofman A, van Gijn J, et al. Hypertension and cerebral white matter lesions in a prospective cohort study. Brain. 2002;125(Pt 4):765–72.
7. Abraham HM, Wolfson L, Moscufo N, Guttmann CR, Kaplan RF, White WB. Cardiovascular risk factors and small vessel disease of the brain: blood pressure, white matter lesions, and functional decline in older persons. J Cereb Blood Flow Metab. 2016;36(1):132–42.
8. Filomena J, Riba-Llena I, Vinyoles E, Tovar JL, Mundet X, Castane X, et al. Short-term blood pressure variability relates to the presence of subclinical brain small vessel disease in primary hypertension. Hypertension. 2015;66(3): 634–40. discussion 445
9. Pavlovic AM, Pekmezovic T, Zidverc Trajkovic J, Svabic Medjedovic T, Veselinovic N, Radojicic A, et al. Baseline characteristic of patients presenting with lacunar stroke and cerebral small vessel disease may predict future development of depression. Int J Geriatr Psychiatry. 2016;31(1):58–65.
10. Toyoda G, Bokura H, Mitaki S, Onoda K, Oguro H, Nagai A, et al. Association of mild kidney dysfunction with silent brain lesions in neurologically normal subjects. Cerebrovasc Dis Extra. 2015;5(1):22–7.
11. Toyoda K. Cerebral small vessel disease and chronic kidney disease. J Stroke. 2015;17(1):31–7.
12. Staals J, Makin SD, Doubal FN, Dennis MS, Wardlaw JM. Stroke subtype, vascular risk factors, and total MRI brain small-vessel disease burden. Neurology. 2014;83(14):1228–34.
13. Ott A, Stolk RP, van Harskamp F, Pols HA, Hofman A, Breteler MM. Diabetes mellitus and the risk of dementia: the Rotterdam study. Neurology. 1999; 53(9):1937–42.
14. Dearborn JL, Schneider AL, Sharrett AR, Mosley TH, Bezerra DC, Knopman DS, et al. Obesity, insulin resistance, and incident small vessel disease on magnetic resonance imaging: atherosclerosis risk in communities study. Stroke. 2015;46(11):3131–6.
15. Alagiakrishnan K, Hsueh J, Zhang E, Khan K, Senthilselvan A. Small vessel disease/white matter disease of the brain and its association with osteoporosis. J Clin Med Res. 2015;7(5):297–302.
16. Lahousse L, Tiemeier H, Ikram MA, Brusselle GG. Chronic obstructive pulmonary disease and cerebrovascular disease: a comprehensive review. Respir Med. 2015;109(11):1371–80.
17. Durgan DJ, Bryan RM Jr. Cerebrovascular consequences of obstructive sleep apnea. J Am Heart Assoc. 2012;1(4):e000091.
18. Makedonov I, Black SE, MacIntosh BJ. Cerebral small vessel disease in aging and Alzheimer's disease: a comparative study using MRI and SPECT. Eur J Neurol. 2013;20(2):243–50.
19. Ortner M, Kurz A, Alexopoulos P, Auer F, Diehl-Schmid J, Drzezga A, et al. Small vessel disease, but neither amyloid load nor metabolic deficit, is dependent on age at onset in Alzheimer's disease. Biol Psychiatry. 2015;77(8):704–10.
20. Kim HJ, Im K, Kwon H, Lee JM, Kim C, Kim YJ, et al. Clinical effect of white matter network disruption related to amyloid and small vessel disease. Neurology. 2015;85(1):63–70.
21. Jang YK, Kwon H, Kim YJ, Jung NY, Lee JS, Lee J, et al. Early- vs late-onset subcortical vascular cognitive impairment. Neurology. 2016;86(6):527–34.
22. Bersano A, Debette S, Zanier ER, Lanfranconi S, De Simoni MG, Zuffardi O, et al. The genetics of small-vessel disease. Curr Med Chem. 2012;19(24):4124–41.
23. Popescu BO, Toescu EC, Popescu LM, Bajenaru O, Muresanu DF, Schultzberg M, et al. Blood–brain barrier alterations in ageing and dementia. J Neurol Sci. 2009;283(1–2):99–106.
24. Ueno M, Chiba Y, Matsumoto K, Murakami R, Fujihara R, Kawauchi M, et al. Blood–brain barrier damage in vascular dementia. Neuropathology. 2016; 36(2):115–24.
25. Srinivasan V, Braidy N, Chan EK, Xu YH, Chan DK. Genetic and environmental factors in vascular dementia: an update of blood brain barrier dysfunction. Clin Exp Pharmacol Physiol. 2016;43(5):515–21.
26. Wang M, Norman JE, Srinivasan VJ, Rutledge JC. Metabolic, inflammatory, and microvascular determinants of white matter disease and cognitive decline. Am J Neurodegener Dis. 2016;5(5):171-77.
27. Tibbling G, Link H, Ohman S. Principles of albumin and IgG analyses in neurological disorders. I. Establishment of reference values. Scand J Clin Lab Invest. 1977;37(5):385–90.
28. Blennow K, Hampel H, Weiner M, Zetterberg H. Cerebrospinal fluid and plasma biomarkers in Alzheimer disease. Nat Rev Neurol. 2010;6(3):131–44.
29. Farrall AJ, Wardlaw JM. Blood–brain barrier: ageing and microvascular disease–systematic review and meta-analysis. Neurobiol Aging. 2009;30(3):337–52.
30. Wallin A, Blennow K, Fredman P, Gottfries CG, Karlsson I, Svennerholm L. Blood brain barrier function in vascular dementia. Acta Neurol Scand. 1990; 81(4):318–22.
31. Wallin A, Sjogren M, Edman A, Blennow K, Regland B. Symptoms, vascular risk factors and blood–brain barrier function in relation to CT white-matter changes in dementia. Eur Neurol. 2000;44(4):229–35.
32. Wallin A, Sjogren M. Cerebrospinal fluid cytoskeleton proteins in patients with subcortical white-matter dementia. Mech Ageing Dev. 2001;122(16):1937–49.
33. Bjerke M, Zetterberg H, Edman A, Blennow K, Wallin A, Andreasson U. Cerebrospinal fluid matrix metalloproteinases and tissue inhibitor of metalloproteinases in combination with subcortical and cortical biomarkers in vascular dementia and Alzheimer's disease. J Alzheimers Dis. 2011;27(3): 665–76.
34. Rosenberg GA, Bjerke M, Wallin A. Multimodal markers of inflammation in the subcortical ischemic vascular disease type of vascular cognitive impairment. Stroke. 2014;45(5):1531–8.

35. Marchi N, Cavaglia M, Fazio V, Bhudia S, Hallene K, Janigro D. Peripheral markers of blood–brain barrier damage. Clin Chim Acta. 2004;342(1–2): 1–12.
36. Levada OA, Trailin AV. [Serum level of S100B as a marker of progression of vascular mild cognitive impairment into subcortical vascular dementia and therapy effectiveness]. Likars'ka sprava/Ministerstvo okhorony zdorov'ia Ukrainy. 2012;2(3–4):53–59.
37. Gao Q, Fan Y, Mu LY, Ma L, Song ZQ, Zhang YN. S100B and ADMA in cerebral small vessel disease and cognitive dysfunction. J Neurol Sci. 2015; 354(1–2):27–32.
38. Rothermundt M, Arolt V, Wiesmann M, Missler U, Peters M, Rudolf S, et al. S-100B is increased in melancholic but not in non-melancholic major depression. J Affect Disord. 2001;66(1):89–93.
39. Dittrich S, Sunyakumthorn P, Rattanavong S, Phetsouvanh R, Panyanivong P, Sengduangphachanh A, et al. Blood–brain barrier function and biomarkers of central nervous system injury in Rickettsial versus other neurological infections in Laos. AmJTrop Med Hyg. 2015;93(2):232–7.
40. Mecocci P, Parnetti L, Romano G, Scarelli A, Chionne F, Cecchetti R, et al. Serum anti-GFAP and anti-S100 autoantibodies in brain aging, Alzheimer's disease and vascular dementia. J Neuroimmunol. 1995;57(1–2):165–70.
41. Blennow K, Wallin A, Ekman R. Neuron specific enolase in cerebrospinal fluid: a biochemical marker for neuronal degeneration in dementia disorders? J Neural Transm Park Dis Dement Sect. 1994;8(3):183–91.
42. Wallin A, Blennow K, Rosengren LE. Glial fibrillary acidic protein in the cerebrospinal fluid of patients with dementia. Dementia. 1996;7(5):267–72.
43. Heneka MT, Golenbock DT, Latz E. Innate immunity in Alzheimer's disease. Nat Immunol. 2015;16(3):229–36.
44. Holmes C. Review: systemic inflammation and Alzheimer's disease. Neuropathol Appl Neurobiol. 2013;39(1):51–68.
45. Aribisala BS, Wiseman S, Morris Z, Valdes-Hernandez MC, Royle NA, Maniega SM, et al. Circulating inflammatory markers are associated with magnetic resonance imaging-visible perivascular spaces but not directly with white matter hyperintensities. Stroke. 2014;45(2):605–7.
46. Satizabal CL, Zhu YC, Mazoyer B, Dufouil C, Tzourio C. Circulating IL-6 and CRP are associated with MRI findings in the elderly: the 3C-Dijon study. Neurology. 2012;78(10):720–7.
47. Shoamanesh A, Preis SR, Beiser AS, Vasan RS, Benjamin EJ, Kase CS, et al. Inflammatory biomarkers, cerebral microbleeds, and small vessel disease: Framingham heart study. Neurology. 2015;84(8):825–32.
48. van Dijk EJ, Prins ND, Vermeer SE, Vrooman HA, Hofman A, Koudstaal PJ, et al. C-reactive protein and cerebral small-vessel disease: the Rotterdam scan study. Circulation. 2005;112(6):900–5.
49. Engelhart MJ, Geerlings MI, Meijer J, Kiliaan A, Ruitenberg A, van Swieten JC, et al. Inflammatory proteins in plasma and the risk of dementia: the rotterdam study. Arch Neurol. 2004;61(5):668–72.
50. Ravaglia G, Forti P, Maioli F, Chiappelli M, Montesi F, Tumini E, et al. Blood inflammatory markers and risk of dementia: the Conselice study of brain aging. Neurobiol Aging. 2007;28(12):1810–20.
51. Miralbell J, Soriano JJ, Spulber G, Lopez-Cancio E, Arenillas JF, Bargallo N, et al. Structural brain changes and cognition in relation to markers of vascular dysfunction. Neurobiol Aging. 2012;33(5):1003.e1009–17.
52. Wersching H, Duning T, Lohmann H, Mohammadi S, Stehling C, Fobker M, et al. Serum C-reactive protein is linked to cerebral microstructural integrity and cognitive function. Neurology. 2010;74(13):1022–9.
53. Bettcher BM, Yaffe K, Boudreau RM, Neuhaus J, Aizenstein H, Ding J, et al. Declines in inflammation predict greater white matter microstructure in older adults. Neurobiol Aging. 2015;36(2):948–54.
54. Vilar-Bergua A, Riba-Llena I, Nafria C, Bustamante A, Llombart V, Delgado P, et al. Blood and CSF biomarkers in brain subcortical ischemic vascular disease: involved pathways and clinical applicability. J Cereb Blood Flow Metab. 2016;36(1):55–71.
55. Tarkowski E, Blennow K, Wallin A, Tarkowski A. Intracerebral production of tumor necrosis factor-alpha, a local neuroprotective agent, in Alzheimer disease and vascular dementia. J Clin Immunol. 1999;19(4):223–30.
56. Tarkowski E, Issa R, Sjogren M, Wallin A, Blennow K, Tarkowski A, et al. Increased intrathecal levels of the angiogenic factors VEGF and TGF-beta in Alzheimer's disease and vascular dementia. Neurobiol Aging. 2002;23(2): 237–43.
57. Ohrfelt A, Andreasson U, Simon A, Zetterberg H, Edman A, Potter W, et al. Screening for new biomarkers for subcortical vascular dementia and Alzheimer's disease. Dement Geriatr Cogn Dis Extra. 2011;1(1):31–42.
58. Ozturk C, Ozge A, Yalin OO, Yilmaz IA, Delialioglu N, Yildiz C. Tet al. The diagnostic role of serum inflammatory and soluble proteins on dementia subtypes: correlation with cognitive and functional decline. Behav Neurol. 2007;18(4):207–15.
59. Olsson B, Hertze J, Lautner R, Zetterberg H, Nagga K, Hoglund K, et al. Microglial markers are elevated in the prodromal phase of Alzheimer's disease and vascular dementia. J Alzheimers Dis. 2013;33(1):45–53.
60. Weekman EM, Wilcock DM. Matrix metalloproteinase in blood–brain barrier breakdown in dementia. J Alzheimers Dis. 2016;49(4):893–903.
61. Rosenberg GA. Matrix metalloproteinase-mediated Neuroinflammation in vascular cognitive impairment of the Binswanger type. Cell Mol Neurobiol. 2016;36(2):195–202.
62. Adair JC, Charlie J, Dencoff JE, Kaye JA, Quinn JF, Camicioli RM, et al. Measurement of gelatinase B (MMP-9) in the cerebrospinal fluid of patients with vascular dementia and Alzheimer disease. Stroke. 2004; 35(6):e159–62.
63. Candelario-Jalil E, Thompson J, Taheri S, Grossetete M, Adair JC, Edmonds E, et al. Matrix metalloproteinases are associated with increased blood–brain barrier opening in vascular cognitive impairment. Stroke. 2011;42(5):1345–50.
64. Hoffman PN, Cleveland DW, Griffin JW, Landes PW, Cowan NJ, Price DL. Neurofilament gene expression: a major determinant of axonal caliber. Proc Natl Acad Sci U S A. 1987;84(10):3472–6.
65. Perrot R, Berges R, Bocquet A, Eyer J. Review of the multiple aspects of neurofilament functions, and their possible contribution to neurodegeneration. Mol Neurobiol. 2008;38(1):27–65.
66. Rosengren LE, Karlsson JE, Karlsson JO, Persson LI, Wikkelso C. Patients with amyotrophic lateral sclerosis and other neurodegenerative diseases have increased levels of neurofilament protein in CSF. J Neurochem. 1996;67(5): 2013–8.
67. Hu YY, He SS, Wang XC, Duan QH, Khatoon S, Iqbal K, et al. Elevated levels of phosphorylated neurofilament proteins in cerebrospinal fluid of Alzheimer disease patients. Neurosci Lett. 2002;320(3):156–60.
68. Norgren N, Karlsson JE, Rosengren L, Stigbrand T. Monoclonal antibodies selective for low molecular weight neurofilaments. Hybrid Hybridomics. 2002;21(1):53–9.
69. Gresle MM, Butzkueven H, Shaw G. Neurofilament proteins as body fluid biomarkers of neurodegeneration in multiple sclerosis. Mult Scler Int. 2011; 2011:315406.
70. Friede RL, Samorajski T. Axon caliber related to neurofilaments and microtubules in sciatic nerve fibers of rats and mice. Anat Rec. 1970;167(4): 379–87.
71. Sjogren M, Blomberg M, Jonsson M, Wahlund LO, Edman A, Lind K, et al. Neurofilament protein in cerebrospinal fluid: a marker of white matter changes. J Neurosci Res. 2001;66(3):510–6.
72. Bjerke M, Andreasson U, Rolstad S, Nordlund A, Lind K, Zetterberg H, et al. Subcortical vascular dementia biomarker pattern in mild cognitive impairment. Dement Geriatr Cogn Disord. 2009;28(4):348–56.
73. Jonsson M, Zetterberg H, van Straaten E, Lind K, Syversen S, Edman A, et al. Cerebrospinal fluid biomarkers of white matter lesions - cross-sectional results from the LADIS study. Eur J Neurol. 2010;17(3):377–82.
74. Norgren N, Rosengren L, Stigbrand T. Elevated neurofilament levels in neurological diseases. Brain Res. 2003;987(1):25–31.
75. Skillback T, Farahmand B, Bartlett JW, Rosen C, Mattsson N, Nagga K, et al. CSF neurofilament light differs in neurodegenerative diseases and predicts severity and survival. Neurology. 2014;83(21):1945–53.
76. Petzold A, Keir G, Warren J, Fox N, Rossor MN. A systematic review and meta-analysis of CSF neurofilament protein levels as biomarkers in dementia. Neurodegener Dis. 2007;4(2–3):185–94.
77. Bjerke M, Jonsson M, Nordlund A, Eckerstrom C, Blennow K, Zetterberg H, et al. Cerebrovascular biomarker profile is related to white matter disease and ventricular dilation in a LADIS Substudy. Dement Geriatr Cogn Dis Extra. 2014;4(3):385–94.
78. Brettschneider J, Petzold A, Schottle D, Claus A, Riepe M, Tumani H. The neurofilament heavy chain (NfH) in the cerebrospinal fluid diagnosis of Alzheimer's disease. Dement Geriatr Cogn Disord. 2006;21(5–6):291–5.
79. Omlin FX, Webster HD, Palkovits CG, Cohen SR. Immunocytochemical localization of basic protein in major dense line regions of central and peripheral myelin. J Cell Biol. 1982;95(1):242–8.
80. Yin X, Crawford TO, Griffin JW, Tu P, Lee VM, Li C, et al. Myelin-associated glycoprotein is a myelin signal that modulates the caliber of myelinated axons. J Neurosci. 1998;18(6):1953–62.

81. Wallin A, Blennow K, Uhlemann C, Langstrom G, Gottfries CG. White matter low attenuation on computed tomography in Alzheimer's disease and vascular dementia–diagnostic and pathogenetic aspects. Acta Neurol Scand. 1989;80(6):518–23.
82. Kalaria RN, Erkinjuntti T. Small vessel disease and subcortical vascular dementia. J Clin Neurol. 2006;2(1):1–11.
83. Brouns R, De Vil B, Cras P, De Surgeloose D, Marien P, De Deyn PP. Neurobiochemical markers of brain damage in cerebrospinal fluid of acute ischemic stroke patients. Clin Chem. 2010;56(3):451–8.
84. Hjalmarsson C, Bjerke M, Andersson B, Blennow K, Zetterberg H, Aberg ND, et al. Neuronal and glia-related biomarkers in cerebrospinal fluid of patients with acute ischemic stroke. J Cent Nerv Syst Dis. 2014;6:51–8.
85. Fredman P, Wallin A, Blennow K, Davidsson P, Gottfries CG, Svennerholm L. Sulfatide as a biochemical marker in cerebrospinal fluid of patients with vascular dementia. Acta Neurol Scand. 1992;85(2):103–6.
86. Tullberg M, Mansson JE, Fredman P, Lekman A, Blennow K, Ekman R, et al. CSF sulfatide distinguishes between normal pressure hydrocephalus and subcortical arteriosclerotic encephalopathy. J Neurol Neurosurg Psychiatry. 2000;69(1):74–81.
87. Jonsson M, Zetterberg H, Rolstad S, Edman A, Gouw AA, Bjerke M, et al. Low cerebrospinal fluid sulfatide predicts progression of white matter lesions: the LADIS study. Dement Geriatr Cogn Disord. 2012;34(1):61–7.
88. Han X, Fagan AM, Cheng H, Morris JC, Xiong C, Holtzman DM. Cerebrospinal fluid sulfatide is decreased in subjects with incipient dementia. Ann Neurol. 2003;54(1):115–9.
89. Tarkowski E, Tullberg M, Fredman P, Wikkelso C. Correlation between intrathecal sulfatide and TNF-alpha levels in patients with vascular dementia. Dement Geriatr Cogn Disord. 2003;15(4):207–11.
90. Zetterberg H, Lautner R, Skillback T, Rosen C, Shahim P, Mattsson N, et al. CSF in Alzheimer's disease. Adv Clin Chem. 2014;65:143–72.
91. Cavedo E, Lista S, Khachaturian Z, Aisen P, Amouyel P, Herholz K, et al. The road ahead to cure Alzheimer's disease: development of biological markers and Neuroimaging methods for prevention trials across all stages and target populations. J Prev Alzheimers Dis. 2014;1(3):181–202.
92. McKhann GM, Knopman DS, Chertkow H, Hyman BT, Jack CR Jr, Kawas CH, et al. The diagnosis of dementia due to Alzheimer's disease: recommendations from the National Institute on Aging-Alzheimer's Association workgroups on diagnostic guidelines for Alzheimer's disease. Alzheimers Dement. 2011;7(3):263–9.
93. Dubois B, Feldman HH, Jacova C, Hampel H, Molinuevo JL, Blennow K, et al. Advancing research diagnostic criteria for Alzheimer's disease: the IWG-2 criteria. Lancet Neurol. 2014;13(6):614–29.
94. Mori H, Hosoda K, Matsubara E, Nakamoto T, Furiya Y, Endoh R, et al. Tau in cerebrospinal fluids: establishment of the sandwich ELISA with antibody specific to the repeat sequence in tau. Neurosci Lett. 1995;186(2–3):181–3.
95. Kapaki E, Paraskevas GP, Zalonis I, Zournas C. CSF tau protein and beta-amyloid (1–42) in Alzheimer's disease diagnosis: discrimination from normal ageing and other dementias in the Greek population. Eur J Neurol. 2003; 10(2):119–28.
96. Paraskevas GP, Kapaki E, Liappas I, Theotoka I, Mamali I, Zournas C, et al. The diagnostic value of cerebrospinal fluid tau protein in dementing and nondementing neuropsychiatric disorders. J Geriatr Psychiatry Neurol. 2005;18(3):163–73.
97. Tato RE, Frank A, Hernanz A. Tau protein concentrations in cerebrospinal fluid of patients with dementia of the Alzheimer type. J Neurol Neurosurg Psychiatry. 1995;59(3):280–3.
98. Andreasen N, Minthon L, Davidsson P, Vanmechelen E, Vanderstichele H, Winblad B, et al. Evaluation of CSF-tau and CSF-Abeta42 as diagnostic markers for Alzheimer disease in clinical practice. Arch Neurol. 2001;58(3):373–9.
99. Andreasen N, Vanmechelen E, Van de Voorde A, Davidsson P, Hesse C, Tarvonen S, et al. Cerebrospinal fluid tau protein as a biochemical marker for Alzheimer's disease: a community based follow up study. J Neurol Neurosurg Psychiatry. 1998;64(3):298–305.
100. Jia JP, Meng R, Sun YX, Sun WJ, Ji XM, Jia LF. Cerebrospinal fluid tau, Abeta1-42 and inflammatory cytokines in patients with Alzheimer's disease and vascular dementia. Neurosci Lett. 2005;383(1–2):12–6.
101. Stefani A, Bernardini S, Panella M, Pierantozzi M, Nuccetelli M, Koch G, et al. AD with subcortical white matter lesions and vascular dementia: CSF markers for differential diagnosis. J Neurol Sci. 2005;237(1–2):83–8.
102. Leszek J, Malyszczak K, Janicka B, Kiejna A, Wiak A. Total tau in cerebrospinal fluid differentiates Alzheimer's disease from vascular dementia. Med Sci Monit. 2003;9(11):CR484–8.
103. Paraskevas GP, Kapaki E, Papageorgiou SG, Kalfakis N, Andreadou E, Zalonis I, et al. CSF biomarker profile and diagnostic value in vascular dementia. Eur J Neurol. 2009;16(2):205–11.
104. Vandermeeren M, Mercken M, Vanmechelen E, Six J, van de Voorde A, Martin JJ, et al. Detection of tau proteins in normal and Alzheimer's disease cerebrospinal fluid with a sensitive sandwich enzyme-linked immunosorbent assay. J Neurochem. 1993;61(5):1828–34.
105. Vigo-Pelfrey C, Seubert P, Barbour R, Blomquist C, Lee M, Lee D, et al. Elevation of microtubule-associated protein tau in the cerebrospinal fluid of patients with Alzheimer's disease. Neurology. 1995;45(4):788–93.
106. Kaerst L, Kuhlmann A, Wedekind D, Stoeck K, Lange P, Zerr I. Cerebrospinal fluid biomarkers in Alzheimer's disease, vascular dementia and ischemic stroke patients: a critical analysis. J Neurol. 2013;260(11):2722–7.
107. Hermann P, Romero C, Schmidt C, Reis C, Zerr I. CSF biomarkers and neuropsychological profiles in patients with cerebral small-vessel disease. PLoS One. 2014;9(8):e105000.
108. Wallin A, Nordlund A, Jonsson M, Blennow K, Zetterberg H, Ohrfelt A, et al. Alzheimer's disease-subcortical vascular disease spectrum in a hospital-based setting: overview of results from the Gothenburg MCI and dementia studies. J Cereb Blood Flow Metab. 2016;36(1):95–113.
109. Rosenberg GA, Prestopnik J, Adair JC, Huisa BN, Knoefel J, Caprihan A, et al. Validation of biomarkers in subcortical ischaemic vascular disease of the Binswanger type: approach to targeted treatment trials. J Neurol Neurosurg Psychiatry. 2015;86(12):1324–30.
110. Lewczuk P, Esselmann H, Otto M, Maler JM, Henkel AW, Henkel MK, et al. Neurochemical diagnosis of Alzheimer's dementia by CSF Abeta42, Abeta42/Abeta40 ratio and total tau. Neurobiol Aging. 2004;25(3):273–81.
111. Chasseigneaux S, Allinquant B. Functions of Abeta, sAPPalpha and sAPPbeta : similarities and differences. J Neurochem. 2012;120(Suppl 1):99–108.
112. Rosen C, Andreasson U, Mattsson N, Marcusson J, Minthon L, Andreasen N, et al. Cerebrospinal fluid profiles of amyloid beta-related biomarkers in Alzheimer's disease. NeuroMolecular Med. 2012;14(1):65–73.
113. Kohriyama T, Yamaguchi S, Tanaka E, Yamamura Y, Nakamura S. Coagulation and fibrinolytic parameters as predictors for small-vessel disease revealed by magnetic resonance imaging of the brain. Rinsho Shinkeigaku. 1996;36(5):640–7.
114. Wiseman S, Marlborough F, Doubal F, Webb DJ, Wardlaw J. Blood markers of coagulation, fibrinolysis, endothelial dysfunction and inflammation in lacunar stroke versus non-lacunar stroke and non-stroke: systematic review and meta-analysis. Cerebrovasc Dis. 2014;37(1):64–75.
115. Ritz MF, Grond-Ginsbach C, Kloss M, Tolnay M, Fluri F, Bonati LH, et al. Identification of inflammatory, metabolic, and cell survival pathways contributing to cerebral small vessel disease by postmortem gene expression microarray. Curr Neurovasc Res. 2016;13(1):58–67.
116. Kilpatrick TJ, Matkovic Z, Davis SM, McGrath CM, Dauer RJ. Hematologic abnormalities occur in both cortical and lacunar infarction. Stroke. 1993; 24(12):1945–50.
117. Bath PM, Blann A, Smith N, Butterworth RJ. Von Willebrand factor, P-selectin and fibrinogen levels in patients with acute ischaemic and haemorrhagic stroke, and their relationship with stroke sub-type and functional outcome. Platelets. 1998;9(3–4):155–9.
118. Salobir B, Sabovic M, Peternel P, Stegnar M, Grad A. Classic risk factors, hypercoagulability and migraine in young women with cerebral lacunar infarctions. Acta Neurol Scand. 2002;105(3):189–95.
119. Jood K, Danielson J, Ladenvall C, Blomstrand C, Jern C. Fibrinogen gene variation and ischemic stroke. J Thromb Haemost. 2008;6(6):897–904.
120. Alvarez-Perez FJ, Castelo-Branco M, Alvarez-Sabin J. Usefulness of measurement of fibrinogen, D-dimer, D-dimer/fibrinogen ratio, C reactive protein and erythrocyte sedimentation rate to assess the pathophysiology and mechanism of ischaemic stroke. J Neurol Neurosurg Psychiatry. 2011;82(9):986–92.
121. Beer C, Blacker D, Hankey GJ, Puddey IB. Association of clinical and aetiologic subtype of acute ischaemic stroke with inflammation, oxidative stress and vascular function: a cross-sectional observational study. Med Sci Monit. 2011;17(9):CR467–73.
122. Zhang B, Zhang W, Li X, Pu S, Yin J, Yang N, et al. Admission markers predict lacunar and non-lacunar stroke in young patients. Thromb Res. 2011;128(1):14–7.
123. Vischer UM. Von Willebrand factor, endothelial dysfunction, and cardiovascular disease. J Thromb Haemost. 2006;4(6):1186–93.
124. Isenegger J, Meier N, Lammle B, Alberio L, Fischer U, Nedeltchev K, et al. D-dimers predict stroke subtype when assessed early. Cerebrovasc Dis. 2010; 29(1):82–6.

125. Kario K, Matsuo T, Kobayashi H, Hoshide S, Shimada K. Hyperinsulinemia and hemostatic abnormalities are associated with silent lacunar cerebral infarcts in elderly hypertensive subjects. J Am Coll Cardiol. 2001;37(3):871–7.
126. Kearney-Schwartz A, Rossignol P, Bracard S, Felblinger J, Fay R, Boivin JM, et al. Vascular structure and function is correlated to cognitive performance and white matter hyperintensities in older hypertensive patients with subjective memory complaints. Stroke. 2009;40(4):1229–36.
127. Nagai M, Hoshide S, Kario K. Association of prothrombotic status with markers of cerebral small vessel disease in elderly hypertensive patients. Am J Hypertens. 2012;25(10):1088–94.
128. Colombatti R, De Bon E, Bertomoro A, Casonato A, Pontara E, Omenetto E, et al. Coagulation activation in children with sickle cell disease is associated with cerebral small vessel vasculopathy. PLoS One. 2013;8(10):e78801.
129. Salmaggi A, Gelati M, Dufour A, Corsini E, Pagano S, Baccalini R, et al. Expression and modulation of IFN-gamma-inducible chemokines (IP-10, Mig, and I-TAC) in human brain endothelium and astrocytes: possible relevance for the immune invasion of the central nervous system and the pathogenesis of multiple sclerosis. J Interf Cytokine Res. 2002;22(6):631–40.
130. de Leeuw FE, de Kleine M, Frijns CJ, Fijnheer R, van Gijn J, Kappelle LJ. Endothelial cell activation is associated with cerebral white matter lesions in patients with cerebrovascular disease. Ann N Y Acad Sci. 2002;977:306–14.
131. Deanfield JE, Halcox JP, Rabelink TJ. Endothelial function and dysfunction: testing and clinical relevance. Circulation. 2007;115(10):1285–95.
132. Han JH, Wong KS, Wang YY, Fu JH, Ding D, Hong Z. Plasma level of sICAM-1 is associated with the extent of white matter lesion among asymptomatic elderly subjects. Clin Neurol Neurosurg. 2009;111(10):847–51.
133. Rouhl RP, Damoiseaux JG, Lodder J, Theunissen RO, Knottnerus IL, Staals J, et al. Vascular inflammation in cerebral small vessel disease. Neurobiol Aging. 2012;33(8):1800–6.
134. Craggs LJ, Hagel C, Kuhlenbaeumer G, Borjesson-Hanson A, Andersen O, Viitanen M, et al. Quantitative vascular pathology and phenotyping familial and sporadic cerebral small vessel diseases. Brain Pathol. 2013;23(5):547–57.
135. Lammie GA. Hypertensive cerebral small vessel disease and stroke. Brain Pathol. 2002;12(3):358–70.
136. Giwa MO, Williams J, Elderfield K, Jiwa NS, Bridges LR, Kalaria RN, et al. Neuropathologic evidence of endothelial changes in cerebral small vessel disease. Neurology. 2012;78(3):167–74.
137. Hainsworth AH, Oommen AT, Bridges LR. Endothelial cells and human cerebral small vessel disease. Brain Pathol. 2015;25(1):44–50.
138. Hassan A, Hunt BJ, O'Sullivan M, Bell R, D'Souza R, Jeffery S, et al. Homocysteine is a risk factor for cerebral small vessel disease, acting via endothelial dysfunction. Brain. 2004;127(Pt 1):212–9.
139. Pavlovic AM, Pekmezovic T, Obrenovic R, Novakovic I, Tomic G, Mijajlovic M, et al. Increased total homocysteine level is associated with clinical status and severity of white matter changes in symptomatic patients with subcortical small vessel disease. Clin Neurol Neurosurg. 2011;113(9):711–5.
140. Hainsworth AH, Yeo NE, Weekman EM, Wilcock DM. Homocysteine, hyperhomocysteinemia and vascular contributions to cognitive impairment and dementia (VCID). Biochim Biophys Acta. 2016;1862(5):1008–17.
141. Kondziella D, Gothlin M, Fu M, Zetterberg H, Wallin A. B-type natriuretic peptide plasma levels are elevated in subcortical vascular dementia. Neuroreport. 2009;20(9):825–7.
142. Mirza SS, de Bruijn RF, Koudstaal PJ, van den Meiracker AH, Franco OH, Hofman A, et al. The N-terminal pro B-type natriuretic peptide, and risk of dementia and cognitive decline: a 10-years follow-up study in the general population. J Neurol Neurosurg Psychiatry. 2016;87(4):356–62.
143. Schneider AL, Rawlings AM, Sharrett AR, Alonso A, Mosley TH, Hoogeveen RC, et al. High-sensitivity cardiac troponin T and cognitive function and dementia risk: the atherosclerosis risk in communities study. Eur Heart J. 2014;35(27):1817–24.
144. Pikula A, Boger RH, Beiser AS, Maas R, DeCarli C, Schwedhelm E, et al. Association of plasma ADMA levels with MRI markers of vascular brain injury: Framingham offspring study. Stroke. 2009;40(9):2959–64.
145. Tsai NW, Chang YT, Huang CR, Lin YJ, Lin WC, Cheng BC, et al. Association between oxidative stress and outcome in different subtypes of acute ischemic stroke. Biomed Res Int. 2014;2014:256879.
146. Wallin A, Ohrfelt A, Bjerke M. Characteristic clinical presentation and CSF biomarker pattern in cerebral small vessel disease. J Neurol Sci. 2012;322(1–2, 192):–16.
147. Blennow K, Wallin A, Fredman P, Karlsson I, Gottfries CG, Svennerholm L. Blood–brain barrier disturbance in patients with Alzheimer's disease is related to vascular factors. Acta Neurol Scand. 1990;81(4):323–6.
148. Frolich L, Kornhuber J, Ihl R, Fritze J, Maurer K, Riederer P. Integrity of the blood-CSF barrier in dementia of Alzheimer type: CSF/serum ratios of albumin and IgG. Eur Arch Psychiatry Clin Neurosci. 1991;240(6):363–6.
149. Mroczko B, Groblewska M, Zboch M, Kulczynska A, Koper OM, Szmitkowski M, et al. Concentrations of matrix metalloproteinases and their tissue inhibitors in the cerebrospinal fluid of patients with Alzheimer's disease. J Alzheimers Dis. 2014;40(2):351–7.
150. Horstmann S, Budig L, Gardner H, Koziol J, Deuschle M, Schilling C, et al. Matrix metalloproteinases in peripheral blood and cerebrospinal fluid in patients with Alzheimer's disease. Int Psychogeriatr. 2010;22(6):966–72.
151. Peskind ER, Griffin WS, Akama KT, Raskind MA, Van Eldik LJ. Cerebrospinal fluid S100B is elevated in the earlier stages of Alzheimer's disease. Neurochem Int. 2001;39(5–6):409–13.
152. Petzold A, Jenkins R, Watt HC, Green AJ, Thompson EJ, Keir G, et al. Cerebrospinal fluid S100B correlates with brain atrophy in Alzheimer's disease. Neurosci Lett. 2003;336(3):167–70.
153. Craig-Schapiro R, Perrin RJ, Roe CM, Xiong C, Carter D, Cairns NJ, et al. YKL-40: a novel prognostic fluid biomarker for preclinical Alzheimer's disease. Biol Psychiatry. 2010;68(10):903–12.
154. Huang CW, Tsai MH, Chen NC, Chen WH, Lu YT, Lui CC, et al. Clinical significance of circulating vascular cell adhesion molecule-1 to white matter disintegrity in Alzheimer's dementia. Thromb Haemost. 2015;114(6):1230–40.
155. Gubandru M, Margina D, Tsitsimpikou C, Goutzourelas N, Tsarouhas K, Ilie M, et al. Alzheimer's disease treated patients showed different patterns for oxidative stress and inflammation markers. Food Chem Toxicol. 2013;61: 209–14.
156. Rosenberg GA, Wallin A, Wardlaw JM, Markus HS, Montaner J, Wolfson L, et al. Consensus statement for diagnosis of subcortical small vessel disease. J Cereb Blood Flow Metab. 2016;36(1):6–25.
157. Ravid R. The uniqueness of biobanks for neurological and psychiatric diseases: potentials and pitfalls. Pathobiology. 2014;81(5–6):237–44.

Posterior reversible encephalopathy syndrome in association with exacerbation of chronic obstructive pulmonary disease

Sushil Khanal* and Subhash Prasad Acharya

Abstract

Background: Posterior reversible encephalopathy syndrome (PRES) is a reversible clinical and neurological entity. There are varieties of comorbid conditions which are associated with PRES. Chronic obstructive pulmonary disease (COPD) is a rare predisposing factor for the development of PRES.

Case presentation: A 55 year old female who was being treated for acute exacerbation of COPD developed altered sensorium and multiple episodes of seizure. Characteristic imaging findings and associated clinical symptoms led us to a diagnosis of PRES in our patient.

Conclusion: Association of PRES and COPD is a rare entity. The diagnosis of PRES should be brought to mind if there is encephalopathy or seizure in COPD exacerbation.

Keywords: Chronic obstructive pulmonary disease, Posterior reversible encephalopathy syndrome, Encephalopathy, Seizure

Background

Posterior Reversible Encephalopathy Syndrome (PRES) is characterized by headache, seizure, altered mental status and visual disturbances. It is a clinical and radiological entity and typically causes reversible changes in the posterior circulation system of the brain [1]. The association of PRES has been described frequently with number of medical conditions like hypertensive encephalopathy, eclampsia, and the use of cytotoxic and immunosuppressant drugs [2]. To the best of our knowledge, there are few case reports of PRES in the background of Chronic obstructive pulmonary disease (COPD). Here, we present a case of a 55 year old female with COPD exacerbation developing the characteristics features of PRES.

Case presentation

A 55 year old female patient was being treated at local hospital for 3 days symptoms suggestive of acute exacerbation of COPD. She was referred to our center for further management after she developed multiple episodes of seizure followed by loss of consciousness on the first day of hospital admission. The patient's relatives revealed that she had history of COPD for last 5 years but was not compliant to inhaler medications. Her family history was unremarkable. She has been a smoker for the last 30 years. No other significant history was available.

On examination, the patient was drowsy, and was not obeying commands. She had a temperature of 37.6 °C, blood pressure of 130/80 mmHg, pulse rate of 96/min and respiratory rate of 26/min. She had widespread expiratory wheeze. While the patient was regaining consciousness, she reported of headache and a decreased vision. An ocular examination revealed normally reactive pupil and fundus. Cranial nerves examination was unremarkable. Motor and sensory function examination was normal. There was no any clinical sign of meningeal irritation.

Her laboratory tests on admission were as follows: hemoglobin, 17 g/dl; white blood cells, 12640 /Cumm; platelets, 155000 /Cumm; urea, 37 mg/ dl; creatinine

* Correspondence: khanaliom@gmail.com
Department of Critical Care, Grande International Hospital (GIH), Kathmandu, Nepal

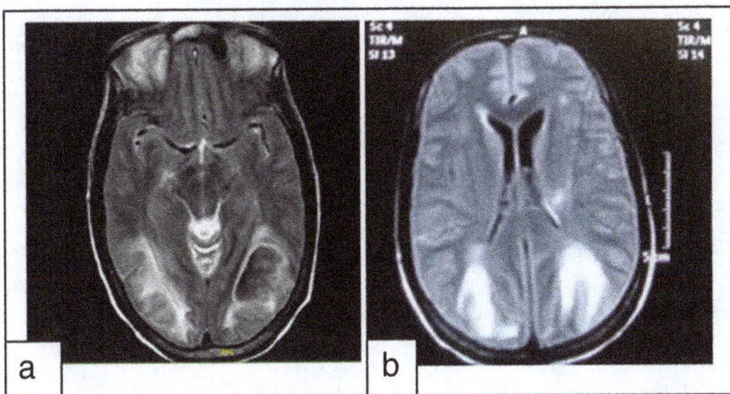

Fig. 1 MRI findings (T2 sequence (**a**), FLAIR (**b**)) showing the diffuse confluent white matter hyperintensities in bilateral parieto- occipital region

0.3 mg/dl; Na, 132 meq/L; K,4.6 meq/L. Chest X-radiography revealed emphysematous changes. Arterial blood gas finding showed the pH, 7.56; pCO_2, 46.2; pO_2, 81.0; HCO_3, 41.5. Magnetic Resonance Imaging (MRI) demonstrated hyperintense lesions in the bilateral parieto-occipital region consistent with PRES (Fig.1).

Our patient was treated with salbutamol and ipratropium nebulisation, hydrocortisone, levetiracetam and other supportive care. The patient was continuously monitored for hemodynamic stability in Intensive Care Unit (ICU) for 2 days and was later transferred to a general ward. The patient continued to improve clinically and was discharged home on the sixth day of hospitalization without any respiratory and neurological symptom.

Discussion and conclusion

Posterior reversible encephalopathy syndrome (PRES) has been described as a clinical syndrome of headache, altered level of consciousness, visual changes, and seizure. There is a characteristic neuroimaging finding of posterior cerebral white matter edema in PRES. Although pathogenesis of PRES is unclear, it is likely to be the consequences of disordered cerebral autoregulation and endothelial dysfunction [1].

A variety of clinical conditions like hypertensive emergency, renal disease, pre-eclampsia/eclampsia and use of immunosuppressive agents are commonly associated with the development of PRES. There are very few case reports linking the relation of PRES with COPD [3, 4]. Increased level of circulating tumor necrosis factor alpha (TNFα), interleukin-1 (IL-1) and endothelin-1 (ET-1) in COPD causes endothelial dysfunction in cerebral arteries. Infection during COPD exacerbation also raises the levels of IL-1, TNFα and ET-1. This may be the most probable pathophysiology behind the development of PRES during COPD exacerbation [4].

Differential diagnosis of PRES include other neurologic conditions, such as stroke, venous thrombosis, toxic or metabolic encephalopathy, demyelinating disorders, vasculitis, or encephalitis. As there is limited history and broad differential diagnosis, early neuroimaging is crucial for the diagnosis of PRES [5]. Typical MRI findings in PRES are of bilateral white-matter abnormalities in vascular watershed areas in the posterior regions of both cerebral hemispheres, affecting mostly the occipital and parietal lobes [6].

The predilection of posterior brain regions in PRES is not well understood. One possibility involves the regional heterogeneity of the sympathetic innervation of the intracranial arterioles, with better development of sympathetic autoregulation in the anterior circulation than in the posterior circulation [7]. Removal of precipitating factors seem to enhance the full recovery of PRES within a period of days to weeks in most of the cases. However, radiologic improvement lags behind clinical recovery [8, 9].

In Conclusion, there is high rate of admission of COPD in the Intensive Care unit. Although the association of COPD and PRES is rare entity, the differential diagnosis of PRES should be kept in the mind whenever there is encephalopathy or seizure in COPD exacerbation.

Abbreviations

COPD: Chronic obstructive pulmonary disease; ET-1: Endothelin-1; ICU: Intensive care unit; IL-1: Interleukin-1; MRI: Magnetic resonance imaging; PRES: Posterior reversible encephalopathy syndrome; TNFα: Tumor necrosis factor alpha

Acknowledgements

The authors thank Department of Critical Care (Grande International Hospital, Kathmandu).

Funding

Not Applicable

Authors' contributions

Both authors read and approved the final manuscript.

Competing interests

The authors declare that they have no competing interests.

References

1. Hinchey J, Chaves C, Appignani B, Breen J, Pao L, Wang A, et al. A reversible posterior leukoencephalopathy syndrome. N Engl J Med. 1996;334:494–500.
2. Chambers KA, Cain TW. Postpartum blindness: two cases. Ann Emerg Med. 2004;43:243–6.
3. Tanaka H, Yamamoto D, Uchiyama T, Ohashi T. Posterior reversible encephalopathy syndrome in a woman with chronic obstructive pulmonary disease. Intern Med. 2017;56(9):1119–20.
4. Dardis C, Craciun R, Schell R. Posterior reversible encephalopathy syndrome in the setting of COPD:proposed pathogenesis. Med Hypotheses. 2013;80:197–200.
5. Ay H, Buonanno FS, Schaefer PW, Le DA, Wang B, Gonzalez RG, Koroshetz WJ. Posterior leukoencephalopathy without severe hypertension: utility of diffusion-weighted MRI. Neurology. 1998;51:1369–76.
6. Bartynski W. Posterior reversible encephalopathy syndrome, part 1: fundamental imaging and clinical features. AJNR Am J Neuroradiol. 2008;29:1036–42.
7. Beausang-Linder M, Bill A. Cerebral circulation in acute arterial hypertension-protective effects of sympathetic nervous activity. Acta Physiol Scand. 1981; 111(2):193.
8. Lee VH, Wijdicks EF, Manno EM, Rabinstein AA. Clinical spectrum of reversible posterior leukoencephalopathy syndrome. Arch Neurol. 2008; 65(2):205.
9. Roth C, Ferbert A. Posterior reversible encephalopathy syndrome: long-term follow-up. J Neurol Neurosurg Psychiatry. 2010;81(7):773.

21

A case report of delayed cortical infarction adjacent to sulcal clots after traumatic subarachnoid hemorrhage in the absence of proximal vasospasm

Christian Schinke[1,3], Viktor Horst[2], Ludwig Schlemm[1,2,4,5], Matthias Wawra[1], Michael Scheel[6], Jed A. Hartings[7] and Jens P. Dreier[1,2,3,8,9*]

Abstract

Background: Cortical ischemic lesions represent the predominant pathomorphological pattern of focal lesions after aneurysmal subarachnoid hemorrhage (aSAH). Autopsy studies suggest that they occur adjacent to subarachnoid blood and are related to spasm of small cortical rather than proximal arteries. Recent clinical monitoring studies showed that cortical spreading depolarizations, which induce cortical arterial spasms, are involved in lesion development. If subarachnoid blood induces adjacent cortical lesions, it would be expected that (i) they also develop after traumatic subarachnoid hemorrhage (tSAH), and (ii) lesions after tSAH can occur in absence of angiographic vasospasm, as was found for aSAH.

Case presentation: An 86-year-old woman was admitted to our hospital with fluctuating consciousness after hitting her head during a fall. The initial computed tomography (CT) was significant for tSAH in cortical sulci. On day 8, the patient experienced a secondary neurological deterioration with reduced consciousness and global aphasia. Whereas the CT scan on day 9 was still unremarkable, magnetic resonance imaging (MRI) on day 10 revealed new cortical laminar infarcts adjacent to sulcal blood clots. Proximal vasospasm was ruled out using MR and CT angiography and Doppler sonography. CT on day 14 confirmed the delayed infarcts.

Conclusions: We describe a case of delayed cortical infarcts around sulcal blood clots after tSAH in the absence of proximal vasospasm, similar to results found previously for aSAH. As for aSAH, this case suggests that assessment of angiographic vasospasm is not sufficient to screen for risk of delayed infarcts after tSAH. Electrocorticography is suggested as a complementary method to monitor the hypothesized mechanism of spreading depolarizations.

Keywords: Traumatic subarachnoid hemorrhage, Delayed ischemic neurological deficits, Cortical spreading depolarization

Background

In autopsy studies, cortical ischemic lesions are the predominant pattern of parenchymal damage both in patients with aneurysmal subarachnoid hemorrhage (aSAH) [1, 2] and in the non-human primate model of aSAH [3]. The cortical lesions typically occur adjacent to subarachnoid blood clots. They showed no relationship with angiographic vasospasm of the large cerebral arteries in either humans or non-human primates [1–3]. It has been suggested that the most likely explanation for these infarcts is vasospasm of cortical resistance arteries and arterioles caused by blood products [2]. Vasospasm in these small vessels cannot be resolved using digital subtraction angiography (DSA).

The autopsy observations are consistent with the clinical finding that thick layers of subarachnoid blood on admission computed tomography (CT) scans are among the

* Correspondence: jens.dreier@charite.de
[1]Department of Neurology, Charité - Universitätsmedizin Berlin, Freie Universität Berlin, Humboldt-Universität zu Berlin, Berlin Institute of Health, Berlin, Germany
[2]Center for Stroke Research Berlin, Charité - Universitätsmedizin Berlin, Freie Universität Berlin, Humboldt-Universität zu Berlin, Berlin Institute of Health, Berlin, Germany
Full list of author information is available at the end of the article

most important predictors of infarction and unfavorable outcome after aSAH [4]. If adjacent cortical lesions are induced by subarachnoid blood, it would be expected that (i) they also develop after traumatic subarachnoid hemorrhage (tSAH), and (ii) lesions after tSAH can occur in absence of angiographic vasospasm, as was found for aSAH [5–8]. In fact, both early and delayed ischemic lesions have been described after tSAH [9]. However, to our knowledge, it has not been documented that delayed lesions can develop without angiographic vasospasm. Here, we report a case of tSAH in which delayed cortical infarcts developed around sulcal blood clots in the absence of proximal vasospasm.

Case presentation

An 86-year-old woman was admitted from an outside institution to our neurological intensive care unit with fluctuating consciousness after hitting her head during a fall. Four weeks before admission, she was in normal health for her age with a history of arterial hypertension. Because of atrial fibrillation, she was treated with rivaroxaban 20 mg once daily. Two weeks before hospitalization, she experienced pain in her lower abdomen accompanied by a feeling of illness and fatigue which she self-medicated with aspirin. She experienced nose bleeding but continued to take aspirin. She was then admitted to an external clinic after falling. During the first in-hospital night, she fell out of bed and struck her head. Thereafter, consciousness decreased and she was transferred to the neurocritical care unit of our institution. She presented with dysarthria and mild motor aphasia, but language comprehension was fully preserved. In addition, mild right-sided hemiparesis was noted. Most of the time, she was awake but intermittently somnolent. Body temperature was 37.6 °C. Routine laboratory tests revealed prolonged prothrombin time, increased international normalized ratio (INR), increased CRP, leukocytosis and corresponding signs of a urinary tract infection. She was treated with prothrombin complex concentrate and antibiotics.

The initial computed tomography (CT) on day 0 showed contusions in the left frontal and temporal lobes and tSAH. Figure 1a shows this first CT scan with subarachnoid blood in two sulci of the left frontal cortex. A contre-coup injury was found in the right posterior cranial fossa with an epidural hematoma and corresponding tSAH. In addition, a small intra-parenchymal hemorrhage was observed in the right basal ganglia. Arterial aneurysms or arteriovenous malformation were ruled out using CT angiography (CTA). Blood was also detected in the fourth ventricle, but signs of disturbed cerebrospinal fluid circulation were not seen. Accordingly, the patient did not receive external ventricular drainage. Further CT scans on days 1, 3 and 5 showed neither increase of the epidural hematoma nor development of an occlusive hydrocephalus. They revealed only the progressive decrease of Hounsfield units within the blood-related hyperdensities. Nimodipine was not given because there is currently no recommendation for its use after tSAH [9].

The patient was alert and in an improved general condition when she was transferred to the normal ward on day 7. On day 8, however, the patient experienced a secondary deterioration of her neurological status, as characterized by reduced consciousness and global aphasia, with loss of ability to speak or understand. Whereas the CT scan on day 9 was still unremarkable, the MRI scan on day 10 revealed new cortical laminar infarcts adjacent to the sulcal clots (Fig. 1 c and d). The infarcts included both Broca and Wernicke areas. Transcranial Doppler sonography (TCD) on day 10 showed normal mean velocities of the posterior cerebral arteries (right PCA 29 cm/s, left PCA 23 cm/s) and normal pulsatility indices. The bone window was not sufficient to assess velocities of the middle cerebral arteries (MCA). Neither MR angiography (MRA) on day 10 nor CTA on day 14 showed any signs of proximal vasospasm (Fig.1 e and f). However, the CT scan on day 14 revealed the same infarcts as the MRI scan on day 10 (Fig. 1 b). Over the following week, the patient improved again. She was able to respond to simple commands when she was transferred to clinical rehabilitation.

Discussion and conclusions

In addition to contusions and an epidural hematoma, this patient experienced tSAH with sulcal blood clots and initial focal neurological deficits. After initial improvement, this was succeeded by a secondary neurological deterioration with global aphasia on day 8. Accordingly, an MRI on day 10 showed new infarcts around sulcal blood clots. In contrast to the CT scan on day 9, the CT scan on day 14 also showed the new infarcts. No signs of proximal vasospasm were found using MRA, CTA and TCD.

A limitation of the study is that, despite serial use of multiple diagnostic procedures, there is a theoretical possibility that proximal vasospasm occurred but escaped detection. For example, the bone windows for TCD examination were sufficient to assess the PCAs but not the MCAs. It is also possible that proximal vasospasm occurred in connection with new infarct development between days 9 and 10 but resolved rapidly and was not detected by MRA on day 10. However, this scenario is unlikely since proximal vasospasm after aSAH, as assessed by either TCD or DSA, typically resolves only after day 16 [10, 11]. Another consideration is that while CTA and MRA are reliable noninvasive methods to assess proximal diameters of the basal cerebral arteries, they are inferior to DSA for evaluation of the more distal arterial branches [12, 13]. Accordingly, we cannot exclude that vasospasm occurred in these more distal branches in our patient. Nonetheless, several lines of

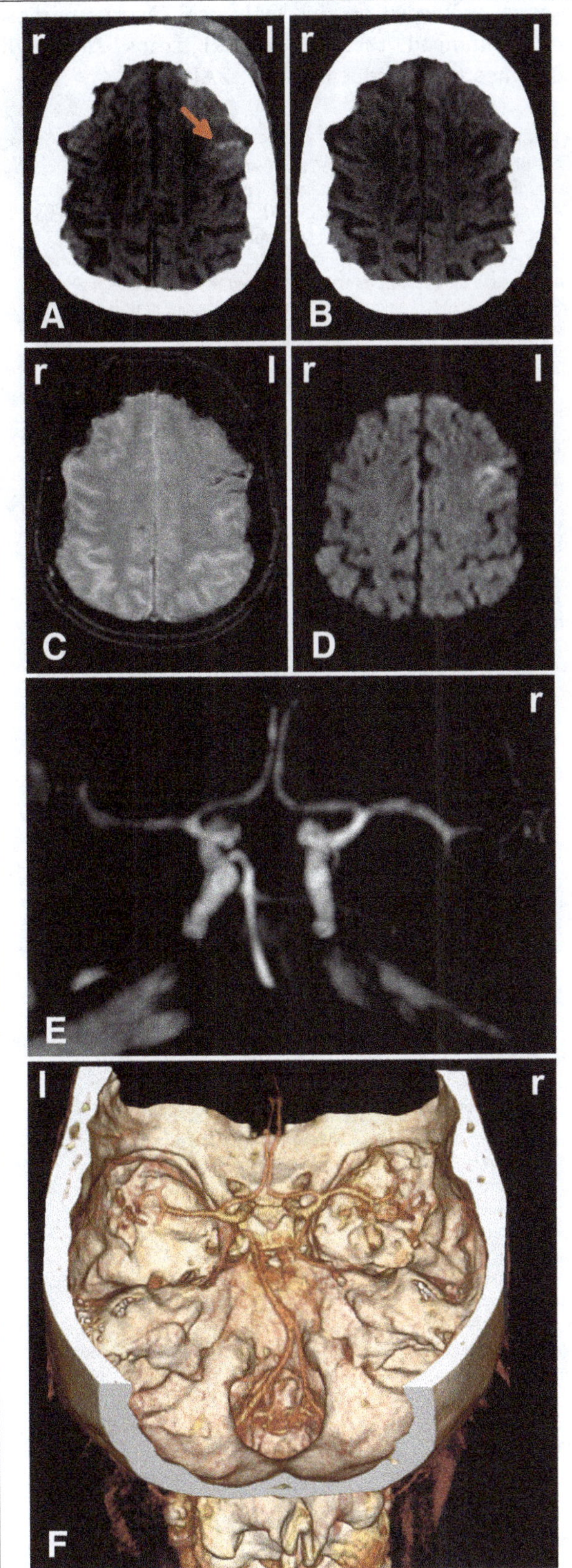

Fig. 1 Development of a cortical infarct around sulci filled with subarachnoid blood. (**a**) is a representative image of the initial CT scan on day 0. It shows subarachnoid blood in two sulci of the left frontal cortex (arrow). In addition, a left-sided hematoma exterior of the head marks the area of the impact. (**b**) Whereas the subsequent CT scans on days 1, 3, 5 and 9 showed no new infarcts, the follow-up CT scan on day 14 revealed a new hypodensity confined to the cortical gray matter around the sulci that had shown subarachnoid blood in the CT scan on day 0. This lesion was consistent with the new infarct seen on the MRI scan of day 10. (**c**) The T2* weighted image of the MRI on day 10 revealed that the subarachnoid blood was still present in the sulci in which it had been seen on the initial CT scan, although the hyperdensity had disappeared on later CT scans. (**d**) The DWI on day 10 showed a hyperintensity typical of a new infarct around the sulci with subarachnoid blood. This DWI hyperintensity corresponded to an ADC reduction (not shown). The synopsis of images (**a**) – (**d**) provides evidence for delayed cortical laminar necrosis adjacent to the sulcal clot in the left frontal cortex. (**e**) The MRA on day 10 and (**f**) the CTA on day 14 did not show any evidence of proximal vasospasm

evidence suggest that cortical ischemic lesions after aSAH are primarily the consequence of spasm in the cortical microvessels that lie beyond the resolution of DSA, as explained below [14, 15].

Cortical ischemic lesions similar to those reported here were observed by Stoltenburg-Didinger and Schwarz in 106 of 139 (76%) autopsy cases of ruptured aneurysms [2]. Notably, intravascular thrombi occurred in only 4 of the 106 autopsy cases with infarcts, and it was concluded that these thrombi did not precipitate the infarcts, but rather resulted from microcirculatory disorders secondary to the developing necrosis. Endothelial swelling was also excluded as an etiologic factor since this occurs temporarily and would only obstruct the lumina of capillaries, not arteries or arterioles. Compression was unlikely as a potential cause since subarachnoid clots would lead to venous prior to arterial compression due to the thinner vessel wall of veins. Venous compression would result in primarily hemorrhagic infarcts, but the cortical infarcts were always anemic. Finally, no relationship was found between the cortical lesions and angiographic vasospasm of the large cerebral arteries in either humans or non-human primates [1–3]. The only consistent finding in the autopsies of both patients and monkeys was that the cortical lesions typically occurred adjacent to subarachnoid blood clots, suggesting that blood products are involved in their pathogenesis [2, 3]. In the pathoanatomical descriptions, the cortical infarcts were of different shape and size. Most of them were bell-shaped, corresponding to the territory of small perforating arteries, or laminar, corresponding to the territories of rectangular branches of cortical arteries. It was suggested that the most likely explanation for these infarcts is spasm of the cortical arteries [2].

The first experimental evidence that subarachnoid blood clots can cause focal cortical necrosis was provided almost

70 years ago by Iwanowski and Olszewski, who published a study on 'subpial cerebral siderosis' [16]. After injections of blood into the subarachnoid space, the dogs in this study developed neurological deficits on the following days, and pathologic changes included the occurrence of cortical laminar necrosis. A similar result was recently found in the swine sulcal clot model, in which subarachnoid blood alone was sufficient to cause adjacent cortical infarcts [17]. Notably, their development was associated with spreading depolarizations (SD), in agreement with previous rat studies showing that subarachnoid blood products induce SDs. A key aspect of SDs in the presence of blood products is that they induce an inverse neurovascular response, known as spreading ischemia, in contrast to the arteriolar dilation and spreading hyperemia observed in response to SD in normal cortex [18, 19]. Thus, SDs in the presence of blood products initiated severe long-lasting spasm of cortical arteries with consequent spreading ischemia. Spreading ischemia alone was sufficient to cause cortical infarcts that have similar pathologic morphology as observed in patients with aSAH. Subsequently, SDs and spreading ischemias were described in patients with aSAH [20] and also those with tSAH [21]. Thus, in the wake of both aSAH and tSAH, inverse neurovascular coupling in response to SDs might acutely exacerbate the microarterial spasm resulting from cortical exposure to blood products. The idea that these mechanisms can contribute to the development of new infarcts was recently confirmed in a study of 11 patients with aSAH [22]. In this study, subdural opto-electrodes were used to monitor cortical tissue at risk for development of delayed infarcts. Typically ischemic episodes started with a cluster of repetitive SDs and progressively prolonged spreading ischemias. The SDs eventually became terminal, without recovery, and were followed by a negative ultraslow potential (NUP) that is thought to reflect the progression from persistent depolarization to cell death in an increasing fraction of neurons. Accordingly, NUP-displaying electrodes were significantly more likely to overlie a developing infarction than those not displaying a NUP. During the NUP, the median duration of spreading ischemia was 40 min, CBF fell from 57 to 26%, and tissue partial pressure of oxygen abruptly decreased from 13 to 3 mmHg.

In conclusion, the present case suggests that proximal vasospasm is not a *conditio* sine qua non for the development of delayed infarcts after tSAH, similar to results found previously for aSAH. A multidisciplinary international research group has previously recommended that the presence of angiographic vasospasm should not be a criterion to diagnose delayed infarcts after aSAH [23]. The present results suggest the same for delayed infarcts after tSAH. Although aSAH and tSAH differ in the mechanism of primary injury (aneurysm rupture vs. trauma), we suggest that they may share common mechanisms of secondary injury [24, 25]. Further systematic research is needed on this topic, and for this purpose, we recommend that serial MRI scans should be performed more frequently after tSAH.

Abbreviations

ADC: apparent diffusion coefficient; aSAH: aneurysmal subarachnoid haemorrhage; CRP: C-reactive protein; CT: computed tomography; CTA: computed tomography angiography; DWI: diffusion weigthed imaging; INR: international normalized ratio; MCA: middle cerebral artery; MRA: magnetic resonance angiography; MRI: magnetic resonance imaging; NUP: negative ultraslow potential; PCA: posterior cerebral artery; SD: spreading depolarization; TCD: transcranial Doppler sonography; tSAH: traumatic subarachnoid hemorrhage

Acknowledgements

Dr. Dreier was supported by grants of the DFG (DFG DR 323/5-1 and DFG DR 323/10-1), the Bundesministerium für Bildung und Forschung (BMBF) Center for Stroke Research Berlin 01 EO 0801 and FP7 no 602150 CENTER-TBI. We acknowledge support from the German Research Foundation (DFG) and the Open Access Publication Fund of Charité – Universitätsmedizin Berlin.

Funding

Dr. Dreier was supported by grants of the DFG (DFG DR 323/5–1 and DFG DR 323/10–1), the Bundesministerium für Bildung und Forschung (BMBF) Center for Stroke Research Berlin 01 EO 0801 and FP7 no 602150 CENTER-TBI.

Authors' contributions

CS and MW were involved in direct patient care. CS and JD were the main contributors of writing the manuscript. JH reviewed the article and gave intellectual input to the background and discussion. LS was involved in patient examination while VH and MS provided and edited the figure. All three gave intellectual input to the discussion. All authors read and approved the final manuscript.

Competing interest

The authors declare that they have no competing interests.

Author details

[1]Department of Neurology, Charité - Universitätsmedizin Berlin, Freie Universität Berlin, Humboldt-Universität zu Berlin, Berlin Institute of Health, Berlin, Germany. [2]Center for Stroke Research Berlin, Charité - Universitätsmedizin Berlin, Freie Universität Berlin, Humboldt-Universität zu Berlin, Berlin Institute of Health, Berlin, Germany. [3]Department of Experimental Neurology, Charité - Universitätsmedizin Berlin, Freie Universität Berlin, Humboldt-Universität zu Berlin, Berlin Institute of Health, Berlin, Germany. [4]Berlin Institute of Health (BIH), Berlin, Germany. [5]London School of Economics and Political Science, London, UK. [6]Department of Neuroradiology, Charité - Universitätsmedizin Berlin, Freie Universität Berlin, Humboldt-Universität zu Berlin, Berlin Institute of Health, Berlin, Germany. [7]Department of Neurosurgery, University of Cincinnati (UC) College of Medicine, Cincinnati, OH, USA. [8]Bernstein Center for Computational Neuroscience Berlin, Berlin, Germany. [9]Einstein Center for Neurosciences Berlin, Berlin, Germany.

References

1. Neil-Dwyer G, Lang DA, Doshi B, Gerber CJ, Smith PW. Delayed cerebral ischaemia: the pathological substrate. Acta Neurochir. 1994;131(1–2):137–45.
2. Stoltenburg-Didinger G, Schwarz K. Brain lesions secondary to subarachnoid hemorrhage due to ruptured aneurysms. In: Cervós-Navarro J, Ferszt R, editors. Stroke and microcirculation. New York: Raven Press; 1987. p. 471–80.

3. Schatlo B, Dreier JP, Glasker S, Fathi AR, Moncrief T, Oldfield EH, et al. Report of selective cortical infarcts in the primate clot model of vasospasm after subarachnoid hemorrhage. Neurosurgery. 2010;67(3):721–8 discussion 8-9.
4. van Norden AG, van Dijk GW, van Huizen MD, Algra A, Rinkel GJ. Interobserver agreement and predictive value for outcome of two rating scales for the amount of extravasated blood after aneurysmal subarachnoid haemorrhage. J Neurol. 2006;253(9):1217–20.
5. Dreier JP, Sakowitz OW, Harder A, Zimmer C, Dirnagl U, Valdueza JM, et al. Focal laminar cortical MR signal abnormalities after subarachnoid hemorrhage. Ann Neurol. 2002;52(6):825–9.
6. Woitzik J, Dreier JP, Hecht N, Fiss I, Sandow N, Major S, et al. Delayed cerebral ischemia and spreading depolarization in absence of angiographic vasospasm after subarachnoid hemorrhage. J Cereb Blood Flow Metab. 2012;32(2):203–12.
7. Weidauer S, Vatter H, Beck J, Raabe A, Lanfermann H, Seifert V, et al. Focal laminar cortical infarcts following aneurysmal subarachnoid haemorrhage. Neuroradiology. 2008;50(1):1–8.
8. Brown RJ, Kumar A, Dhar R, Sampson TR, Diringer MN. The relationship between delayed infarcts and angiographic vasospasm after aneurysmal subarachnoid hemorrhage. Neurosurgery. 2013;72(5):702–7 discussion 7-8.
9. Perrein A, Petry L, Reis A, Baumann A, Mertes P, Audibert G. Cerebral vasospasm after traumatic brain injury: an update. Minerva Anestesiol. 2015; 81(11):1219–28.
10. Vora YY, Suarez-Almazor M, Steinke DE, Martin ML, Findlay JM. Role of transcranial Doppler monitoring in the diagnosis of cerebral vasospasm after subarachnoid hemorrhage. Neurosurgery. 1999;44(6):1237–47 discussion 47-8.
11. Coyne TJ, Loch Macdonald R, Christopher WM. Angiographic vasospasm in a contemporary series of patients with aneurysmal subarachnoid haemorrhage. Journal of clinical neuroscience : official journal of the Neurosurgical Society of Australasia. 1994;1(2):106–10.
12. Mills JN, Mehta V, Russin J, Amar AP, Rajamohan A, Mack WJ. Advanced imaging modalities in the detection of cerebral vasospasm. Neurol Res Int. 2013;2013:415960.
13. Kerkeni H, Schatlo B, Dan-Ura H, Remonda L, Muroi C, Diepers M, et al. Proximal arterial diameters on CT angiography and digital subtraction angiography correlate both at admission and in the vasospasm period after aneurysmal subarachnoid hemorrhage. Acta Neurochir Suppl. 2015; 120:171–5.
14. Ohkuma H, Manabe H, Tanaka M, Suzuki S. Impact of cerebral microcirculatory changes on cerebral blood flow during cerebral vasospasm after aneurysmal subarachnoid hemorrhage. Stroke. 2000;31(7):1621–7.
15. Dreier JP. The role of spreading depression, spreading depolarization and spreading ischemia in neurological disease. Nat Med. 2011;17(4):439–47.
16. Iwanowski L, Olszewski J. The effects of subarachnoid injections of iron-containing substances on the central nervous system. J Neuropathol Exp Neurol. 1960;19:433–48.
17. Hartings JA, York J, Carroll CP, Hinzman JM, Mahoney E, Krueger B, et al. Subarachnoid blood acutely induces spreading depolarizations and early cortical infarction. Brain. 2017;140(10):2673–90.
18. Dreier JP, Korner K, Ebert N, Gorner A, Rubin I, Back T, et al. Nitric oxide scavenging by hemoglobin or nitric oxide synthase inhibition by N-nitro-L-arginine induces cortical spreading ischemia when K+ is increased in the subarachnoid space. J Cereb Blood Flow Metab. 1998;18(9):978–90.
19. Dreier JP, Petzold G, Tille K, Lindauer U, Arnold G, Heinemann U, et al. Ischaemia triggered by spreading neuronal activation is inhibited by vasodilators in rats. J Physiol. 2001;531(Pt 2):515–26.
20. Dreier JP, Major S, Manning A, Woitzik J, Drenckhahn C, Steinbrink J, et al. Cortical spreading ischaemia is a novel process involved in ischaemic damage in patients with aneurysmal subarachnoid haemorrhage. Brain. 2009;132(Pt 7):1866–81.
21. Hinzman JM, Andaluz N, Shutter LA, Okonkwo DO, Pahl C, Strong AJ, et al. Inverse neurovascular coupling to cortical spreading depolarizations in severe brain trauma. Brain. 2014;137(Pt 11):2960–72.
22. Luckl J, Lemale CL, Kola V, Horst V, Khojasteh U, Oliveira-Ferreira AI, et al. The negative ultraslow potential, electrophysiological correlate of infarction in the human cortex. Brain. 2018;141(6):1734–52.
23. Vergouwen MD, Vermeulen M, van Gijn J, Rinkel GJ, Wijdicks EF, Muizelaar JP, et al. Definition of delayed cerebral ischemia after aneurysmal subarachnoid hemorrhage as an outcome event in clinical trials and observational studies: proposal of a multidisciplinary research group. Stroke. 2010;41(10):2391–5.
24. Balanca B, Meiller A, Bezin L, Dreier JP, Marinesco S, Lieutaud T. Altered hypermetabolic response to cortical spreading depolarizations after traumatic brain injury in rats. J Cereb Blood Flow Metab. 2017;37(5):1670–86.
25. Dreier JP, Fabricius M, Ayata C, Sakowitz OW, William Shuttleworth C, Dohmen C, et al. Recording, analysis, and interpretation of spreading depolarizations in neurointensive care: review and recommendations of the COSBID research group. J Cereb Blood Flow Metab. 2017;37(5):1595–625.

First three cases of scalp temperature change in symptomatic areas affected by nummular headache

Yonghui Liu and Tianlu Wei*

Abstract

Background: Nummular headache is a distinct headache disorder characterized by a rounded or elliptical symptomatic area that is typically 2 to 6 cm in diameter and does not change in shape or size with time. Although the pathomechanism is still not clear, nummular headache is thought to be a primary headache disorder. To date, more than 250 cases have been reported; the symptoms of this disease vary, but no cases with scalp temperature changes in the symptomatic areas have been reported yet. In this study, we present three patients with a new manifestation of nummular headache, in which the symptomatic areas of the scalp were colder or warmer than normal areas; we believe that our work might be helpful for medical practitioners and researchers.

Case presentation: The temperature differences between the symptomatic areas and the normal areas were tested in three patients with nummular headache accompanied by changes in scalp temperature. Three patients' symptomatic areas were either colder or warmer than the normal areas. In every case, we took measurements from the painful site and from the opposite side of the head. The margin of error was 0.01 °C, and the difference was statistically significant ($P < 0.01$).

Conclusion: We firmly believe that our study will provide an enriched understanding of the variation in clinical manifestations of nummular headache. Our observations might also have clinical implications regarding the pathomechanism of this disease, which remains largely unclear at present.

Keywords: Nummular headache, Coin-shaped cephalalgia, Paraesthesia

Background

Nummular headache, or coin-shaped cephalalgia, is a headache disorder characterized by pain in a round or oval/elliptical shaped area of the head; this disorder was first described in 2002 by Pareja in a series of 13 patients, in whom the symptomatic area did not change in shape or size over time [1]. Since 2002, more than 250 cases have been reported in the literature [2]. With the increasing attention being paid to nummular headache, new clinical manifestations have been reported, such as bifocal [3–5] and even multifocal localization [6, 7], trophic change [7, 8], menstruation-related timing [9], and occurrence secondary to subtentorial meningioma [10]. To date, however, the literature still contains no articles that describe scalp temperature changes in the symptomatic areas. To provide more information about nummular headache, we report herein that we have encountered three cases with scalp temperature changes in the symptomatic areas in our clinical practice. These observations might have implications regarding the pathogenesis of nummular headache.

* Correspondence: weitianlu90@126.com
Department of Encephalopathy, The First Affiliated Hospital of Guangxi University of Chinese Medicine, Nanning 530023, China

Case presentation

Case 1

A 74-year-old female presented at our headache clinic with a 2-year history of headache that felt cold in the symptomatic area, which was confined to an ellipse 3 cm in diameter in the left parietal region. The headache consisted of stabbing pain of mild intensity. The episodes of pain lasted approximately 3 to 5 min each and occurred 2 to 3 times every week, with the intensity fluctuating around 2 to 3 on a 10-point visual analogue scale (VAS). There were no other complaints and no related focal neurological symptoms. The patient had no known family history of migraine, stroke, psychiatric disorders or dementia. She had a 5-year history of Type 2 diabetes. She had no cutaneous abnormalities in the painful area and had normal routine blood analyses, erythrocyte sedimentation rate and cerebral computed tomography. During the course of diagnosis and treatment, the patient's headaches had occurred 4 times in the same area, and she complained of a cold sensation in the symptomatic skin. The symptomatic area was colder than the normal area, as estimated by touch and measured by an infrared thermometer. The recorded temperatures are presented in Table 1. As of a two-week follow-up visit, the patient had achieved good relief with gabapentin.

Case 2

A 46-year-old male driver visited our outpatient headache clinic and complained of a twenty-year history of focal episodic pain located in a circumscribed area on the right temple. We learned that this patient had no personal or family history of migraine, stroke, hypertension or psychiatric disorders. The patient's neurological examination was normal, with neither tenderness nor trophic changes inside the painful area. Blood tests and an MRI scan of the brain were also normal. The patient complained of an occasionally annoying hot sensation that appeared in the symptomatic area every time the pain attacked. Other than minor benefits from acupuncture and gabapentin, the intensity of the pain did not change with time. During the man's visit to our clinic, we tested his scalp temperature using an infrared thermometer and recorded the results. We followed up with the patient over the next month and recorded the temperature the of the symptomatic area; here, we have opted to report only the records from the four most recent time points (Table 1).

Case 3

A 38-year-old female patient complained of a two-month history of headache; the painful area was perfectly circular and confined to a diameter of approximately 3 cm on the posterior occipital part of the head. The pain was pulsating, sometimes stabbing, with the intensity fluctuating around 5 on a 10-point VAS. The attacks of pain differed in duration, sometimes lasting 5 min and sometimes lasting a whole day; fortunately, the intensity of the pain did not affect the patient's life quality and did not cause a mood disorder. In addition, the patient complained that she had a hot sensation in the symptomatic area every time the pain attacked, particularly in the summer, and she could feel an obvious distinction between the symptomatic area and normal areas by touch. We tested the symptomatic area with an infrared thermometer and recorded the temperature every time when the patient visited our outpatient headache office. We reported the last four data points in Table 3. However, she had no other accompanying symptoms and no related focal neurological symptoms. She had a few years' history of alcohol intake. She had no related family history of stroke, migraine, heart disease or psychiatric disorders. In the two months preceding her visit, the patient was given acupuncture and ibuprofen, which elicited a good response, but the frequency of the attacks did not change. The patient needed to take medicine or undergo acupuncture treatment whenever the pain attacked. The patient's neurological examination was normal, with neither tenderness nor trophic changes in the painful area. Blood tests and an MRI scan of the brain were also normal.

Table 1 Scalp temperature between symptomatic area and normal area

	Case1		Case 2		Case 3	
	Sym	Nor	Sym	Nor	Sym	Nor
1	35.8	36.4	37.3	36.8	37.4	36.8
2	36.1	36.5	37.4	36.7	37.3	36.7
3	35.5	36.5	37.4	36.8	37.4	36.8
4	35.5	36.5	37.3	36.6	37.5	36.8

P<0.01,the difference is statistically significant
Note: unit: °C。 Sym refers symptomatic area. Nor refers normal area
All measurements were made by reseacher

Discussion and conclusions

Here, we are the first to report three cases of scalp temperature changes in symptomatic areas affected by nummular headache, which may provide an enriched understanding of the variation in clinical manifestations of nummular headache. Scalp temperature changes are a form of paraesthesia, which may have clinical implications for its peripheral pathogenesis. The exact pathogenesis of nummular headache has not been clearly defined. Studies have advanced two main hypotheses: a peripheral mechanism and a central mechanism. Pareja and his colleagues have classified nummular headache as a localized neuralgia stemming from epicranial tissues – specifically, neuralgia affecting a terminal branch of one of the cutaneous nerves of the scalp [11]. The skin and hair changes in the symptomatic area also reflect a peripheral nerve lesion or, alternatively, an autoimmune process [12, 13]. In an extensive case series, Cuadrado and his colleagues reported that nummular headache was associated with a local increase in pain sensitivity to mechanical stimulation (reduced pressure pain thresholds [PPTs]) confined to the symptomatic area [14]. Although the pain is asserted to originate from epicranial tissues including the skull, scalp, vessels, and nerves [15–17], some nummular headaches have been described as "symptomatic nummular headaches", which implies that they might be secondary to underlying structural lesions or other causes, such as subtentorial meningioma

[10], pituitary lesion [18], or arachnoid cysts [19]. These observations represent the secondary form of nummular headache. Some researchers have also reported that nummular headache may arise from intracranial lesions or stress, both of which need to be ruled out when this type of headache appears [19]. Aside from these pathogenetic hypotheses, some researchers have suggested that nummular headache is caused by psychiatric disturbances [15]. However, other researchers have excluded the possibility of psychological factors as a cause of nummular headache disorder, and it is important to note that depression and anxiety are not symptoms of nummular headache disorder. Patients suffering from nummular headache disorder showed mood states similar to those of a healthier person [20]. We have discussed the pathogenesis of nummular headache, and we believe the observed changes in scalp temperature might be a clue in this mystery. However, we could not absolutely exclude the central hypothesis or the possibility of a complex pathogenesis involving both peripheral and central mechanisms. Further studies are still needed to help unveil the mystery.

In the initial report by Pareja in 2002, nummular headache was established to be a primary disease with clear-cut clinical features including a single, circumscribed location and mild to moderate pain. The three cases that we report in this paper involved paraesthesia, with the affected areas of the scalp being colder or warmer than the normal areas. This finding might support a peripheral mechanism of nummular headache. However, we could not definitively exclude the central hypothesis [21], and future studies with larger samples and follow-up designs may reveal a central mechanism as the cause of nummular headache. The ultimate judgement must be made by the appropriate healthcare professional(s) responsible for decisions regarding specific clinical procedures and treatment plans.

Abbreviations

MRI: Magnetic Resonance Imaging; PPTs: Pressure Pain Thresholds; VAS: Visual Analogue Scale

Acknowledgements

Not applicable.

Funding

Not applicable.

Authors' contributions

Study concept and design: YHL. Acquisition of data: YHL. Analysis and interpretation of data: YHL. Drafting of the manuscript: TLW. Critical revision of the manuscript for important intellectual content: YHL. All authors read and approved the final manuscript.

Competing interests

The authors declare that they have no competing interests.

References

1. Pareja JA, Caminero AB, Serra J, et al. Numular headache: a coin-shaped cephalgia. Neurology. 2002;58(11):1678–9.
2. Schwartz DP, Robbins MS, Grosberg BM. Nummular headache update. Curr Pain Headache Rep. 2013;17(6):340.
3. Cuadrado ML, Valle B, Fernandez-de-las-Penas C, et al. Bifocal nummular headache: the first three cases. Cephalalgia. 2009;29(5):583–6.
4. Guerrero AL, Cuadrado ML, Garcia-Garcia ME, et al. Bifocal nummular headache: a series of 6 new cases. Headache. 2011;51(7):1161–6.
5. Rocha-Filho PA. Nummular headache: two simultaneous areas of pain in the same patient. Cephalalgia. 2011;31(7):874.
6. Rodriguez C, Herrero-Velazquez S, Ruiz M, et al. Pressure pain sensitivity map of multifocal nummular headache: a case report. J Headache Pain. 2015;16:523.
7. Porta-Etessam J, Lapena T, Cuadrado ML, et al. Multifocal nummular headache with trophic changes. Headache. 2010;50(10):1612–3.
8. Pareja JA, Cuadrado ML, Fernandez-de-las Penas C, et al. Nummular headache with trophic changes inside the painful area. Cephalalgia. 2008;28(2):186–90.
9. Robbins MS, Grosberg BM. Menstrual-related nummular headache. Cephalalgia. 2010;30(4):507–8.
10. Guillem A, Barriga FJ, Gimenez-Roldan S. Nummular headache secondary to an intracranial mass lesion. Cephalalgia. 2007;27(8):943–4.
11. Pareja JA, Montojo T, Alvarez M. Nummular headache update. Curr Neurol Neurosci Rep. 2012;12(2):118–24.
12. Alkhalifah A, Alsantali A, Wang E, et al. Alopecia areata update: part I. clinical picture, histopathology, and pathogenesis. J Am Acad Dermatol. 2010;62(2): 177–88 quiz 89-90.
13. Ahmed Z, Banik RL, Paul HK, et al. Histopathological changes in different stages of alopecia areata. Mymensingh Med J. 2010;19(1):100–5.
14. Cuadrado ML, Valle B, Fernandez-de-las-Penas C, et al. Pressure pain sensitivity of the scalp in patients with nummular headache: a cartographic study. Cephalalgia. 2010;30(2):200–6.
15. Cohen GL. Nummular headache: what denomination? Headache. 2005; 45(10):1417–8 author reply 8.
16. Moon J, Ahmed K, Garza I. Case series of sixteen patients with nummular headache. Cephalalgia. 2010;30(12):1527–30.
17. Pareja JA, Pareja J, Barriga FJ, et al. Nummular headache: a prospective series of 14 new cases. Headache. 2004;44(6):611–4.
18. Chui C, Chen WH, Yin HL. Nummular headache and pituitary lesion: a case report and literature review. Ann Indian Acad Neurol. 2013;16(2):226–8.
19. Guillem A, Barriga FJ, Gimenez-Roldan S. Nummular headache associated to arachnoid cysts. J Headache Pain. 2009;10(3):215–7.
20. Fernandez-de-Las-Penas C, Penacoba-Puente C, Lopez-Lopez A, et al. Depression and anxiety are not related to nummular headache. J Headache Pain. 2009;10(6):441–5.
21. Dai W, Yu S, Liang J, et al. Nummular headache: peripheral or central? One case with reappearance of nummular headache after focal scalp was removed, and literature review. Cephalalgia. 2013;33(6):390–7.

Intra-familial phenotypic heterogeneity in a Sudanese family with *DARS2*-related leukoencephalopathy, brainstem and spinal cord involvement and lactate elevation

Ashraf Yahia[1,9,12], Liena Elsayed[1*], Arwa Babai[2], Mustafa A. Salih[3], Sarah Misbah El-Sadig[4,8], Mutaz Amin[1], Mahmoud Koko[5], Rayan Abubakr[2], Razaz Idris[2], Shaimaa Omer M.A. Taha[6], Salah A. Elmalik[13], Alexis Brice[11,12], Ammar Eltahir Ahmed[7,8] and Giovanni Stevanin[10,12]

Abstract

Background: Leukoencephalopathy with brainstem and spinal cord involvement and lactate elevation (LBSL, OMIM #611105) is a genetic disease of the central nervous system characterized by lower limb spasticity, cerebellar ataxia and involvement of the dorsal column. The disease is caused by mutations in the *DARS2* gene but has never been reported in sub-Saharan Africa so far.

Case presentation: Two siblings, aged 18 years and 15 years, from a consanguineous family presented with pyramidal signs and symptoms since infancy and developmental delay. Whole exome sequencing of the proband identified two compound heterozygous variants (NM_018122.4:c.1762C > G and c.563G > A) in *DARS2*. Sanger sequencing confirmed the presence of the mutations and their segregation in *trans* in both patients and in their elder sister (aged 20 years), who showed only brisk reflexes and mild lower limb spasticity. Surprisingly, in contrast to her subtle clinical presentation, the elder sister had abnormal MRI features and serum lactate levels comparable to her ill sisters.

Conclusion: This report illustrates intra-familial phenotypic variation in LBSL and provides an example of a marked dissociation between the clinical and radiological phenotypes of the disease. This may have implications for the detection of mutation carriers in LBSL.

Keywords: LBSL, *DARS2*, Clinico-radiological dissociation, Intra-familial phenotypic heterogeneity, Africa

Background

Leukoencephalopathy with brainstem and spinal cord involvement and lactate elevation (LBSL, OMIM # 611105) is a genetic disease of the central nervous system characterized by lower limb spasticity, cerebellar ataxia and involvement of the dorsal column [1]. The clinical presentation is variable both in age at onset (early childhood or adulthood) and in associated features (learning difficulty, epilepsy, mental deterioration and others) [2]. Brain magnetic resonance imaging (MRI) shows diffuse cerebral white matter changes with signal abnormalities in the dorsal column and lateral corticospinal tracts in addition to spectroscopic findings of increased lactate [1].

LBSL is an autosomal recessive disease caused by mutations in *DARS2* [3]. This gene, located on chromosome 1, has 17 exons and encodes the mitochondrial aspartyl-tRNA synthetase [3]. Defects in this gene in neurons impair the translation of mitochondrial mRNAs, leading to mitochondrial dysfunction and progressive cell loss [4]. We report here the identification of two compound heterozygous rare variants (NM_018122.4:c.1762C > G and c.563G > A) segregating in a Sudanese family with a wide clinical spectrum of

* Correspondence: doctorlbo@hotmail.com
[1]Department of Biochemistry, Faculty of Medicine, University of Khartoum, Khartoum, Sudan
Full list of author information is available at the end of the article

LBSL and a marked dissociation between clinical and radiological phenotypes in one of the affected siblings.

Case presentation

Two siblings, aged 18 years and 15 years, from a Sudanese family (individuals 2043 and 2044) presented with pyramidal features since infancy (Table 1). Both patients were the outcome of uncomplicated normal vaginal deliveries and developed normally before the initial symptoms of the disease. Patient 2043 developed her symptoms from the age of 8 months after an attack of fever complicated by febrile convulsions. Initially, she manifested floppiness, which later turned into spasticity. Speech and walking were delayed (achieved at ages 3–4 and 6 years, respectively). At the age of 10 months she had three attacks of seizures, which were later controlled by carbamazepine. Spasticity progressed over time and currently the patient can only walk with support. In patient 2044, the disease started at the age of 4 months with initial floppiness followed by spasticity and delayed motor development as well, but without any history of convulsions or precipitating febrile illness. Speech developed normally. Her motor disability was analogous to that of her sister. Examination of the lower limbs showed severe spasticity, hyperreflexia and "up-going" plantar reflex in both patients. Whereas patient 2043 showed severe proximal and distal lower limb weakness, patient 2044 manifested only moderate proximal weakness. Due to the severe spasticity, heel on shin test was not applicable. Upon examination of the upper limbs, the two patients showed increased reflexes with normal tone and a normal finger-to-nose test. Ocular cerebellar signs (nystagmus, slow saccades and interrupted pursuit) were present in both patients. There were no extrapyramidal signs.

Table 1 Clinical characteristics of the described genetically affected siblings

Patient ID	2042	2043	2044
Gender	Female	Female	Female
Age at examination	20 years	18 years	15 years
Age at onset	–	8 months	4 months
Initial sign / symptom	Hypertonia and hyperreflexia detected during the sampling session	Floppiness	Floppiness
Delayed motor development	–	+	+
Delayed speech	–	+	–
Epilepsy	–	+	–
Cognitive impairment	–	–	–
Degree of motor disability	No functional handicap but signs at examination	Walk with support / unable to run	Walk with support / unable to run
Muscle wasting (UL & LL)	–	–	–
UL hypertonia	–	–	–
UL motor deficit	–	–	–
UL hyperreflexia	+	+	+
LL hypertonia	+	+	+
LL motor deficit	–	Severe	Moderate
LL hyperreflexia	+	+	+
Sensory impairment	–	–	–
Dysarthria	–	+	+
Ocular cerebellar signs	–	+	+
Dysmetria	–	–	–
Optic atrophy	–	–	–
Clinical summary	Pyramidal features	Pyramidal features, seizures, delayed speech, ocular cerebellar signs and dysarthria	Pyramidal features, ocular cerebellar signs and dysarthria
MRI changes in brain and spinal cord	+	+	+
Serum lactate level in mmol/L (reference range 0.5–2.2 mmol/L)	6.13	6.8	5.97

UL upper limb, *LL* lower limb, – absent, + present

Sensory nervous system and fundus examinations were normal. Both patients had normal cognitive functions and they were able to graduate from high school and attend university. Brain MRIs of patients 2043 and 2044 showed abnormal high signal intensity in the periventricular white matter and dentate nuclei bilaterally together with thinning of corpus callosum and cerebral and cerebellar atrophy (Fig. 1). Spinal MRI showed signal changes with dorsal spinal cord atrophic changes in both these affected sisters.

Four first-degree relatives were assessed for inclusion as controls in the genetic analysis: the parents (2040 and 2041), an elder sister (2042), and a younger sister (2045). They underwent routine clinical examination to rule out the possibility of subtle abnormalities. The examination was normal in the parents and the younger sister. The

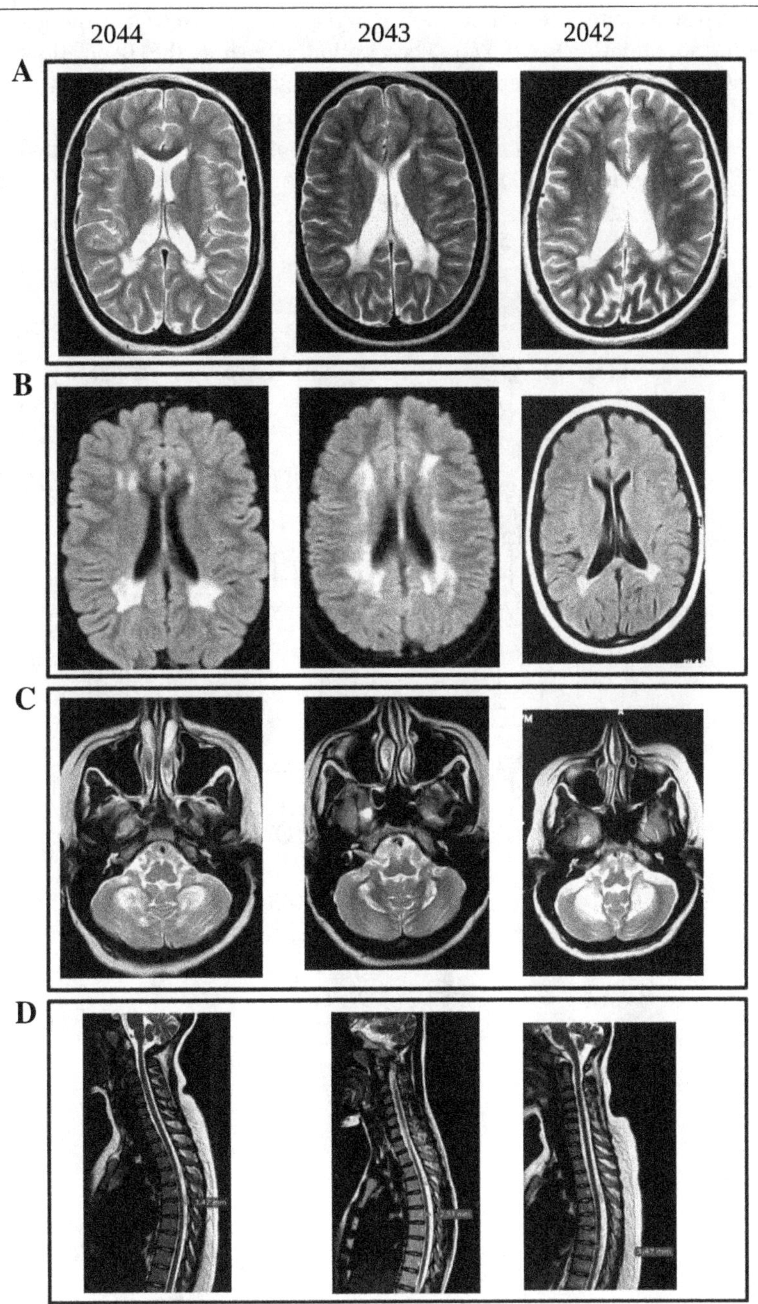

Fig. 1 Brain and spinal cord MRIs of the three patients. MRIs of subjects 2044, 2043 and 2042 ordered from left to right. **a** and **b** Axial T2 and fluid-attenuated inversion recovery (FLAIR) sections of brain MRIs showing abnormal periventricular white matter high signal intensities in the three subjects. **c** Axial T2 MRIs through the cerebellar hemispheres demonstrate mild cerebellar atrophy in the three subjects. **d** Sagittal T2 MRIs of the spinal cord show spinal cord atrophic changes in the three subjects

elder sister showed brisk reflexes in both upper and lower limbs and mild spasticity in the lower limbs but no other clinically detectable abnormality (Table 1).

DNA was extracted from saliva samples. Whole exome sequencing was performed in the proband (patient 2043) and revealed two compound heterozygous rare variants in the *DARS2* gene (NM_018122.4: c.1762C > G and NM_018122.4: c.563G > A; p.(Leu588Val) and p.(Arg188 Gln), respectively). The variants were predicted as pathogenic using three pathogenicity prediction tools (SIFT [5], PolyPhen-2 [6] and MutationTaster [7]). The variant c.1762C > G (rs972404343) was reported as "likely pathogenic" in the ClinVar database [8]; it was absent from both the ExAC and gnomAD databases [9]. The second variant, c.563G > A (rs182811621), was not reported in the ClinVar database but had very low allele frequencies in the ExAC and gnomAD databases (0.00001 and 0.000004, respectively) [9]. Sanger sequencing (Fig. 2) identified the father and mother as heterozygous carriers of the single variant c.1762C > G and c.563G > A, respectively, and validated the presence of both variants in patients 2043 and 2044. Additionally, subject 2042, who had only mild signs on examination, was found to harbor both variants.

To further investigate the genotype-phenotype correlation as well as the association between the clinical and radiological findings, brain and spinal MRIs were obtained for patient 2042. Interestingly, she presented similar features to her affected siblings in the form of periventricular white matter, dentate nuclei, medulla

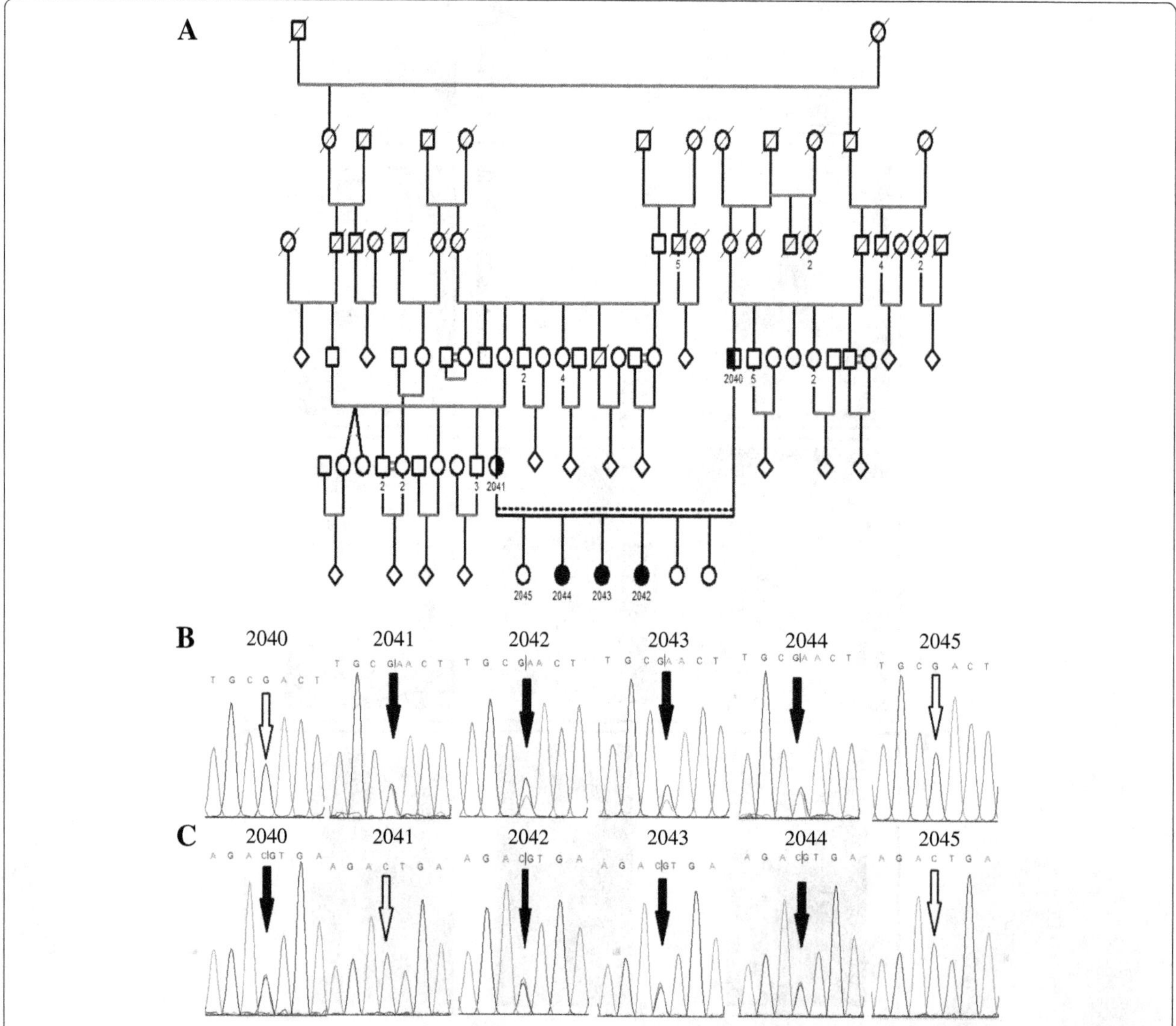

Fig. 2 Pedigree and segregation analysis. Segregation analysis shows compound heterozygous pattern of disease inheritance. **a** Family pedigree. **b** and **c** Electropherograms showing the segregation pattern of c.563G > A and c.1762C > G (black arrows), in (**b**) and (**c**), respectively; in subjects 2040, 2041 (parents), 2045 (healthy sister), 2042, 2043 and 2044 (patients). White arrows point to wild type variants at the genomic positions of interest. The variant c.563G > A is inherited from the mother (2041) while the variant c.1762C > G is inherited from the father

oblongata and cervical spinal cord areas of signal changes and cerebral and spinal cord atrophic changes (Fig. 1). Biochemical investigations showed an elevated serum lactate level (reference range: 0.5–2.2 mmol/L) in patients 2043 and 2044 (6.8 mmol/L and 5.97 mmol/L, respectively) and in patient 2042 (6.13 mmol/L) as well. Currently, the younger patients are on regular physiotherapy. No further medical intervention has been undertaken in the minimally affected elder sister.

Discussion and conclusion

Compound heterozygous mutations are implicated in the majority of LBSL cases [10]. There is a wide variety in the clinical presentation of patients [10]. In addition, there is no apparent genotype-phenotype correlation nor is there a correlation between the degree of mitochondrial aspartyl-tRNA synthetase dysfunction and disease severity [11]. In this report, we showed that patients in the same family with the same compound heterozygous mutations can vary in their clinical presentations from an apparently healthy individual (with findings limited to brisk reflexes incidentally recognized at age 20 years) to disabled patients. Additionally, we highlighted the marked dissociation that can occur between clinical phenotype and MRI findings in LBSL. To the best of our knowledge, such a dissociation has only previously been reported in two sisters diagnosed with asymptomatic LBSL due to compound heterozygous mutations in *DARS2* [12]. On the other hand, the dissociation between clinical and radiological phenotypes has been reported in other forms of leukodystrophies [13, 14]. However, the biological basis of this dissociation has yet to be unraveled. In our opinion biochemical, radiological or genetic screening of healthy siblings of LBSL patients could be of value to rule out the presence of the disease. Detecting asymptomatic/minimally symptomatic patients is of value in premarital counseling, especially in countries where consanguineous marriage is common. Studies that are more comprehensive could determine the sensitivity, specificity and cost-effectiveness of such screening methods. Our study is the first to report cases of LBSL from sub-Saharan Africa. Nevertheless, functional studies are still needed to confirm the pathogenicity of the reported variants.

In conclusion, LBSL can show marked phenotypic variability even within the same family. This variable expressivity may complicate the detection of the causative variants in the context of genetic counseling.

Abbreviations

FLAIR: Fluid-attenuated inversion recovery; LBSL: Leukoencephalopathy, brainstem and spinal cord involvement and lactate elevation; MRI: Magnetic resonance imaging; OMIM: Online mendelian inheritance in man

Acknowledgements

Not applicable.

Funding

This study was financially supported by the Agence Nationale pour la Recherche (to GS), the European Union (H2020, to GS) and the E-rare program (to GS). AY is a recipient of a Campus France and University of Khartoum fellowship. MAS was supported by the Deanship of Scientific Research, King Saud University, Riyadh, Saudi Arabia, via research group project number RGP-VPP-301. The funding bodies had no role in the design of the study, in the collection, analysis and interpretation of data or in writing the manuscript.

Authors' contributions

Study design and conception: GS, AEA, LE and AB2, acquisition of phenotypic and biological data: SME, MAS, AY, LE, SAE, AB1, RA, RI and SOMAT, bioinformatic analysis: AY, LE and MK, interpretation of MRIs: SOMAT, phenotypic-genotypic correlations and writing the first draft: AY, AB1 and MA, review and critique: SME, MAS, GS, AEA, AB2, MK, LE, RA, SAE, SOMAT and RI. All authors read and approved the final manuscript. All authors agreed to be accountable for all aspects of the work in ensuring that questions related to the accuracy or integrity of any part of the work are appropriately investigated and resolved.

Competing interests

The authors declare that they have no competing interests.

Author details

[1]Department of Biochemistry, Faculty of Medicine, University of Khartoum, Khartoum, Sudan. [2]Institute of Endemic Diseases, University of Khartoum, Khartoum, Sudan. [3]Division of Pediatric Neurology, Department of Pediatrics, College of Medicine, King Saud University, Riyadh, Saudi Arabia. [4]Department of Medicine, Faculty of Medicine, University of Khartoum, Khartoum, Sudan. [5]Department of Neurology & Epileptology, Hertie Institute for Clinical Brain Research, University of Tübingen, Tübingen, Germany. [6]Department of Radiology, Dar Al Elaj specialized hospital, Khartoum, Sudan. [7]Department of Physiology, Faculty of Medicine, University of Khartoum, Khartoum, Sudan. [8]Department of Neurology, Soba University Hospital, Khartoum, Sudan. [9]Department of Biochemistry, Faculty of Medicine, National University, Khartoum, Sudan. [10]Ecole Pratique des Hautes Etudes, EPHE, PSL Research University, Paris, France. [11]Department of Genetics, APHP, Pitié-Salpêtrière Hospital, Paris, France. [12]Institut du Cerveau et de la Moelle épinière, INSERM U1127, CNRS UMR7225, Sorbonne Universités UMR_S1127, 75013 Paris, France. [13]Department of Physiology, College of Medicine, King Saud University, Riyadh, Saudi Arabia.

References

1. Van Der Knaap MS, Van Der Voorn P, Barkhof F, Van Coster R, Krägeloh-Mann I, Feigenbaum A, et al. A new leukoencephalopathy with brainstem and spinal cord involvement and high lactate. Ann Neurol. 2003;53(2):252–8.
2. van Berge L, Hamilton EM, Linnankivi T, Uziel G, Steenweg ME, Isohanni P, et al. Leukoencephalopathy with brainstem and spinal cord involvement and lactate elevation: clinical and genetic characterization and target for therapy. Brain. 2014;137(Pt 4):1019–29.
3. Scheper GC, van der Klok T, van Andel RJ, van Berkel CGM, Sissler M, Smet J, et al. Mitochondrial aspartyl-tRNA synthetase deficiency causes leukoencephalopathy with brain stem and spinal cord involvement and lactate elevation. Nat Genet. 2007;39(4):534–9.
4. Aradjanski M, Dogan SA, Lotter S, Wang S, Hermans S, Wibom R, et al. DARS2 protects against neuroinflammation and apoptotic neuronal loss, but is dispensable for myelin producing cells. Hum Mol Genet. 2017; 26(21):4181–9.
5. Sim N-L, Kumar P, Hu J, Henikoff S, Schneider G, Ng PC. SIFT web server: predicting effects of amino acid substitutions on proteins. Nucleic Acids Res. 2012;40(Web Server issue):W452–7.
6. Adzhubei I, Jordan DM, Sunyaev SR. Predicting functional effect of human missense mutations using PolyPhen-2. Curr Protoc Hum Genet 2013 Jan; Chapter 7:Unit7.20.
7. Schwarz JM, Cooper DN, Schuelke M, Seelow D. MutationTaster2: mutation prediction for the deep-sequencing age. Nat Methods. 2014;11(4):361–2.

8. Landrum MJ, Lee JM, Riley GR, Jang W, Rubinstein WS, Church DM, et al. ClinVar: public archive of relationships among sequence variation and human phenotype. Nucleic Acids Res. 2014;42(Database issue):D980–5.
9. Karczewski KJ, Weisburd B, Thomas B, Solomonson M, Ruderfer DM, Kavanagh D, et al. The ExAC browser: displaying reference data information from over 60 000 exomes. Nucleic Acids Res. 2017;45(D1):D840–5.
10. Finsterer J, Zarrouk-Mahjoub S. Phenotypic spectrum of DARS2 mutations. J Neurol Sci. 2017;376:117–8.
11. van Berge L, Kevenaar J, Polder E, Gaudry A, Florentz C, Sissler M, et al. Pathogenic mutations causing LBSL affect mitochondrial aspartyl-tRNA synthetase in diverse ways. Biochem J. 2013;450(2):345–50.
12. Labauge P, Dorboz I, Eymard-Pierre E, Dereeper O, Boespflug-Tanguy O. Clinically asymptomatic adult patient with extensive LBSL MRI pattern and DARS2 mutations. J Neurol. 2011;258(2):335–7.
13. Di Bella D, Pareyson D, Savoiardo M, Farina L, Ciano C, Caldarazzo S, et al. Subclinical leukodystrophy and infertility in a man with a novel homozygous CLCN2 mutation. Neurology. 2014;83(13):1217–8.
14. Abrams CK, Scherer SS, Flores-Obando R, Freidin MM, Wong S, Lamantea E, et al. A new mutation in GJC2 associated with subclinical leukodystrophy. J Neurol. 2014;261(10):1929–38.

To be active through indoor-climbing: an exploratory feasibility study in a group of children with cerebral palsy and typically developing children

Mark Schram Christensen[1,3], Thor Jensen[1], Camilla B. Voigt[2], Jens Bo Nielsen[1,2] and Jakob Lorentzen[1,2*]

Abstract

Background: Cerebral Palsy (CP) is the most common cause of motor disabilities in children and young adults and it is also often associated with cognitive and physiological challenges. Climbing requires a multifaceted repertoire of movements, participants at all levels of expertise may be challenged functionally and cognitively, making climbing of great potential interest in (re)habilitation settings. However, until now only few research projects have investigated the feasibility of climbing as a potential activity for heightening physical activity in children with CP and the possible beneficial effects of climbing activities in populations with functional and/or cognitive challenges. The aim of this study was therefore to test the feasibility of an intensive 3 weeks indoor-climbing training program in children with CP and typically developing (TD) peers. In addition we evaluated possible functional and cognitive benefits of 3 weeks of intensive climbing training in 11 children with cerebral palsy (CP) aged 11–13 years and six of their TD peers.

Method: The study was designed as a feasibility and interventional study. We evaluated the amount of time spent being physically active during the 9 indoor-climbing training sessions, and climbing abilities were measured. The participants were tested in a series of physiological, psychological and cognitive tests: two times prior to and one time following the training in order to explore possible effects of the intervention.

Results: The children accomplished the training goal of a total of nine sessions within the 3-week training period. The time of physical activity during a 2:30 h climbing session, was comparably high in the group of children with CP and the TD children. The children with CP were physically active on average for almost 16 h in total during the 3 weeks. Both groups of participants improved their climbing abilities, the children with CP managed to climb a larger proportion of the tested climbing route at the end of training and the TD group climbed faster. For the children with CP this was accompanied by significant improvements in the Sit-to-stand test ($p < 0.01$), increased rate of force development in the least affected hand during an explosive pinch test and increased muscular-muscular coherence during a pinch precision test ($p < 0.05$). We found no improvements in maximal hand or finger strength and no changes in cognitive abilities or psychological well-being in any of the groups.

(Continued on next page)

* Correspondence: jlo@elsassfonden.dk
[1]Center for Neuroscience, Section for Integrative Neuroscience, University of Copenhagen, Panum Institute, Building 33.3, Nørre Allé 20, DK-2200 Copenhagen N, Denmark
[2]Elsass Instituttet, Holmegårdsvej 28, DK-2920 Charlottenlund, Denmark
Full list of author information is available at the end of the article

(Continued from previous page)

Conclusions: These findings show that it is possible to use climbing as means to make children with CP physically active. The improved motor abilities obtained through the training is likely reflected by increased synchronization between cortex and muscles, which results in a more efficient motor unit recruitment that may be transferred to daily functional abilities.

Keywords: Cerebral Palsy, Children, Climbing, Motor skills, peer socialization

Background

Cerebral palsy (CP) is the most common cause of motor disabilities in children and young adults and it is also often associated with cognitive and psychological challenges [1, 2]. As a consequence, children with CP show less participation in social activities than their typically developed (TD) peers [3, 4]. This low early socialization is also predictive of social isolation later in life [5], which emphasizes the necessity of facilitating the motor and cognitive development of the children as early as possible. Besides individual physical therapy, children with CP should have the possibility to take part in leisure sports activities in groups of children with and without disabilities.

Performing intensive sports activities may facilitate the motor and cognitive development of the children and ensure a strengthening of their social integration, and should therefore be made available for children with CP.

Climbing involves strength, endurance [6], postural stability [7], technique, balance, coordination [8], route finding [9, 10] and attention [11], as well as a number of psychological aspects beyond fear [12], which put high demands on the participant. Independent of the participant's level of expertise, all of the above mentioned physical and psychological abilities can continuously be challenged in climbing, because there are infinite possibilities of increasing the physical demands and challenge the participants. This is possible in climbing both on artificial climbing walls as well as during outdoor rock climbing.

Because climbing on artificial climbing walls at the same time can be considered safe in terms of number of injuries pr. 1000 h of activity [13, 14] and be mentally and physically challenging, we consider the activity ideal as a challenging way of training mental and physical abilities at the same time. Artificial climbing walls provide several possibilities for varied activities: lead sports climbing, top robe climbing and bouldering. Lead sports climbing is a safe way of climbing, if the necessary precautions are taken, where the participant clicks the safety rope into carabiners while climbing, but it provides the possibility of falling into free air for several meters before the robe catches the climber, which can give rise to mentally challenging situations [15], but may depend on climbing ability level. Top rope climbing is a very safe activity, where the safety rope always go through a safety anchor above the climbing wall. Here the focus can be on the difficulty of the movement rather than fear of falling. Bouldering, where climbing is performed above mattresses to a maximum height of 2.5–3 m without a safety rope, provides an easy way to train specific movements without the need of time consuming rope work, but requires some skills in falling appropriately. The therapeutic benefits of climbing has been studied in patients with physical disabilites [16, 17], mental disorders [18] and neurological disorders [19], where improvements after climbing was found to a similar degree or even higher than conventional therapy, but there may exist possible confounds in many of the studies of the potential therapeutic benefits of climbing (see Buechter &Fechtelpeter 2011 [20]). Studies of effects of climbing in children and adolescents [21, 22], has shown improvements in self-efficacy [22], increases in motor activity [23] and improvements in grip strength and upper body endurance, among other parameters [21]. Despite the possible benefits of climbing injuries have been observed in particular in upper extremities such as shoulders and fingers [14], but with proper warm up and precautions made to minimize certain types of grips [24] reductions in injury rates is expected.

Climbing, can be a sports activity for almost every child, including children with physical disability and cognitive deficit. For children with severe physical disability specific climbing platforms has been developed (see for instance http://www.ep-uk.com/configurations/disabled_-climbing.html). The children had to understand the intention of moving against gravity by climbing, and the fact of falling by losing the grips. Fear of high, severe joint deformities, acute inflammatory joint diseases or increased risk for bone fractures needed further evaluation if climbing is an optimal sport for these children.

One of the main challenges in modern western societies is the lack of physical activity among children and in particular children with physical disabilities. Not only are children with physical disabilities less mobile, which makes it more difficult for them to participate in sports activities in general, they may also experience social stigmatization making it less likely that non-disabled children are going to engage in play and sports with them [5]. Climbing is considered an activity where the participants show a high degree of endogenous motivation to participate [25], which also means that competition between participants become less important compared with for instance team ball sports [25]. This makes climbing an activity where the individual level of expertise becomes less important, and where the individual's relative progress becomes more important. The possibility of adjusting difficulty so it matches the individual's level of expertise combined with both the natural pauses in-between climbing ascents and the obvious visible progress of gripping one more hold or reaching the top, makes climbing a very social sport, where participants can exchange knowledge on how to improve. Furthermore, because of the diversity of ways of climbing, training can be focused on very different aspects of physical skills, such as balance, strength, agility, flexibility, endurance, fear, attention and decision making. This makes it possible to individualize training and target specific needs, such as improving strength in a paretic arm, all within the same settings in a climbing gym, with few adjustments of climbing holds. Henceforth, we have considered climbing an ideal activity where physical disabilities may become less disabling for maintaining interaction with TD peers.

In this study, we investigated the feasibility of climbing training as a mean to activate children with CP and we further explored possible functional, physiological, cognitive and psychological changes following 3 weeks of intensive climbing training in children with CP and a group of TD. We anticipated that the climbing gym, together with skilled instructors, in combination with the notion of climbing as an endogenously motivated activity [25] in 3 weeks of intensive climbing training would I) facilitate a high level of activity among children with CP., II) improve hand coordination and increased pinch grip strength.,III) improve cognitive skills related to spatial working memory and, IV) improve the participant's own evaluation of their physical abilities as well as skills in general. In order to test these predictions and further investigate possible changes caused by 3 weeks of climbing, we combined a set of physiological, functional, cognitive and psychological test to explore possible changes within the respective domains and shed light on possible physiological mechanisms that may change after intensive climbing training.

Methods

Participants

Seventeen children from the age of 11 to 13 years with (N = 11) and without (N = 6) cerebral palsy were recruited to this non randomized, non-blinded feasibility and intervention study. The children with CP were recruited according to their CP diagnosis regardless of CP type or functional level. The only exclusion criteria was severe functional dysfunction that made climbing impossible. Four of the participants knew each other prior to project (TD + CP, CP + CP). Seven of the children with CP attended mainstream school and 4 attended a school with a special program for children with physical and cognitive disabilities. All children in the TD group attended normal school.

The parents gave written and informed consent before the children participated in the study. The study was approved by the local ethics committee of the capital region of Copenhagen (H-B-2009-017). The study was performed in accordance with the Helsinki Declaration.

The participants were recruited through online advertisements. All the participants were unfamiliar with climbing training as an organized sport, a few of the participants had tried an indoor climbing wall before, but none were regular users.

Table 1 provides an overview of the participants including a note on the group that they were assigned to, based on the medical evaluation performed.

Medical evaluation

Neurological examinations were made of all participants by an experienced physiotherapist specialized in child neurology. This examination included test of reflexes, muscle tone, muscle strength, range of motion and gross motor function. History of surgery for in relation to treatments and current antispastic drug use in children with CP were recorded (see under Results).

Intervention

The climbing facility was a climbing gym with approximately 600 m^2 of climbing walls with walls and routes up to 12 m of height. The gym was reserved for this particular purpose during the hours that this intervention took place, which meant that the instructors and participants were the only ones present in the gym during the intervention. The gym was formerly the main climbing gym for the Danish Mountain and Climbing Club, but the club had moved to new larger (2000 m^2) facilities. This older and smaller gym was mainly used for climbing activities with school classes. The first climbing day was performed in the larger facilities of a commercial climbing gym belonging to the Danish Mountain and Climbing Club, where the participants were provided with climbing shoes, which they used throughout the climbing period. During the first day other climbers were present in the commercial climbing gym. Nine days of climbing were planned within a period of 17 days, week 1 & 2: climbing on Monday, Tuesday and Friday,

Table 1 Overview of the participants

Participant	Age (y)	Sex	Height (cm)	Weight[a] (kg)	Group	Electrophysiologically Tested hand[b]	Tested leg	GMFCS
P01	11–13	F	140–150	40–50	CP	L[c]	L	1
P02	11–13	M	140–150	30–40	CP	R[c]	L	2
P03	11–13	M	150–160	40–50	CP	R[c]	R	1
P04	11–13	F	140–150	30–40	CP	R[c]	R	1
P05	11–13	M	140–150	30–40	CP	R[c]	R	1
P06	11–13	M	140–150	30–40	CP	L[c]	L	1
P07	11–13	F	130–140	30–40	CP	L[c]	L	1
P08	11–13	M	130–140	20–30	CP	L[c]	L	1
P09	11–13	M	130–140	20–30	CP	R[c]	R	1
P10	11–13	F	150–160	40–50	CP	L[c]- > R	L- > R	1
P16	11–13	M	150–160	30–40	CP	R[c]	R	1
Mean ± SD	11.6 ± 0.8	: 4 M: 7	145 ± 9.6	35.2 ± 7.5	CP (N = 11)		-	-
P11	11–13	F	140–150	40–50	TD	L- > R	L- > R	Ø
P12	11–13	F	150–160	50–60	TD	R	R	Ø
P13	11–13	M	150–160	40–50	TD	R	R	Ø
P14	11–13	F	140–150	30–40	TD	R	R	Ø
P15	11–13	M	140–150	40–50	TD	R	R	Ø
P17	11–13	F	170–180	60–70	TD	R	R	Ø
Mean ± SD	11.8 ± 0.9	F: 4 M: 2	153 ± 7	46.9 ± 13.2	TD(N = 6)	-	-	-

[a)] Measure of weight is based on the average of three measurement performed in connection with the HUR balance test at the three test rounds. [b)] Based on a combined evaluation of the hand and pinch strength measurements from pre test 1 and 2 and the clinical evaluation used for sorting data for statistical analyses [c)]Based on the participants most disabled hand for the CP group according to their own judgment, under the assumption that we would expect more room for improvement. The evaluation is then only used to sort left and right hand strength and RFD measures to measure performance changes after the climbing intervention

week 3: Climbing on Monday, Tuesday and Wednesday. All climbing was performed in the afternoon after school hours. Each climbing day consisted of approximately 2.5 h of physical activity. The 2.5 h were each time split into approx. 30 min of warm up exercises specifically focused on climbing. Subsequently the participants were split into two half with an approximately equal number of children with CP and TD participants in each group, where one group started with bouldering exercises, The other half of the participants were engaged in wall climbing with a top rope as safety. In order to avoid long waiting times during the top rope session, 3–4 instructors were allocated for the top rope practice, and one instructor was responsible for the bouldering session. After approximately 1 h, the two groups swapped activity. Each climbing day ended with a wrap up where the participants told what they had learned during the day. The intervention was planned as a sports activity, where the focus for the participants was to improve their climbing performance and experience that they learned new skills. Without focusing on specific needs of the individual participant with disabilities, we hoped that the focus of climbing performance also would give rise to therapeutical benefits, but intentionally without focusing on these specifically. This intentional lack of focus on therapeutical benefits was made, because we believe such a focus would remove the intrinsic enjoyment of climbing when applying external goals, see for instance [25]. The mixture of bouldering and top rope climbing provided a good foundation for a great diversity of dynamic and static movements, that challenged the participants motor skills and muscle endurance, demanding their full attention. Implementing both types of climbing also helped getting the participants to stay active and engaged longer, both physically by climbing and mentally by figuring out the routes and bouldering problems.

Three to five climbing instructors were present each day at the climbing gym during the intervention to supervise the 17 participants. The instructors were: one exercise physiologist (BSc), climbing instructor (level 3) and route setter; one neuroscientist, climbing instructor and researcher in this study, one school teacher and climbing instructor, one exercise physiologist student (M.Sc.), climber and researcher in this study, and one physiotherapist and PhD student on a project on CP and climber. The instructors did not have previous experience working with children with CP, but most of them had experience with climbing with children. The supervision consisted of constructive feedback and technical advice (e.g. active use of the legs and toes, advice on how to approach the different forms of holds such as jugs (large positive grips) and crimps (grips only held by the fingertips)) on how the participants could position their body, hands and feet in order to overcome obstacles and hard passages on the wall. Participants were also encouraged to help each other performing the different drills, and point out challenges to each other, when the instructors were not available for 1:1 coaching. During the 2 days with performance measurements (see next section) participants were cheering each other and encouraging one another to do their best. The participants were also engaged in observational learning when watching each other climbing, which have been shown to enhance motor skill learning by initiating formation of cognitive representation in memory that can be enacted and refined during overt practice, further enhancing consolidation of as much information as possible [26, 27]. Furthermore, we hoped that the vicarious experiences through observation of peers (e.g. the children with CP watching other children with CP climb) could promote a sense of personal efficacy for climbing, as it has been shown that observing or visualizing people similar to oneself perform successfully often raise efficacy beliefs in the observer [28].

To enhance social learning and strengthen group dynamics the instructors created a relaxed and playful atmosphere. It has been observed in previous studies that the feeling of relatedness (the feeling of being connected to others) enhances motivation and promote engagement in physical therapy [29–31]. With that in mind a high extent of peer socialization between the children with CP and TD group was emphasized to promote positive attitudes and acceptance instead of alienation between groups. We hoped that through positive relations the groups could inspire each other to a higher degree of task persistence and thereby facilitate the participants' intrinsic motivation (the inherent tendency to seek out new challenges, to explore and to learn [29]) towards the climbing intervention. Furthermore, it was of great importance that the climbing instructors acted as relational key figures for the children, to establish a secure relational basis that provided the foundation for growth-orientated activity participation. Therefore, the instructors implemented and supervised games with emphasis on social interaction among the children as a fundamental part of the climbing sessions to break down physical and mental barriers by having fun.

The warm-up exercises included group- and pair-plays, where all participants were playing with each other. The exercises included chain-catch, were initially two persons had to catch the others, and when one had been captured (he/she) had to hold hands thereby acting as a unity or a chain capturing the remaining participants. The participants also had to climb on each other's bodies and roll across a line of participants.

The climbing exercises included top rope climbing, which is an individual endeavor. However, the instructors strongly encouraged the participants to cheer each other. The instructors continuously adjusted the selection of routes to the different participants according to whether they needed a challenge (choosing a route more difficult than the instructor and participant expected was possible or a good experience (choosing an easy route to gain confidence)).

The bouldering exercises included climbing on problems defined by the instructors. The instructors tried to select problems that were just above the abilities of the participant, in order to challenge them. Often the participants were put into small groups of 3–4 participants working on the same problem, which encouraged them to share ideas on how to perform the movements. The bouldering exercises also included purely movement based tasks, like holding the hands on two pre specified holds and then trying to touch as many holds as possible with the feet. The instructors also designs exercises where specific aspects of climbing techniques were challenged, such as focus on foot-placement on small holds and holding on to edges in various orientations.

Each climbing session was also finished with all participants sitting together and telling what they had learned during the session, and explaining whether they had been able to climb better than expected.

Test procedures

All the physiological, cognitive and psychological tests were performed at the Elsass Institute by an experienced physiotherapist specialized in child neurology or one of the two exercise physiologists that performed all assessments. The 17 participants were tested three times in all of the mentioned tests, unless otherwise stated. Two test rounds were performed prior to the intervention separated by approximately 14 days, and the 17 participants performed each test round within a period of 4–5 days on normal working/school days. The third test round was conducted the following week immediately after the last day of intervention. All the participants attended school and testing was performed such that it fitted within the participant's normal week schedules.

Each test day lasted approximately 3 h in total for each participant. During each test day the order of tests were mixed.

Performance measurements

On day 3 and day 8 each participant was video-filmed on one climbing route using top rope as safety. The participants were filmed on the same route on day 3 and 8 in order to monitor progress in their climbing abilities. A route was selected by the instructors for each participant, which was judged to be just above the individual participant's current (on day 3) climbing abilities, based on subjective evaluations by the instructors from the first 2 days of climbing. The routes were selected among 4 different routes in the climbing gym and were either 12 m or 7 m from ground level to the anchor (top point of the route) ranging in difficulty from grade 4a to 5c + (French sport climbing grading system (https://en.wikipedia.org/wiki/Grade_(climbing))). The video was subsequently used for quantification of climbing performance as measured by 1) total time on the route (from time when both feet were off the ground until the participant was holding the last hold on the wall (before he/she was lowered down)), 2) height of route climbed before decision to stop (and lowered down), 3) number of breaks (i.e. When weight was carried by the safety rope), 4) number of erroneous holds being body weight baring used by the hands, and 5) number of erroneous holds being body weight baring used by the feet.

Climbing speed (m/min) was calculated based on the total time (1) on the route and the total height climbed on the wall (2). Climbing success was calculated as fraction of route climbed. Based on the video recording the high point of climbing (2) was divided by the total height of the route (7 or 12 m). Two participants (TDs) were unfortunately not present during the last climbing days due to illness and therefore no video was recorded of them at day 8 (see also Compliance, below). Therefore performance measurements from these two participants are omitted.

On one of the 9 climbing days the children wore an electronic activity measurement device (SenseWear armband, Temple Healthcare pty Ltd., Bowral, New South wales Australia). The device estimates, based on recordings from accelerometers, thermometers and galvanic skin responses, the amount of activity performed by the wearer of the armband. Because each of the climbing days consisted of the same types of activities, the measurement of the individual participant's activity from the 1 day they carried the armband, was used as a best estimate of their activity level during the climbing days. In order to calculate the total time that the participants in each group on average performed physical activity, we multiplied the time the individual performed physical activity with the number of days they were present for the climbing training. In order to calculate the group average, the total times were added and divided by the number of participants in each group.

During the three test sessions we obtained subjective reports of the amount of activity made during the last week from each participant using a modified version of the International Physical Activity Questionnaire (IPAQ).

Physiological test

Pinch precision task

Electromyographic (EMG) activity of the hand musculature was recorded from 2 channels. Pairs of non-polarized bipolar electrodes (diameter 0.5 cm; Blue sensor, Ambu, Ølstykke, Denmark) placed on the hand over the first dorsal interosseus m. (FDI) and abductor pollicis brevis m. (APB) (interelectrode distance 1.0 cm). Before placement of the electrodes, thorough abrasion of the skin was performed to ensure the best possible signal transduction. The EMG signal were amplified (HiZx10), filtered (band pass, 5 Hz to 1 kHz), sampled at 2000 Hz and stored on a PC for off-line analysis (CED 1401,+ with Signal 5.09 software, Cambridge Electronic Design, Cambridge, UK).

To reduce electrical noise of the EMG recordings of the hand muscles a ground electrode was mounted at the distal end of ulnaris (styloid process). To eliminate electrical inferences (50 Hz noise) two Humbugs (a humbug to filtrate each EMG channel separately due to the possible different noise on the channels) were implemented in the experimental setup (Quest scientific instruments, Vancouver, Canada). Subsequent to the mounting of the electrodes the participants were instructed to perform a maximal contraction on the load cell with the thumb and index finger followed by relaxation of the hand to ensure that the EMG signal for the respective channels were of sufficient quality and stabilized over time.

The dynamic strain gauge amplifier (Dacell, Korea) connected to the load cell was adjusted to gain 800 and The EMG signal for FDI and APB muscles of the selected hand were recorded during the 90 × 7 s. frames of the visuo-motor tracking task.

The participants performed a precision grip task with the thumb and index finger where they had to make a light isometric finger pinch hold for 5 s 90 times (90 frames lasting 7 sec.) without rest with guidance from visual force feedback from the computer screen. The force level of the ramp plateau was set to 5.5 N lasting 5 s with an up-going and down-going slope lasting 0.25 s. The onset of the ramp was varied randomly between 4 different onset times. The force was measured with a load cell (gain ×800) (UU2-K30, Dacell, Korea) elevated slightly on a foam platform to place the hand in a more natural possession for performing the pinch grip. The pinch test task is depicted in Fig. 1a and b in Larsen et al. (2016) [32], with the exception that we in this study used a static pinch instead of a dynamic

Pinch strength task

Pinch strength was tested in the same setup as used for the Pinch precision task, except that force gain was set at ×200 in order to prevent saturation of the signal. Participants performed 3 maximal voluntary contractions (MVCs) with each hand using only their index finger and thumb. After countdown from 3 to 2-1-go participants were instructed to perform a finger pinch as forcefully as possible. Visual feedback of the force was

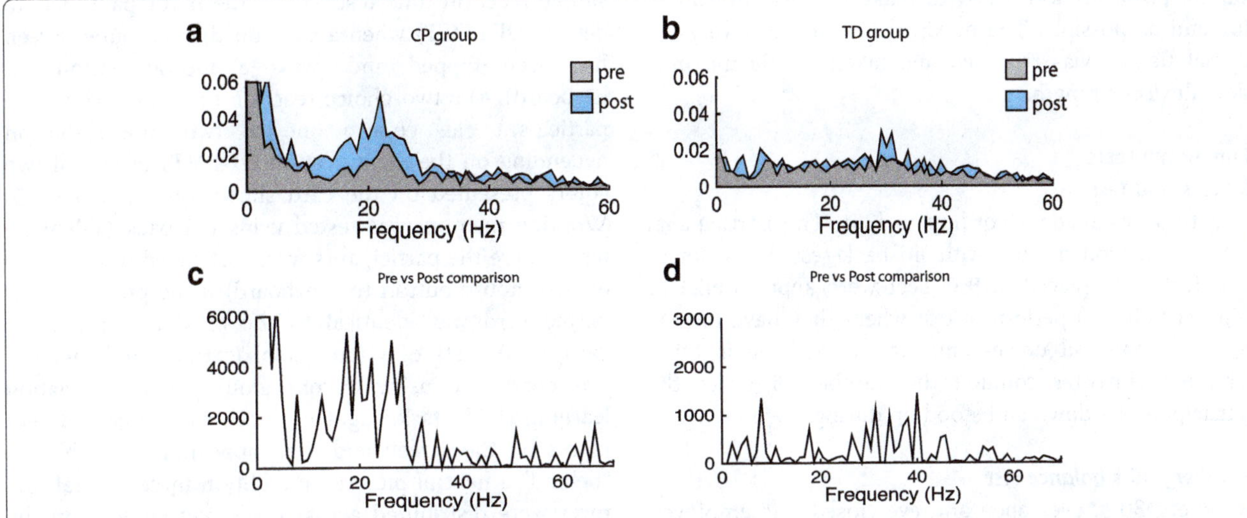

Fig. 1 Changes in FDI_APB coherence following 3 weeks of climbing training. **a-d**. EMG_{APB}-EMG_{FDI} coherence. Pooled Inter-muscular coherence data from EMG_{APB}-EMG_{FDI} for the children with CP (*N* = 10, P16 included in the analysis, P7 excluded according to missing data) and TD (*N* = 6) group respectively. Coherence is calculated from 3.5 s hold phase in 90 trials. A and B shows pooled coherence pre (light gray) and post (light blue) climbing. **c** and **d** show the χ^2 extended test for differences of coherence. Note that the χ^2 values give the statistical differences between the measurements and that peak values of χ^2 values may indicate both an increase and decrease in coherence. It is therefore not possible to determine from the bottom line of graphs which of the measurements was the largest. This can only be determined from the above graph. The dashed horizontal lines in all plots denote the 95% confidence limits χ^2

provided. After the first MVC a horizontal cursor was placed indicating the maximal exerted force and was used as target (to exceed) for the next trials. At least 1 min of rest was provided between trials.

Pinch rate-of-force-development (RFD)

Pinch RFD was tested in the same setup as used for the precision task and strength task, except that force gain was set at ×200 in order to prevent saturation of the signal. Two vertical cursors was placed on the screen with a separation of 1.5 s. The participants were instructed to perform a brisk forceful pinch within the two vertical cursors. If the participant failed to remain relaxed before the first vertical cursor, the trial was repeated. The aim was to perform three valid trials with each hand.

Hand strength

The test of whole hand strength was carried out with an analog hand-dynamometer (North Coast Medical, Gilroy, California, USA). The dynamometer was adjusted to the correct hand size and the participants were instructed to hold the dynamometer with their arm adjacent to the body and elbow flexed approximately 90°. Subsequent to a short introduction and familiarization of the task, the participants performed 3 trials with each hand as forcefully as possible. The experimenter noted the force (measured in kg).

In this test both the least affected and most affected hand were tested. For the TD group this separation was done based on hand dominance.

Ankle contraction

Test of ankle coordination was performed on measures of EMG-EMG coherence within two recording channels. Pairs of non-polarized bipolar electrodes (diameter 0.5 cm; Blue sensor, Ambu, Ølstykke, Denmark) were placed above the TA muscle while participants performed 2 min of static ankle dorsi flexion at 10% of MVC against a constant resistance provided by the experimenter. Signals were amplified and converted into digital signals in a similar way as for the pinch task, but recorded in Spike2 software (Cambridge Electronic Design, Cambridge, UK).

Ankle passive stiffness

Test of ankle stiffness was performed using a hand held dynamometer (PSAD). The test was performed according to the description provided by Willerslev-Olsen et al. [33]

Ankle range of motion

Test of ankle ROM was performed using a hand held dynamometer (PSAD). The test was performed according to the description provided by Willerslev-Olsen et al. [33].

Ankle strength

Test of ankle dorsiflexion strength was performed using a hand held dynamometer (PSAD) [34]. The handheld dynamometer was during the test placed in a secure stable position while the tested person (positioned in supine position) was asked to make a dorsal flexion as forceful as possible. The maximal forced created by the dorsal flexors was recorded and taken as the maximal dorsiflexion strength.

Functional tests

Sit-to-stand test

The test was made according to [35]. The participants were placed on a stool with no back-rest. Hips, knees and feet were placed in 90°. Feet were kept parallel to hip. Participants perform a test where they have to perform as many sit down-stand ups as possible in 30 s. The experimenter counted the number of times the participant sat down and stood up during the 30 s.

Romberg 30 s balance test

Romberg 30 s, eyes open and eye closed was employed on all participants. The participants were placed without shoes and no support on a force platform (HUR BT4 balance trainer, HUR, Helsinki, Finland). Heels were held approximately 2 cm separated with an angle of 30° between the medial sides of the feet. The arms were kept relaxed at the side of the body. Prior to the test height and weight of the participant was obtained. The outcome measure is the C90 areas measured in mm^2, which is the area within which the center of gravity is held for 90% of the test time, as reported previously in [36]. Data from one measurement from one participant was lost due to a technical failure. One participant's data were excluded from analysis, because the participant almost fell asleep standing with.

Cognitive and psychological tests

CogState

CogState is a set of computerized tests that can be assembled from a large battery of various cognitive tests. The tests were conducted on a laptop computer in a quiet room. The instructions to each test was read aloud by the experimenter. Each test was preceded by a short training test. In this project we combined the following tests into a battery that lasted approximately 20–25 min. The tests were: **1)** a visuo-motor skill test **(CHASE)**, where the participant has to chase a moving object inside a 10 × 10 grid of locations for 30 s using clicks with a computer mouse, the outcome measure is number of correct clicks pr. sec. **2)** a test of visuo-spatial memory in the Groton Maze learning test **(MAZE)** where participants has to find a hidden path (maze) from upper left corner to lower right corner in a 10 × 10 grid of locations by revealing, using a mouse click, whether a specific location is within the correct hidden path. In the first trial participants explore the maze and in the subsequent 5 rounds they have to remember the path and move through the path as quickly as possible. **3)** a simple reaction time test, where the participants has to detect **(DETECT)** when a card on the computer screen has been flipped and press a mouse button (or keyboard). **4)** a two-choice reaction time task, where the participant can choose one of two mouse button depending on the identification **(IDENT)** of one of two colors presented on the card shown on the screen. **5)** Working memory was tested using a 1-back **(1-BACK)** task, where the participants were instructed to press one of two mouse button (or keyboard) if the presently displayed card was identical to the previously presented card. **6)** A tests of visuo-spatial learning and memory was conducted using a continuous paired association learning **(PAL)** task: Eight objects was located different places on the screen and their appearance was hidden "behind" a neutral picture, in addition three neutral pictures were distributed across the screen as well, in the center of the screen one of the eight objects was shown, and the participant had to click on the location of that specific object. Five rounds were completed; one round required that all eight objects had been correctly located. When a wrong object location was clicked, the appearance of the objects clicked was revealed. 7) Finally, a delayed recall of the Groton maze-learning test **(MAZE-delay)** was employed at the end of the test session.

Depending on which of the seven test was analyzed, speed (number of clicks pr. s.), reaction times, number of errors or accuracy, or overall normalized scores were calculated (in-build function of the software) and used for statistical tests.

Evaluation of personal and social competencies

In order to explore psychological changes following 3 weeks of climbing training on personal and social competencies, we employed the questionnaire "Sådan er jeg" for 4th–9th grade school children where the participants rate on a 4 point scale how they experience themselves in 72 questions [37]. The questions are ordered into five domains: Physical abilities (14 questions), skills and abilities (14 questions), mental well-being (16 questions), relation to parents (14 questions), and relation to others (14 questions). The ratings were converted into an integer scale (−2, −1, 1, 2) depending on the positive or negative content of the question and a total sum (within or across the five domains) was calculated as raw scores. The raw scores for each domain and the total scores were also transformed into stanine scores (1–9) based on a material of approximately 400 school children (Table 2).

Analysis of electrophysiological data

EMG and coherence analysis

All surface EMG recordings of the FDI and APB muscles were analyzed offline using Matlab 2014b (Mathworks, MA, USA). Electrical recordings for one participant

Table 2 Overview of tests performed

Assessment	Outcome measurement	Comments
Physical activity		
Activity estimates	Amount of physical activity estimated as Total time with meaurement, total physcal acivity, very vigorous, vigorous, modrate, light and sedentary in [hh:mm:ss]	The SenseWear armband has been evaluted in children with relatively good results [58]
Climbing performance		
Route fraction	Fraction [0–1] of specific test climbing route climbed	Height on route is vaild method to access climbing performance and used in lead climbing competitons. We did not emoply disqialification if erroneous holds very used. Measurements a reliable to within 0.5 m, i.e. between 1/14 and 1/24 of the route fraction.
Speed	Estimate of [m/min] climbed of the test climbing route based calculated as the time from start to highest point on route incl. Breaks divided by the estiamated amount of meters climbed from ground to highest point on route.	Time on route is used in climbing competitions to separte climber reaching the same hold on a route. Our measurements were based on total tome on route incl. Breaks, and may therefore not reflect actual climbing speed, but the time spend on the route in total, we believe reflect climbing peformance to some extend. Measurements of time on route are reliable to within 1 s.
Errors (Hands / Feet)	Count [#] of number of times a hold *not* part of the test route was used either with the hands or the feet.	This measurement may not directly access climbing performance.
Functional tests		
Sit-to-stand	Count [#] of sit-stands on 30s	This test is usually done in elderly but also in children with CP to access lower body strenght. Minimum Detectable Change in children with CP is 1.8 rep/30s (based on estimates from [59] where a 5 times STS was performed).It is a reliable and valid test to measure functional strength in children with spastic diplegia [59]
Romberg	Area of sway [mm] of center of gravity in 30s with eyes open and closed	The test reflect balance abilites.
Physiological tests		
Hand strength	Whole hand pinch strength in [N]	The test acceses whole hand strength. The mesurements are reliable to within 5 N.
Pinch strength	Index-tumb finger pinch strength in [N]	The test acceses finger strength. The mesurements are highly reliable.
RFD 0–30 ms	Rate of force increase [N/s] in the first 30 ms after onset of a fast pinch	RFD measurements are the golden standard to measure explosive strength. Our equipment has high reliability.
RFD 0–50 ms	Rate of force increase [N/s] in the first 50 ms after onset of a fast pinch	Do
RFD 0–100 ms	Rate of force increase [N/s] in the first 100 ms after onset of a fast pinch	Do
RFD 0–200 ms	Rate of force increase [N/s] in the first 200 ms after onset of a fast pinch	Do
Coherence		
Finger pinch	Synchronisation of muscle activity between FDI and APB muscles measured as coherence $C(\lambda)_{FDI\text{-}ABF} = \lvert f_{FDI\text{-}ABP}(\lambda)\rvert/(f_{FDI\text{-}FDI}(\lambda) f_{APB\text{-}APB}(\lambda)$. Statistics is done on calculations of log transforms of areas under $C(\lambda)$ in the interval $\lambda = 15–30$ Hz	The assessment partly reflect synchronisation between cortex and muscles, and is therefore an estimate of efficient of efficient motor unit recruitment [60].
Ankle Dorsiflexion	Synchronisation of TA muscle activity between two electrodes TA1 and TA2 measured as coherence $C(\lambda)_{FDI\text{-}ABF} = \lvert f_{TA1\text{-}TA2}(\lambda)\rvert/(f_{TA1\text{-}TA1}(\lambda) f_{TA2\text{-}TA2}(\lambda)$. Statistics is done on calculations of log transforms of areas under $C(\lambda)$ in the interval $\lambda = 15–30$ Hz	The assessment partly reflect synchronisation between cortex and muscles, and is therefore an estimate of efficient of efficient motor unit recruitment [60].
Ankle joint		
Stiffness	Nm/degree	The evaluation of ROM and the ankle stiffness was performed by moving the foot from a plantar flexed position to a maximal dorsal flexed position while
ROM	Range of motion in degrees	

Table 2 Overview of tests performed *(Continued)*

		the participant trying to relax. The movements were made at a slow velocity (<20/s)
Strength	Nm/degree	The maximal force registered during a static contraction was used to reflect strength.
Cognitive tests		
Detection	Reaction time [ms], accuracy [% correct], normalized score [AU]	The assessment tests reaction time as a basic psychomotor function. The measurements based on computer registrations are very reliable.
Identification	Reaction time [ms], accuracy [% correct], normalized score [AU]	The assessment tests choice reaction time and reflects attention. The measurements based on computer registrations are very reliable.
1-back	Reaction time [ms], accuracy [% correct], normalized reaction time [AU], normalized accuracy	The assessment reflect working memory capacities. The measurements based on computer registrations are very reliable.
Chase	Clicks pr. sec. [#]	Test the ability to use a computer mouse. The measurements based on computer registrations are very reliable.
Maze	Total number of error [#], normalized score [AU]	The assessment refect visual spatial memory and is a measurement of executive functions.The measurements based on computer registrations are very reliable.
PAL	Number of errors [#]	The assessments tests paired associative learning. The measurements based on computer registrations are very reliable.
Psychological		
Overall	Normalized scores [0–9]	The assessment is a self-evaluation test which has tested in more than 1500 school children.
Physical abilities	Normalized scores [0–9]	Do
Skills and abilities	Normalized scores [0–9]	Do
Mental well-being	Normalized scores [0–9]	Do
Relationship to parents	Normalized scores [0–9]	Do
Relationship to others	Normalized scores [0–9]	Do

during pretest 2 (P7) were not obtained due to contamination of the signal of the FDI channel and therefore not available for further analysis. The coherence data were epoched in four different time intervals of 3.5 s duration during the tonic pinch grip (corresponding to the four different levels (L) of the ramp plateau; L1 = (1.5–5 s.), L2 = (1.75–5.25 s.), L3 = (2–5.5 s.), L4 = (2.25–5.75 s.)). As preprocessing steps before undertaking population analysis the epoched data were notch filtered to reduce 50 Hz noise, normalized to have unit variance, full wave rectified to maximize the information regarding timing of motor unit action potentials [38–41] and possible contamination of electrical cross-talk were removed for all EMG data by visual inspection. Only EMG amplitudes above approximately 1/2 of the mean EMG amplitudes were used for further analysis, in order to remove low amplitude cross talk between muscles (the Matlab application software Peakfinder was used for this purpose, http://www.mathworks.com/matlabcentral/fileexchange/25500-peakfinder-x0%2D-sel%2D-thresh%2D-extrema%2D- includeendpoints–interpolate-). Power spectra were constructed from sections of data (of 3.5 s. duration) taken at a fixed offset time with respect to trigger points in accordance with the ramp cycle levels mentioned earlier (4 cycles: [1.5–5 s.], [1.75–5.25], [2–5.5], [2.25–5.75]) [42].

Normalized signals are assumed to be realizations of stationary zero mean time series, denoted by x and y. Power spectra were constructed from sections of data taken at a fixed offset time with respect to a trigger point in each trial. Estimates of the power spectra were constructed by averaging periodograms across all trials. $F_{xx}(\lambda)$ and $f_{yy}(\lambda)$ represent the Fourier transforms of processes x, and y, at frequency λ. The cross spectrum between x and y is denoted by $f_{xy}(\lambda)$, and is estimated in a similar manner. Two functions were then used to characterize the signals' correlation structure: coherence, and cumulant density. Coherence estimates are bounded measures of association defined over the range [0, 1]. The cumulant density provides an unbounded time-domain representation of the EMG-EMG correlation structure analogous to the motor unit cross-correlogram and is defined as the inverse Fourier transform of the cross-spectrum [43]. For the present data, coherence estimates provide a measure of the fraction of activity in one EMG (APB) signals that can be predicted be the activity in the other EMG (FDI) signal. In this way, the coherence in this particular experiment is an estimate for the common input to the two muscles (inter-muscular (IM) coherence). In order to summarize the correlation structure across participants, the individual coherence and cumulant density estimates were pooled providing a single time or frequency domain measure [44]. The interpretation of pooled estimates of spectrum, coherence and cumulant is similar to those obtained for individual records, except any inferences related to the population as a whole. The individual coherence and cumulant density were likewise pooled across participants to provide single time and frequency domain measures and the $\chi 2$ extended difference of coherence test were used to make statistical inferences regarding the difference of coherence between the EMG signals of the FDI and APB muscle [42]. EMG from two separate sets of TA electrodes were imported into Matlab. The procedure for analysis was the same as for the EMG^{APB}-EMG^{FDI} analysis except that the data was generated during a 2 min static contraction and not a concatenation of several epochs of static contraction.

Analysis of pinch RFD

Force was measured using a hand held pinch device with a strain gauge providing voltage output corresponding linearly to the applied isometric force. Force onset was calculated using an initial visual inspection of the force measured. A time point prior to visible force onset was identified and a stable force baseline 500 ms prior to that point was calculated. Actual force onset was then calculated as the time point after the visually identified point that exceeded 2 times standard deviation of the 500 ms force baseline.

Analysis of MVC

All MVC data was exported from Signal as Matlab files and analyzed using Matlab 2014b. A customized Matlab script provided information regarding the peak values of the participants' trials to each experimental session (pretest1, prestest 2 and posttest). The trial with the highest MVC value for the left and right hand respectively to each of the sessions was used for further analysis. The peak magnitude of the MVC data, originally measured in Volt, was converted into N.

Analysis of RFD

RFD data was converted into Matlab files and analyzed in Matlab 2014. A customized matlab script was designed and the RFD performed by the voluntary contraction of the thumb and index finger was calculated at different time points (30, 50, 100 and 200 ms) following onset of contraction (which was defined as the time point when the force measurement exceed 2 x SD of the baseline force level. A time point just before the force increase was set by visual inspection which was used to calculate the baseline force 500 ms before the time point set by visual inspection. When the force exceed 2 x SD of the baseline after the time point set by visual inspection, onset of the RFD task was defined). RFD for each participant (3 trials for left and right hand respectively) was first analyzed by visual inspection and all trials contaminated by activity prior to the actual contraction (resulting in upward deflection of baseline force) were discarded. The RFD for the retained trials was then obtained from the slope of the force-time curve (Δforce/Δtime) between time periods of 0-30 ms, 0-50 ms, 0-100 ms, and 0-200 ms relative to the onset of contraction, which is used to express the rate of rise in contractile force [45]. The trial with the highest RFD (N/s) for each hand was used and the mixed linear model described earlier was employed.

Statistical tests

Analysed data from the different tests were imported into R-studios (RStudio Team (2015) RStudio: Integrated Development for R. RStudio, Inc., Boston, MA URL *http://www.rstudio.com/*.) for further statistical analysis. A linear mixed model was used to investigate the effect of the climbing intervention on coherence by testing the specific interactions between group and intervention time and the differences between the values for pretest2 vs. the posttest in the CP and TD group. The large variability between participants was accounted for by including the 'participant' in the model as random effect, reparametrized interaction between group and time as fixed effects and age, height, gender as fixed effects. For all linear mixed models, Normal Quantile-Quantile plots were made, and analyses were rejected if these did not visually display an approximate linear relationship. In addition, residual plots were inspected visually in order to ensure near normal distributions.

In order to test specific hypotheses concerning the effect of the climbing intervention on the two groups we tested differences between pretest 2 and postest in the children with CP and in the TD group, and in order to test for unspecific learning effects due to multiple exposure to the same test, we tested the differences between pretest 1 and 2 in the children with CP and in the TD group.

Correlations were tested using a Pearson's product-moment correlation.

Statistical trends $^{o})$ $p < 0.1$, as well as statistical significant results $^{*})$ $p < 0.05$, $^{**})$ $p < 0.01$, $^{***})$ $p < 0.001$ are indicated when tested.

Results

Participants, physical activity and compliance

Four children with CP had tendon lengthening surgery 2–6 years prior the intervention and no children received antispastic medication.

All children with CP were diagnosed with bilateral CP except one participant that was diagnosed as unilateral CP. All children with CP were ambulant and categorized with GMFCS 1 except in one case with GMFCS 2. No walking aids were used by any of the children with CP but in 6 of the children ankle orthoses were used during daytime, but not during the climbing training. No hand or elbow orthoses were used in the group of children with CP.

The neurological examination revealed generally reduced ability to produce force bilaterally in dorsal flexors, plantar flexors, elbow flexors and elbow extensors. Spasticity was identified (>/= 1 on the MAS scale) in the plantar flexors in 7 cases and elbow flexors in 3 cases. Reduced range of motion was identified (dorsal flexion <20 degrees) in the ankle joint in 6 cases whereas no reduction in elbow was found in any of the cases.

The TD children all had normal age related strength, normal range of motion in all joints-, reflex activity and walking ability.

The primary outcome of this study is that children with CP perform an equal amount of physical activity as their TD peers without having to perform training interventions that are specialized for children with physical disabilities.

Table 3 summarizes the amount of time that was spent doing physical activity during the climbing training sessions. As the results indicate, both groups wore the armband approximately the same duration (within 2 min) and performed the same amount of physical activity.

Nine of the 11 children with CP took part in all 9 climbing days, one child with CP missed 1 day due to a logistic problem, another child with CP cancelled one climbing day due to a school arrangement. Three of the TD participants took part in all climbing days and three took part in 6 of the 9 climbing days. Cancellations in the TD group were due to illness, logistics or other arrangements, not lack of interest in the training.

Using the individual's own time spent doing physical activity, which on average was 1:45 h. We calculated the total time of physical activity performed during the climbing sessions. The children with CP performed on average 16:05 h of physical activity during the climbing specific training and the TD group performed on average 13:01 h of physical activity taking into consideration how often each individual was present at the training. The IPAQ questionnaire disclosed that all children except two (one child with CP and one TD) made the climbing training as addition to their normal activities.

The measures of the performance during the climbing intervention test climbing route is summarized in Table 3. These results show that the children with CP improved climbing performance by the fraction of the test route climbed. However, the children with CP also increased their number of erroneous hand and footholds used during the test climb. The TD group improved climbing speed.

Adverse events

During a warm up play on one of the last days of climbing one of the TD participants accidentally sprained the wrist in a collision with one of the other participants.

Functional tests

Significant improvement was seen after the climbing intervention in number of times the children with CP were able to perform a sit-to-stand movement (pre intervention mean 20.2 SD 4.6, median 19 IQR 17; post intervention mean 23.5 SD 5.8, median 25 IQR 18.5; $p < 0.01$). In order to investigate whether the improvement in Sit-to-Stand was related to climbing performance, we performed correlation analyses of the change in Sit-to-Stand with the change in climbing performance (Climbing speed and fraction of route climbed) from pretest 2 to posttest in the children with CP. Neither of the two correlation analyses revealed significant relationships. No significant improvements were observed in the Romberg 30 s tests. Further details can be found in the Additional file 1: S1.

Physiological tests

Strength measurements

We found significant improvements in the children with CP for the pinch grip RFD calculations of the least affected hand as a result of the climbing intervention in the time intervals 0-50 ms ($p < 0.05$), 0-100 ms ($p < 0.01$) and 0-200 ms ($p < 0.05$). No significant

Table 3 Amount of time that was spent doing physical activity during the climbing training sessions

	Total duration	Physical activity	Very vigorous	Vigorous	Moderate	Light	Sedentary
All (*N* = 17)	02:32:42	**01:45:32**	00:00:04	00:14:39	01:30:49	00:46:42	00:00:28
CP (*N* = 11)	02:33:38	**01:45:27**	00:00:05	00:14:27	01:30:55	00:48:00	00:00:11
TD (*N* = 6)	02:31:00	**01:45:40**	00:00:00	00:15:00	01:30:40	00:44:20	00:01:00

Estimates of duration of physical activity based on measures from the SenseWear armband, all number indicates average duration (hh:mm:ss) of estimated physical activity. The total duration indicates how long time the participants wore the armband. All participants wore the armband at one of the climbing days improvements were found for whole hand-and pinch strength (MVC) for any of the groups. Further details can be found in the Additional file 1: S2 and S3.

Pinch coherence

Results of the EMG-EMG coherence analysis for m. FDI and m. APB are summarized in Fig. 1. We have displayed the pooled coherence for the children with CP in 1A and the TD group in 1B. Here we observed an increase in coherence for the children with CP in a spectrum of frequencies spanning ~10 - ~30 Hz when comparing pre and post intervention. This was not the case for the TD group. The χ^2 difference is depicted in Fig. 1b for the children with CP and 1C for the TD group, showing pronounced, above the confidence interval, increase in EMG-EMG coherence during the pinch precision task. To further investigate the coherence results the difference in log normalized area under the coherence curve in the 15–30 Hz beta band was calculated and showed significant ($z = 2.819$, $p = 0.0184$) increases in the children with CP, when tested in a mixed linear model.

Ankle contraction

Results of the EMG-EMG coherence analysis during the 2 min of static ankle dorsi flexion are summarized in Fig. 2. We have displayed the pooled coherence for the children with CP (2A) and the TD group (2B). Comparisons of pre and post intervention in the ~10 - ~30 Hz range shows a trend towards a difference in pooled coherence for the children with CP but not for the TD group. The χ^2 difference confirms a slight, above the confidence interval, increase in EMG-EMG coherence for the children with CP, especially around the 20 Hz bin. To further investigate the changes in coherence from pretest2 to posttest we calculated the log normalized area under the coherence curve and tested it in a mixed linear model in the 15–30 Hz beta band. This confirmed the trend ($z = 1.95$, $p = 0.0994$) of coherence increases in the children with CP, but did not obtain significant difference.

Ankle joint measurements

Unfortunately the PSAD device did not work properly on Pretest2 and we therefore only compared the measurements of ankle joint stiffness and ankle joint range of motion from Pretest1 with the Posttest. These measurements showed a significant improvement in range of motion (ROM) ($p < 0.05$) for the children with CP but not for the TD group. No significant differences were observed in ankle joint stiffness for any of the groups. Further details can be found in the Additional file 1: S4.

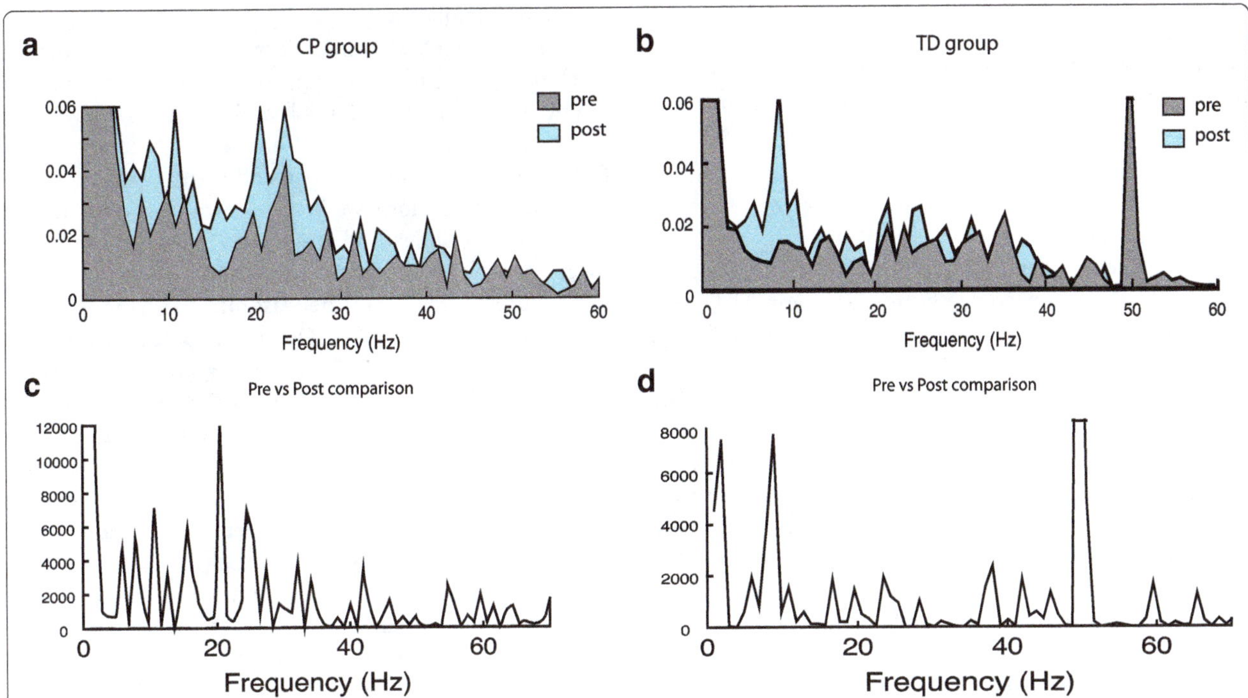

Fig. 2 Changes in TA-TA coherence following 3 weeks of climbing training. TA-TA coherence. Pooled Intra-muscular coherence data from EMG_{TA} -EMG_{TA} pretest 2 and post climbing training for the CP (*N* = 11) group and TD group (*N* = 6) are shown in the top panel. **a** and **b** shows pooled coherence pre (light gray) and post (light blue) climbing. **c** and **d** show the χ^2 extended test for differences of coherence and reveal the difference between the two test sessions. Test of the coherence for the TA measurements revealed modest differences in χ^2 values in a wide frequency band for the children with CP with a peak in the 20 Hz bin

Ankle strength

Ankle strength was measured as torque around the ankle joint using the PSAD. Only data from pretest 1 and posttest was acquired and compared. The linear mixed model of TA strength did not reveal a significant difference between the pretest and posttest in the children with CP or the TD group. Further details can be found in the Additional file 1: S5.

Cognitive and psychological tests

CogState computerized tests was used to assess speed and accuracy in a detection task, and identification task (two choice reaction time task), in a 1-back working memory task, in a continuous paired association learning task and in a maze learning task.

The linear mixed model of the combined detection score did not reveal a significant difference between the pretest 2 and post test in the cardbased CogState computerized tests (the DETECT, IDENT and 1-BACK tasks) or the spatial location based tasks (the CHASE test, the MAZE test, the PAL test and the MAZEdelay test) in any of the groups. Further details can be found in the Additional file 1: S6.

Evaluation of personal and social competencies

The results of the self-reported questionnaire "Sådan er jeg", where the participant should self-report their experience of themselves in 72 questions in 5 different domains did not show significant differences in any of the groups when comparing pre2 and post. Further details can be found in the Additional file 1: S7 (Table 4).

Discussion

Summary of results

We have shown that children with CP can engage in climbing training on equal terms with their TD peers. The children with CP performed equally many hours of physical activity as their TD peers, which amount to more than 5 h per weeks of moderate or vigorous physical activity.

Furthermore, four children with CP and three of the TD children and their parents expressed a wish to continue the climbing training after the 3-weeks ended. On a side note it is also worth mentioning, that three of the children after the 3-week period continued climbing as an organized sport in a local climbing club.

In the present study we have shown that children in the age range of 11 to 13 with and without cerebral palsy can improve climbing abilities with less than 3 weeks of intense climbing training. Furthermore, we have demonstrated that some aspects of physiological measures as well as functional measures can be improved in children with CP with less than 3-weeks of climbing.

In summary, children with CP improved the fraction of the test route climbed, but at the expense of producing more hand placement mistakes while climbing. The children in the TD group did not improve the fraction of route climbed but increased their climbing speed.

With respect to functional improvements, children with CP improved their Sit-to-stand score, a measure used as a general measure of motor abilities.

The physiological tests revealed a significant increase in EMG-EMG coherence in the pinch task for the children with CP after the climbing intervention. Furthermore, the children with CP increased RFD in their least affected hand after the climbing intervention and had increased range of motion in the ankle joint.

None of the cognitive computer tests or the psychological questionnaire revealed any significant changes in either of the two groups when comparing before and after climbing training.

This study extends upon previous studies of biomechanical and physiological effects of sport climbing [7, 46–50]. Previous studies of psychological effects of rock climbing has previously focused on performance anxiety [51–53], attention [11] or the experience of flow [25] but to our knowledge no other studies has focused on effects of climbing training upon other psychological domains.

Functional significance

We have shown that a short intense intervention period of climbing training can improve climbing performance in children with CP GMFCS level I and II. We have also shown that a very basic test of general functional performance reveals improvements after the climbing intervention. Furthermore we have shown that fine motor control of the index and thumb is changed as reflected by an increase in coherence in the most affected hand of the children with CP. In the least affected hand the children with CP improved RFD from 0 to 100 ms. Finally, we have shown that climbing training increase the ankle joint ROM in the children with CP measured on the most affected lower limb. These findings suggest that climbing training have physiological impact on both upper and lower limb physiology and that climbing training can improve aspects of general functionality as measured by the Sit-to-stand test.

The psychological as well as cognitive tests did not reveal any significant improvements. All though climbing training has mental aspects related to management of fear and anxiety and cognitive aspects related to decision making and planning we were not able to see any effects on the employed measurements. This may be due to several reasons. The number of participants was rather small compared to the groups that the psychological test (Sådan er jeg) has been evaluated on.

Table 4 Summary of tests performed

	$CP_{pre; post}$	$CP_{pre \to post}$	$TD_{pre;post}$	$TD_{pre \to post}$
Climbing performance				
Route fraction[a]	0.6(0.23)- > 0.89(0.25)(N = 11)	Z = 4.77, p = 3.7·10^{-6}***	0.74(0.19)- > 0.94(0.13)(N = 4)	Z = 1.81p = 0.127
Speed[a] (m/min)	2.2(0.9)- > 2.9(1.0)(N = 11)	Z = 1.43, p = 0.28	3.9(1.3)- > 5.6(2.0)(N = 4)	Z = 2.86, p = 0.0084**
Errors[a] (#) (Hands / Feet)	2.6(0–9)/4.6(0–8)- > 7.4(0–14)/8.5(0–22)(N = 11)	Z = 3.299, p = 0.0019** / Z = 2.20, p = 0.054°	0.25(0–4/0.5(0–3)- > 0.0(0)/ 0.0(0)(N = 4)	Z = −0.043, p = 0.999 / Z = −0.09, p = 0.995
Functional tests				
Sit-to-stand (#)	20.2(4.6)- > 23.5(5.8)(N = 11)	Z = 3.072, p = 0.0083**	29.0(4.5)- > 30.7(4.5)(N = 6)	Z = 1.044, p = 0.723
Romberg (open / closed)	613(550)- > 504(445)(N = 11)	Z = −1.35, p = 0.509 / z = −0.467, p = 0.979	408(119)- > 754(553)(N = 6)	Z = 0.295, p = 0.996 / Z = 1.917, p = 0.191
Physiological tests				
Hand strength (least / most)	158(58)/114(55)-> 167(51)/128(60)(N = 11)	Z = 1.067, p = 0.708 / Z = 1.715, p = 0.283	216(82)/195(68)-> 227(69)/201(58)(N = 6)	Z = 0.745, p = 0.895 / Z = 0.208, p = 0.999
Pinch strength (least / most)	34.8(6.3)/29.4(8.7)-> 37.5(7.0)/32.2(8.3)(N = 11)	Z = 1.165, p = 0.639 / Z = 1.009, p = 0.746	43.1(12.0)/40.9(12.2)-> 47.3(14.9)/43.1(14.7)(N = 6)	Z = 1.263, p = 0.569 / Z = 0.441, p = 0.983
RFD 0–30 ms (least / most)	59.2(58.6)/50.6(64.4)-> 79.6(68.6)/54.5(68.6)(N = 11)	Z = 1.797 p = 0.242 / Z = 0.714, p = 0.908	69.3(49.0)/41.6(13.3)-> 72.6(29.6)/54.2(25.4)(N = 6)	Z = 0.003, p = 1.0 / Z = 1.493, p = 0.412
RFD 0–50 ms (least / most)	79.0(63.7)/80.0(79.4)-> 109.1(76.6)/90.6(84.8)(N = 11)	Z = 2.317, p = 0.0752° / Z = 1.045, p = 0.723	99.7(66.4)/72.1(28.0)-> 113.6(45.6)/79.6(29.3)(N = 6)	Z = 0.584, p = 0.953 / Z = 0.269, p = 0.997
RFD 0–100 ms (least / most)	110.9(53.1)/109.5(78.5)-> 154.4(56.5)/123.3(76.8)(N = 11)	Z = 2.939, p = 0.0174* / Z = 0.872, p = 0.830	147.5(87.6)/132.3(57.9)-> 171.6(70.9)/133.4(47.5)(N = 6)	Z = 0.989, p = 0.759 / Z = −0.208, p = 0.999
RFD 0–200 ms (least / most)	105.6(36.4)/91.9(45.4)-> 133.9(18.7)-101.4(40.5)(N = 11)	Z = 2.309, p = 0.0768° / Z = 0.733, p = 0.900	133.2(53.9)/123.4(54.6)-> 145.4(60.3)/135.6(49.1)(N = 6)	Z = 0.595, p = 0.9498 / Z = 0.527, p = 0.967
Coherence				
Finger pinch (FDI-APB)	-1.73(0.84)- > −0.89(0.91)(N = 10- > 11)	Z = 2.81, p = 0.0184*	−1.58(0.63)- > −1.49(0.83)(N = 6)	Z = 0.239, p = 0.993
Ankle Dorsiflexion (TA-TA)	-0.96(0.88)- > −0.57(0.98)(N = 11)	Z = 1.951, p = 0.0994°	−1.10(0.45)- > −0.91(0.82)(N = 6)	Z = 0.644, p = 0.7964
Ankle joint				
Stiffness[b]	4.57(1.86) - > 4.08(1.82)(N = 11)	Z = −1.002, p = 0.533	5.05(1.80)- > 5.17(1.18)(N = 5)	Z = 0.379, p = 0.913
ROM[b]	62.5(12.0) - > 67.98(7.76) (N = 11)	Z = 2.764, p = 0.0114*	63.12(6.62)- > 66.16(5.16)(N = 5)	Z = 1.019, p = 0.5214
Strength[c]	25.9(9.5)- > 30.2(12.0)(N = 11)	Z = 1.387, p = 0.304	45.9(17.5)- > 40.7(13.8)(N = 6)	Z = −1.476, p = 0.260
Cognitive tests				
Detection[d]	83.3(10.9)- > 83.1(10.0)(N = 11)	z = −0.048, p = 1.0	98.3(8.5)- > 95.7(7.3)(N = 6)	Z = −0.648, p = 0.933
Identification[d]	87.4(8.0)- > 87.5(9.6)(N = 11)	Z = 0.032, p = 1.0	94,2(6.3)- > 95.3(6.7)(N = 6)	Z = 0.345, p = 0.993
1-back (speed/accuracy)[d]	959(139)/82.3(9.4)-> 962(214)/82.0(7.9)(N = 11)	Z = 0.199, p = 0.999 / Z = −0.190, p = 0.999	768(163)/91.3(12.7)-> 753(198)/91.7(9.4)(N = 6)	Z = 0.473, p = 0.978 / Z = −0.039, p = 1.00
Chase[e]	1.02(0.23)- > 1.15(0.23)(N = 11)	Z = 2.057, p = 0.140	1.54(0.23)- > 1.48(0.22)(N = 6)	Z = −0.646, p = 0.934
Maze[d]	99.6(6.5)- > 103.2(6.4)(N = 11)	Z = 1.721, p = 0.279	101.3(3.7)- > 105.2(5.1)(N = 6)	Z = 1.453, p = 0.438

Table 4 Summary of tests performed *(Continued)*

PAL	45.6(51.1)- > 32.0(62.9)(N = 11)	Z = −1.940, p = 0.181	15.3(15.8)- > 6.5(3.4)(N = 6)	Z = −1.122, p = 0.670
Psychological				
Overall	4.00(2,05)- > 4.63(2.41)(N = 11)	Z = 1.327, p = 0.524	5.5(2.42)- > 6.50(2.07)(N = 6)	Z = 1.484, p = 0.418
Physical abilities	4.64(2.73)- > 4.45(2.73)(N = 11)	Z = −0.342, p = 0.993	5.83(2.93)- > 5.83(2.99)(N = 6)	Z = −0.083, p = 1.000
Skills and abilities	4.54(2.25)- > 4.45(2.38)(N = 11)	Z = −0.216, p = 0.999	4.33(2.5)- > 5.67(2.16)(N = 6)	Z = 1.896, p = 0.198
Mental well-being	4.09(2.21)- > 4.91(2.59)(N = 11)	Z = 1.457, p = 0.436	5.83(1.72)- > 6.67(1.96)(N = 6)	Z = 1.024, p = 0.736
Relationship to parents	3.18(1.89)- > 4.18(2.36)(N = 11)	Z = 1.481, p = 0.420	7.33(1.63)- > 6.83(1.72)(N = 6)	Z = −0.516, p = 0.970
Relationship to others	4.45(2.06)- > 5.27(2.37)(N = 11)	Z = 1.389, p = 0.481	7.67(0.82)- > 7.0(1.55)(N = 6)	Z = −0.804, p = 0.867

Summary of all tests performed and the effect of the climbing intervention. Z-scores and *p*-values are obtained from the employed linear mixed models where four tests have been made, Pre1 vs Pre 2 and Pre 2 vs Post both in the CP and TD group. Only statistics from the pre2 vs post session are presented, but *p*-values are adjusted for multiple comparisons where the pre 1vs pre2 comparison is included. (Least/Most): indicate test of changes in the least or most affected hand. [a] Data from two time points only at day 3 and day 8 of the climbing intervention days. [b] Data from Pre1 and Post only due to technical issue with the measurement device at Pre2 test. [c] Data only from Pre2 and Post. [d] Tests for the combined score-measurements are shown here. The individual test of speed and accuracy are not presented here. None of them revealed significant differences when comparing the effect of the climbing intervention in any of the two groups. [e] The chase test revealed a significant improvement in number of clicks per sec. In the TD group between pre1 and pre2. °) $p < 0.1$, *) $p < 0.05$, **) $p < 0.01$, ***) $p < 0.001$. Correlation analyses was performed between the changes in the Sit-to-stand, ROM, RFD 0-100 ms and Coherence between FDI and APB measurements the improvements in the climbing abilities in the children with CP. However, none of correlations were significant

Clinical significance

Climbing training seems to be a way to engage children with CP in many weekly hours of physical activity in a fun and motivating way that may help improve climbing skills, muscle strength, balance, as well as mental and social skills. Therefore, we propose climbing as an efficient clinical training method with several benefits for children with CP.

This is also what we experienced during the intervention. Although the children had very diverse physical capabilities, they all found routes that suited their different skill-sets. With guidance from the instructors the participants could progress on these routes, often in collaboration with their peers from both the CP and the TD group. The mixture of top rope and bouldering provided a good foundation for the participants to try many different aspects of climbing, and for the instructors it increased the possibilities for setting up playful climbing games where the participants could interact independently of their physical foundation.

The participants self-reliance in relation to their climbing abilities may have improved during the 3 weeks and that the immediate feedback that the nature of climbing provided (e.g. overcoming specific obstacles on the route), may have fueled the children's pursue of their inherent enjoyment rather than external reward or influence. Some of the children even personalized the routes, as one of the children with CP expressed it: He wanted to overcome his 'arch enemy' (the route he progressed on for several weeks). The participants had surprisingly few complaints about the level of their physical exertion, even though the sessions were relatively long and challenged the participants both physically and mentally. This may reflect that the climbing environment and the instructors encouraged the participants to develop the right mindset and self-determination for pushing their limits. In that context, it was enjoyable to see that the children with CP met the challenge with the same enthusiasm as the healthy controls, even though the training was not specifically adapted to the children with CP. Future studies could have even more focus on customizing the climbing training in order to accommodate the specific needs of participants with disabilities. Especially it could be of interest to investigate if climbing training can be used as an effective tool to treat people with even more severe CP. It should also be noted that the clinical significance of climbing has started to be recognized in other patient groups as well (e.g. in people with multiple sclerosis and geriatric patients) [54–56].

Comparison with previous studies

Only very few studies have been conducted looking at effect of (therapeutic) climbing training in children and adolescents [21–23]. We did not find significant changes in hand strenght. The average hand strength measurements reported by pervious studies in youth climbers at a comparable age [21] are within the range which we also observe (between 0.25 and 0.69 (kg/body weight) in the most dominant hand. However, the ranges for the study by Balas is unknown. Balas et al. used 8 weeks of training where we only look at the 3 weeks of training. That may be a reason to why we do not see changes in hand strengt. Balas only observed changes in the group that performed a high volume of climbing. Unfortunately we do not have any reliable way of estimating the amount of climbed meters as Balas et al. had.

With respect to the intervention intensity, previous studies have used climbing once or twice a week for 8 weeks [21] for children that already were climbing, A study of climbing in children with special needs Mazzoni et al. (2009) used 1 hour of climbing once a week for 6 weeks [22]. Therme et al. 1992 used 6 training session (unfortunately, only access to the abstract was available) so further details of the intervention are not possible to obtain [23]. Our intervention protocol was more densely packed, but in terms of total duration pr. day, but also in terms of number of sessions per week (three vs. one or two. However, we do not believe this relatively higher intervention intensity had a major role to play in terms how compliance. For all cases of absentee, reasons such as already planned family arrangements, missing transportation to the climbing gym and illness were given. This relatively high weekly frequency of climbing was used, because the overall duration of the project had to be limited, but future interventions would more ideally be spread over a longer total duration with max 2 training sessions per, week, with a possible gradual increase in weekly frequency.

Perspectives

Children with CP are often confronted with the challenge that they are not disabled enough to participate in adaptive sports, but fall short in traditional competitive sports, which can lead to a loss of motivation and self-confidence [57]. Climbing as an intervention tool has the advantage that the participant competes against him- or herself and the many different routes makes it possible to adjust the level of difficulty according to the requirements of the individual. This provides a basis for successful experiences in a social environment, independent of the level of expertise. Climbers of different levels may climb together or alongside each other with the possibility of the more experienced climbers providing positive feedback to the less experienced, further enhancing good relations between climbers

One can hope that the climbing environment in the future can be an arena for children with CP where they can develop social, mental and motor skills alongside their healthy peers, without the fear of falling short of certain competitive standards. The use of climbing as a tool in physical therapy is still a largely uninvestigated area and therefore much more research should be done on the possible physical, psychological and social benefits of climbing.

Methodological considerations

This study was designed as an exploratory study in order to investigate whether climbing training has the potential to be used as a possible therapeutic intervention, which combines physical and psychological challenges. In order to take into account possible exposure bias to the employed tests, we decided to compare two pre-intervention tests against the pre-post intervention comparison. We tested the differences between the pre1 and pre2 test and only found a significant improvement of the chase test in the CogState test battery for the TD group. All other tests did not show any significant differences between the pre1 and pre2 test. We therefore believe possible learning effect are minimal, and therefore differences between pre2 and post are more likely due to an interventional effect rather than an unspecific learning effect. Some of the employed tests, such as the questionnaire "Sådan er jeg" and the CogState tests may be very general, and not specific enough to test effects of the intervention. In particular we believe the "Sådan er jeg" questionnaire, after having employed it, is not suited for these short term intervention studies. With respect to the CogState tests we hoped to see effects on the MAZE-LEARNING test because the skills that the test resembles are similar to what you learn when trying to memorize a climbing route. The remaining tests in the CogState battery were less climbing-skill related.

The study was designed with the purpose of exploring whether children with CP can engage in climbing training together with their peers and explore possible physiological, psychological and social gains from climbing training. To explore these parameters in the most reliable way, practical issues from the surrounding activities, such as getting to the gym, organizing climbing coaches, etc. was taken care of by the experimenters and not the participant's and their parents to the same degree as "normal" climbing training would require. Therefore, the surrounding circumstances were somewhat easier to cope with for the participants and their parents. We employed a relatively high instructor-to-participant ratio with 3–5 instructors to 17 children. This was done because we wanted to focus on both bouldering and top rope climbing, where the latter requires someone who can belay (hold the rope through a breaking device) the climber. Under normal circumstances, part of a longer climbing training course, belaying would be something that was taught the participants in the beginning or taken care of by parents. But because we wanted to focus on climbing as a physical activity (with it's related aspects) we did not teach belaying techniques during the 3-week session. Furthermore, the activities took place in the early afternoon after school, where the parents of the children were still at work. It has to be considered that the instructors were highly motivated towards the intervention and already prepared that special precautions had to be made in order to properly adjust the climbing training to the children with CP. We therefore acknowledge that this fact potentially could bias the effect of the intervention to favor the children with CP, but when an instructor deals with a participant it would be impossible not to individualize the instruction without paying attention to the individual participant's needs. At the same time the setting of the climbing intervention took place in a safe and inclusive environment, where the instructors facilitated interation between all participants. Therefore, in order to implement children with CP in real life climbing settings, a challenge could be the recruitment of dedicated instructors that are willing to make an extra effort, preferably with some prior knowledge of CP. However, a specialized team has been established for 6 children with CP where they climb once a week in a public climbing gym. Further, the disability level of the children with CP in this study has to be considered. The Children in our study was (with one exception) level 1 on GMFCS scale and therefore had a reasonable level of functional capability. Therefore, another consideration is how well a climbing intervention like ours could be implemented for more severely challenged children with CP.

Statistical considerations

Despite the very small group of participants included in this study, we were able to show some changes in the functional and physiological tests. However, given the large number of tests we performed none of the tests would survive strict Bonferroni correction for multiple comparisons. We have therefore decided to show all tests uncorrected in order to give a better impression of the raw results from the individual tests. We also decided not to correct for multiple comparisons because many of the tests cannot be considered completely independent. As an example, we found high correlations between performance in the computer based chase test and most of the other computer based cognitive tests. Also, tests like the four different RFD measurements are non-independent because they include data from the same time-interval.

Conclusion

These findings show that it is possible to use climbing as a setting for peer socialization (climbing in a mixed group of children with CP and their TD peers) as a motivating and effective training alternative in children with CP. The improved motor abilities obtained through the training is likely reflected by increased synchronization between cortex and muscles, which results in a more efficient motor unit recruitment system that may be transferred to daily functional abilities. It was not possible with this short-lasting intervention to demonstrate larger muscle strength or cognitive or psychological effects of the training.

Additional file

Additional file 1: S1. Functional tests. These data describes the results of the Sit-to-stand- and the Romberg tests. **S2.** Whole Hand strength and pinch strength. These data describes the results of the Hand strength and Pinch strength. **S3.** Pinch rate of force development. These data describes the results of RFD 0-30 ms; RFD 0-50 ms; RFD 0-100 ms; RFD 0-200 ms for the least and most affected arm. **S4.** Ankle joint measurements. These data describes the results of the ankle joint stiffness and ROM measurements. **S5.** Ankle strength measurements. These data describes the results of the ankle strength measurements in TA. **S6.** Cognitive and Psychological test. These data describes the data of cardbased CogState computerized tests and test of the spatial location based tasks. **S7.** Evaluation of personal and social competencies. These data summarize the results of the evaluation of personal and social competencies separated in sections including Overall; Physical abilities; Skills and abilities; Mental well-being; Relation to parents; Relation to others.

Abbrevations

APB: Abductor pollicis brevis; CP: Cerebral palsy; FDI: First dorsal interosseus; MVC: Maximal voluntary contraction; RFD: Rate of force development; ROM: Range of motion; TA: Tibialis anterior; TD: Typically developed

Acknowledgments

This study was funded by the Ludvig and Sara Elsass Foundation. We would like to thank Ulrik Lund for valuable input to the test protocols and expertise as a climbing coach and instructor, Ruth Smith, Marie Kirkegaard, Mie Kristine Jensen, and Eva Østergaard Skaarup for help during data acquisition, Marianne Bakke and Sally Westergaard for inspirational climbing instruction, and Rasmus Frisk for help during the climbing training.

Funding

The study was supported by the Ludvig and Sara Elsass foundation.

Authors' contributions

Study design: MSC, TJ, JBN, JL participated in the design and planning of the study. Data acquisition: MSC, TJ, CV, JL. Data analysis and interpretation: MSC, JBN, TJ. Manuscript writing: MSC, TJ, JL. All authors approved the final version of the manuscript.

Competing interests

The authors declare that they have no competing interests.

Author details

[1]Center for Neuroscience, Section for Integrative Neuroscience, University of Copenhagen, Panum Institute, Building 33.3, Nørre Allé 20, DK-2200 Copenhagen N, Denmark. [2]Elsass Instituttet, Holmegårdsvej 28, DK-2920 Charlottenlund, Denmark. [3]DTU Compute, Department of Applied Mathematics and Computer Science, Technical University of Denmark, Richard Petersens Plads, Building 324, DK-2800 Kgs. Lyngby, Denmark.

References

1. Rosenbaum P, Paneth N, Leviton A, Goldstein M, Bax M, Damiano D, et al. A report: the definition and classification of cerebral palsy April 2006. Dev Med Child Neurol Suppl. 2007;109:8–14.
2. Andersen GL, Irgens LM, Haagaas I, Skranes JS, Meberg AE, Vik T. Cerebral palsy in Norway: prevalence, subtypes and severity. Eur J Paediatr Neurol. 2008;12:4–13.
3. Stevenson CJ, Pharoah POD, Stevenson R. Cerebral palsy -the transition from youth to adulthood. Dev. Med. Child Neurol. 1997;39:336–42.
4. Engel-Yeger B, Jarus T, Anaby D, Law M. Differences in patterns of participation between youths with cerebral palsy and typically developing peers. Am. J. Occup. Ther. 2009;63(1):96–104.
5. Bottcher L. Children with spastic cerebral palsy, their cognitive functioning, and social participation: a review. Child Neuropsychology. 2010;16(3):209–28.
6. Cutts A, Bollen SR. Grip strength and endurance in rock climbers. Proc Inst Mech Eng H. 1993;207:87–92.
7. Bourdin C, Teasdale N, Nougier V. High postural constraints affect the organization of reaching and grasping movements. Exp Brain Res. 1998;122: 253–9.
8. Orth D, Davids K, Seifert L. Coordination in Climbing: Effect of Skill, Practice and Constraints Manipulation. Sports Med. 2015;46:255–68.
9. Cordier P, France MM, Bolon P, Pailhous J. Entropy, degrees of freedom, and free climbing: A thermodynamic study of a complex behavior based on trajectory analysis. Int J Sport Psychol. 1993;24(4):370–8.
10. Cordier P, France MM, Pailhous J, Bolon P. Entropy as a global variable of the learning process. Hum Mov Sci. 1994;13:745–64.
11. Bourdin C, Teasdale N, Nougier V. Attentional demands and the organization of reaching movements in rock climbing. Res Q Exerc Sport. 1998b;69:406–10.
12. Giles D, Draper N, Gilliver P, Taylor N, Mitchell J, Birch L, Woodhead J, Hamlin GBMJ. Current understanding in climbing psychophysiology research. Sports Technology. 2014;7:108-19.
13. Schöffl V, Morrison A, Schwarz U, Schöffl I, Küpper T. Evaluation of injury and fatality risk in rock and ice climbing. Sports Med. 2010;40:657–79.
14. Schöffl VR, Hoffmann G, Küpper T. Acute injury risk and severity in indoor climbing-a prospective analysis of 515,337 indoor climbing wall visits in 5 years. Wilderness Environ Med. 2013;24(3):187-94.
15. Fryer S, Dickson T, Draper N, Blackwell G, Hillier S. A psychophysiological comparison of on-sight lead and top rope ascents in advanced rock climbers. Scand J Med Sci Sports. 2013;23(5):645-50.
16. Engbert K, Weber M. The Effects of Therapeutic Climbing in Patients with Chronic Low Back Pain. Spine. 2011;36:842–9.
17. Kim S-H, Seo D-Y. Effects of a therapeutic climbing program on muscle activation and SF-36 scores of patients with lower back pain. J Phys Ther Sci. 2015;27:743–6.
18. Luttenberger K, Stelzer E-M, Först S, Schopper M, Kornhuber J, Book S. Indoor rock climbing (bouldering) as a new treatment for depression: study design of a waitlist-controlled randomized group pilot study and the first results; 2015. p. 1–10.
19. Marianne Anke S, Sylvie K, Jérôme P, Shahid B, Thomas F, Dieter Georg R, et al. Effect of Long-Term Climbing Training on Cerebellar Ataxia: A Case Series. Rehabilitation Res Practice. 2011;2011:1–8.
20. Buechter RB, Fechtelpeter D. Climbing for preventing and treating healthproblems: a systematic review of randomized controlled trials. Ger Med Sci. 2011;9:Doc19.
21. Baláš J, Strejcová B, Maly T, Mala L, Martin AJ. Changes in upper body strength and body composition after 8 weeks indoor climbing in youth. Isokinet Exerc Sci. 2009;17:173–9.
22. Mazzoni ER, Purves PL, Southward J, Rhodes RE, Temple VA. Effect of indoor wall climbing on self-efficacy and self-perceptions of children with special needs. Adapt Phys Act Q. 2009;26:259–73.
23. Therme P, Mottet D, Bonnon M, Soulayrol R. Training in motor skills and psychopathology. Climbing with psychotic children. Psychiatr Enfant. 1992; 35:519–50.
24. Schweizer A. Sport climbing from a medical point of view. Swiss Med Wkly. 2012;142:w13688.
25. Csikszentmihalyi M. Chapter 6: Deep Play and the Flow Experience in Rock Climbing. In: Beyond Boredom and Anxiety. San Francisco: Jossey Bass, 25th anniversary edition; 2000. p. 1–21.
26. Bandura A. Social foundations of thought and action: A social cognitive theory. USA: Prentice-Hall, Inc; 1986.

27. Weeks DL, Anderson LP. The interaction of observational learning with overt practice: Effects on motor skill learning. Acta psychological. 2000;104.2:259–71.
28. Bandura A. Self-efficacy mechanism in human agency. Am Psychol. 1982;37. 2:122.
29. Ryan RM, Deci EL. Self-determination theory and the facilitation of intrinsic motivation, social development, and well-being. Am Psychol. 2000;55.1:68.
30. Miller L, et al. Mastery motivation: a way of understanding therapy outcomes for children with unilateral cerebral palsy. Disabil Rehabil. 2015;37. 16:1439–45.
31. Poulsen AA, Rodger S, Ziviani JM. Understanding children's motivation from a self-determination theoretical perspective: Implications for practice. Aust Occup Ther J. 2006;53(2):78–86.
32. Larsen LH, Jensen T, Christensen MS, Lundbye-Jensen J, Langberg H, Nielsen JB. Changes in corticospinal drive to spinal motoneurones following tablet-based practice of manual dexterity. Physiol Rep. 2016;4(2). doi:10.14814/phy2.12684.
33. Willerslev-Olsen M, Lorentzen J, Nielsen JB. Gait training reduces ankle joint stiffness and facilitates heel strike in children with Cerebral Palsy. NeuroRehabilitation. 2014;35:643-55.
34. Lorentzen J, Kirk H, Fernandez-Lago H, Frisk R, Scharff Nielsen N, Jorsal M, et al. Treadmill training with an incline reduces ankle joint stiffness and improves active range of movement during gait in adults with cerebral palsy. Disabil Rehabil. 2016 May;30:1–7.
35. Verschuren O, Ketelaar M, Takken T, van Brussel M, Helders PJ, Gorter JW. Reliability of hand-held dynamometry and functional strength tests for the lower extremity in children with cerebral palsy. Disabil Rehabil. 2008;30:1358–66.
36. Lorentzen J, Greve LZ, Kliim-Due M, Rasmussen B, Bilde PE, Nielsen JB. Twenty weeks of home-based interactive training of children with cerebral palsy improves functional abilities. BMC Neurol. 2015;15:75.
37. Ouvinen-Birgerstam, Pirjo 2006 Sådan er jeg : vejledning. Copenhagen, Denmark: Dansk psykologisk Forlag.
38. Myers LJ, Lowery M, O'Malley M, Vaughan CL, Heneghan C, St Clair Gibson A, et al. Rectification and non-linear pre-processing of EMG signals for cortico-muscular analysis. J Neurosci Methods. 2003;124:157–65.
39. Halliday DM, Farmer SF. On the need for rectification of surface EMG. J Neurophysiol. 2010;103:3547. author reply 3548-3549
40. Boonstra TW, Breakspear M. Neural mechanisms of intermuscular coherence: implications for the rectification of surface electromyography. J Neurophysiol. 2012;107:796–807.
41. Ward NJ, Farmer SF, Berthouze L, Halliday DM. Rectification of EMG in low force contractions improves detection of motor unit coherence in the beta-frequency band. J Neurophysiol. 2013;110:1744–50.
42. Jensen T. 2015. Effects of training on corticospinal plasticity in relation to acquisition of finger motor skills.M.Sc. thesis, University of Copenhagen.
43. Halliday DM, Rosenberg JR, Amjad AM, Breeze P, Conway BA, Farmer SF. A framework for the analysis of mixed time series/point process data–theory and application to the study of physiological tremor, single motor unit discharges and electromyograms. Prog Biophys Mol Biol. 1995;64:237–78.
44. Amjad AM, Halliday DM, Rosenberg JR, Conway BA. An extended difference of coherence test for comparing and combining several independent coherence estimates: theory and application to the study of motor units and physiological tremor. J Neurosci Methods. 1997;73:69–79.
45. Aagaard P, Simonsen EB, Andersen JL, Magnusson P, Dyhre-Poulsen P. Increased rate of force development and neural drive of human skeletal muscle following resistance training. J Appl Physiol. 2002;93:1318–26.
46. Macleod D, Sutherland DL, Buntin L, Whitaker A, Aitchison T, Watt I, et al. Physiological determinants of climbing-specific finger endurance and sport rock climbing performance. J Sports Sci. 2007;25:1433–43.
47. Bertuzzi RCDM, Franchini E, Kokubun E, Kiss MAPDM. Energy system contributions in indoor rock climbing. Eur J Appl Physiol. 2007;101:293–300.
48. Brent S, Draper N, Hodgson C, Blackwell G. Journal of Sports Science and Medicine. European J Sport Sci. 2009;9:159–67.
49. Draper N, Dickson T, Blackwell G, Priestley S, Fryer S, Marshall H, et al. Sport-specific power assessment for rock climbing. J Sports Med Phys Fitness. 2011;51:417–25.
50. Baláš J, Panáčková M, Strejcová B, Martin AJ, Cochrane DJ, Kaláb M, Kodejška J, Draper N. The relationship between climbing ability and physiological responses to rock climbing. ScientificWorldJournal. 2014;2014:678387.
51. Aşçi FH, Demirhan G, Koca C, Dinç SC. Precompetitive anxiety and affective state of climbers in indoor climbing competition. Percept Mot Skills. 2006; 102:395–404.
52. Draper N, Jones GA, Fryer S, Hodgson C, Blackwell G. Effect of an on-sight lead on the physiological and psychological responses to rock climbing. JSports Sci Med. 2008;7:492–8.
53. Draper N, Jones GA, Fryer S, Hodgson CI, Blackwell G. Physiological and psychological responses to lead and top rope climbing for intermediate rock climbers. European J Sport Sci. 2009;10:13–20.
54. Velikonja O, et al. Influence of sports climbing and yoga on spasticity, cognitive function, mood and fatigue in patients with multiple sclerosis. Clin Neurol Neurosurg. 2010;112.7:597–601.
55. Kern C, et al. Multiple sclerosis and therapeutic climbing: an interventional long term pilot study indicates beneficial effects. Lausanne: ECSS Lausanne 06 Book of Abstracts; 2006.
56. Fleissner H, et al. Therapeutic climbing improves independence, mobility and balance in geriatric patients. Euro J Ger. 2010;12(1):12–6.
57. Ryan JM, et al. Comparison of patterns of physical activity and sedentary behavior between children with cerebral palsy and children with typical development. Phys Ther. 2015;95(12):1609–16.
58. Lee JM, Kim Y, Bai Y, Gaesser GA, Welk GJ. Validation of the SenseWear mini armband in children during semi-structure activity settings. J Sci Med Sport. 2016 Jan;19(1):41–5.
59. Wang T-Z, Liao H-F, Peng Y-C. Reliability and validity of the five-repetition sit-to-stand test for children with cerebral palsy. Clin Rehabil. 2011;26(7): 664–71.
60. Kilner JM, Baker SN, Salenius S, Jousmäki V, Hari R, Lemon RN. Task-dependent modulation of 15-30 Hz coherence between rectified EMGs from human hand and forearm muscles. J Physiol. 1999;516(Pt 2):559–70.

25

The effects of video game therapy on balance and attention in chronic ambulatory traumatic brain injury

Sofia Straudi[1*], Giacomo Severini[2], Amira Sabbagh Charabati[1], Claudia Pavarelli[1], Giulia Gamberini[1], Anna Scotti[1] and Nino Basaglia[1]

Abstract

Background: Patients with traumatic brain injury often have balance and attentive disorders. Video game therapy (VGT) has been proposed as a new intervention to improve mobility and attention through a reward-learning approach. In this pilot randomized, controlled trial, we tested the effects of VGT, compared with a balance platform therapy (BPT), on balance, mobility and selective attention in chronic traumatic brain injury patients.

Methods: We enrolled chronic traumatic brain injury patients ($n = 21$) that randomly received VGT or BPT for 3 sessions per week for 6 weeks. The clinical outcome measures included: i) the Community Balance & Mobility Scale (CB&M); ii) the Unified Balance Scale (UBS); iii) the Timed Up and Go test (TUG); iv) static balance and v) selective visual attention evaluation (Go/Nogo task).

Results: Both groups improved in CB&M scores, but only the VGT group increased on the UBS and TUG with a between-group significance ($p < 0.05$). Selective attention improved significantly in the VGT group ($p < 0.01$).

Conclusions: Video game therapy is an option for the management of chronic traumatic brain injury patients to ameliorate balance and attention deficits.

Keywords: Gaming, Traumatic brain injury, Balance, Attention deficit, Mobility

Background

Postural instability, due to failures in the complex interactions between the sensory, motor and musculoskeletal systems, is very common in traumatic brain injury (TBI) and persists in one third of survivors years after the trauma [1]. Balance impairment can limit the activities of daily living and active participation in a social life. Similarly, attention deficits are TBI sequelae that affect 39–62% of TBI survivors [2] and might interfere with a person's ability to safely complete motor tasks and learn new activities [3]. Selective attention is pivotal for everyday life to enhance the stimuli that are relevant and suppress the representation of stimuli that are distracting. Thus far, balance outcomes have been tested using different modalities [4–9]. Balance and postural stability improved after conventional physiotherapy based on motor learning principles specifically tailored for treating postural and coordination dysfunctions in an open trial performed with patients with mild-to-moderate TBI [4]. Focusing on specific gait therapies, body weight-support training on a treadmill (BWSTT) was not found to be superior to overground walking [5] or different robotic devices [6]. Other approaches that have been explored include the use of a biofeedback device to improve perception of external perturbations [7], vestibular rehabilitation [8] or a combination of cerebellar intermittent theta burst stimulation (iTBS) and physiotherapy [9]. Nevertheless, this state-of-the-art work in balance

* Correspondence: s.straudi@ospfe.it
[1]Neuroscience and Rehabilitation Department, Ferrara University Hospital, Ferrara, Italy
Full list of author information is available at the end of the article

rehabilitation in TBI cannot be translated into useful evidence-based recommendations, and the use of new interventions such as virtual reality (VR) has been encouraged [10]. In recent years, VR technologies have begun to be used as a treatment tool in rehabilitation given their low-cost, high portability, off-the-shelf nature and ability to deliver engaging, high-repetitive, task-oriented, standardized, active learning therapies [11, 12]. Moreover, VR-based rehabilitation typically provides augmented feedback during training that can contribute to learning motor skills [13]. Virtual reality also increases patient attention and motivation, which are essential components of learning [14]. Indeed, it has been hypothesized that VR efficacy relies on virtual reward-based learning through a dopaminergic facilitation of cortical and subcortical networks [15]. Motivation and rewards can affect attentional processes in healthy subjects [16, 17] and patients with hemispatial neglect [18]. More recently, gaming consoles (e.g., Nintendo Wii, Xbox Kinect) have been introduced in clinical and research settings as a low-cost means of delivering VR training. With Xbox Kinect, patients can see their movement in real time, and the feedback results are more accurate and realistic compared with other devices with external controllers. Moreover, gaming therapy can be delivered at home, promoting self-management strategies to improve motor function and long-term outcomes [19].

There is limited evidence supporting the use of VR rehabilitation on balance and mobility in TBI survivors [20]. The first attempts were made by Sveistrup et al. [21] and Thornton et al. [22]. These authors used the IREX system for balance training. Sveistrup et al. found balance improvements both in VR and conventional exercise groups [21], and Thornton et al. reported greater enthusiasm after VR therapy by TBI patients and caregivers compared with controls [22]. In the past few years, video game therapy (VGT) has been tested in subacute TBI patients undergoing multidisciplinary rehabilitation with positive effects on balance [23] and in chronic TBI patients using customized games [24]. However, the aforementioned studies did not explore the hypothesis that VGT would ameliorate attention through reward-based learning, in addition to motor function. The aims of this exploratory study were to test the effects of a commercially available VGT on balance and selective attention in ambulatory chronic TBI patients compared to a standardized balance platform training (BPT). We hypothesized that the VGT, and in particular "action video games," would improve selective visual attention more so than BPT. In a previous study, video games were shown to improve a patient's ability to focus on a target and to ignore distracting information not present in BPT [25]. In action video games, players constantly receive feedback about the accuracy of their predictions, which is a fundamental step in engaging the reward system [26]. Video game therapy can improve executive attention components such as control of the automatic response, control of goal-directed behavior and the ability to inhibit irrelevant stimuli [25]. Those cognitive components are part of a "top-down" attentional control mechanism that directs attention in a controlled manner that depends on our personal goals and expectations. Our hypothesis is that VGT would activate those cognitive components of learning more so than BPT, leading to an improvement in balance and attention in a convenience sample of TBI patients.

Methods

This exploratory, randomized, controlled study (NCT01883830; April 5 2013) was approved by the Ferrara University Hospital Ethics Committee (Ferrara, Italy), and all subjects signed a consent form prior to participating in any procedures. The subjects were enrolled from patients discharged at home (former patients included in the clinic database) or those patients receiving multidisciplinary inpatient rehabilitation at Ferrara University Hospital. During the multidisciplinary rehabilitation, physical, cognitive, behavioral and vocational therapy were delivered according to the abilities and needs of each patient. However, to reduce possible confounding effects on our measures (balance and selective attention), no additional specific training, except for the research study, was administered for balance and attention. The inclusion criteria included: (i) an age between 18 and 70 years; (ii) a diagnosis of chronic TBI (>12 months); (iii) a balance deficit identified by a Community Balance & Mobility Scale (CB&M) score < 65. The exclusion criteria included: (i) the presence of other neurological diseases; (ii) severe cognitive Levels of Cognitive Functioning (LCF) < 6 or behavioral disorders; (iii) reliance on the use of walking aids. Patients were randomized according to block randomization and allocated into two groups: VGT or BPT. Each patient received three 1-h sessions per week over the course of 6 weeks.

Video game therapy

Video game therapy was delivered with a video game console (X-Box 360 Kinect, Microsoft, Inc., Redmond, WA). Pre-selected games were chosen from "Kinect Adventures" and "Kinect Sports" that encompassed a wide range of motor activities in a standing position. Specifically, balance and mobility-related motor tasks, such as side stepping, lateral weight shifting, jumping, walking (lateral, forward and backward) and arm goal reaching were trained. During the first session, a list of games was tested according to the patients' characteristics, desires and functional level. In the following sessions, games were proposed with a block practice approach. Within each game, progression proceeded over time according to the patients' abilities and successes. Video game therapy provided different types of feedback: visual and augmented (knowledge of both results and performance). Patients exercised for 2–5 min during each game with a rest period if necessary. During the sessions, the patients were carefully supervised by a physiotherapist who monitored the safety of the patients (e.g., risk of falls, impulsive reactions) and provided external feedback.

Balance platform therapy

Balance/rebalancing, postural stability and weight-shifting exercises with and without visual feedback were administered using a balance platform (Biodex Medical Systems, Inc., Shirley, NY) that had been tested previously in multiple sclerosis patients [27]. Each task was trained for about 2 min, and the patients were provided with a rest period between the tasks if necessary. During the first session, the tasks were performed at an "entry level," and the exercise progression was adjusted over time according to the patients' functional level (intermediate and difficult level). Balance platform therapy offered visual feedback and knowledge of performance (augmented feedback). The physiotherapist, as during VGT, provided additional external feedback.

Outcome measures

Clinical, posturographic and cognitive tests were assessed pre- and post-treatment. We selected balance measures that explored a broad range of motor tasks (both static and dynamic), were suitable for assessing ambulatory patients and were less susceptible to a ceiling effect [28–30]. We assessed balance and mobility using the CB&M. This 13-item scale measures challenging motor tasks necessary for mobility in the community. The tasks have components of speed, precision and accuracy such as tandem walking, running, walking while looking laterally, backward walking and descending stairs [28, 29]. Furthermore, we administered the Unified Balance Scale (UBS) to assess each patient's ability to maintain his or her balance, either statically or while performing functional movement. This 27-item scale derives from three well-established balance scales (Berg Balance Scale, Tinetti Scales and Fullerton Advanced Balance Scale) that address five balance domains: quite stance, anticipatory postural adjustments, sensory orientation, external perturbations and stability in gait [30]. We also administered the Timed Up and Go (TUG) test, which measures mobility. We gave patients verbal instructions to stand up from a chair, walk 3 m, cross a line marked on the floor, turn around, walk back and sit down [31].

Selective visual attention (Go/Nogo task)

The Go/Nogo task was taken from a German standard battery used to test attentional functions [32]. This task consists of five types of stimuli: two of them are target stimuli in which the patients were required to press a button, as quickly as possible, if one of the two defined targets is presented. This test measures the selective attention as the time of reaction and the impulsivity as the number of false alarms (a button press when the patient viewed a non-target stimulus).

Static balance

In this test, patients were asked to step on the central region of the force plate, always facing in the same direction, and to assume an up-right posture with their arms lying alongside their legs and the lateral malleoli distance equal to the iliac spine distance. The patients were asked to either keep their eyes open (looking straight ahead at a 3 m distant visual reference) or closed. For each condition, three 90-s trial were recorded, and we allowed a 5-min break between trials. The eyes opened (EO) condition reflected a highly automatic activity, and the eyes closed (EC) condition detected sensory integration deficits [33]. The x and y positions of the center of pressure (COP) of the subjects were calculated from forces and moments measured by the force platform. Parameters related to postural sway and balance were calculated from the COP trajectory during each trial, namely the anteroposterior (AP), mediolateral (ML) and total path lengths and the sway speed.

Statistical analysis

We compared baseline characteristics between the groups to assess the quality of randomization. Pre--post effects within groups were investigated using the Wilcoxon matched-pairs signed-rank test, and between-groups differences were explored using the Wilcoxon rank-sum test. Statistical analysis was performed using STATA 13.1 software (College Station, TX: StataCorp LP). Significance was recognized for $p < 0.05$.

Results

We enrolled 21 ambulatory chronic TBI patients (17 males, 4 females) with a median age of 36 (12 IQR) years; one patient dropped out for personal reasons. The cohort's median duration since TBI was 4 years (7 IQR). The study flow diagram is shown in Fig. 1.

The clinical and demographic characteristics of the patients are summarized in Table 1. The two groups were similar in demographic and clinical characteristics except for time since TBI ($p = 0.02$).

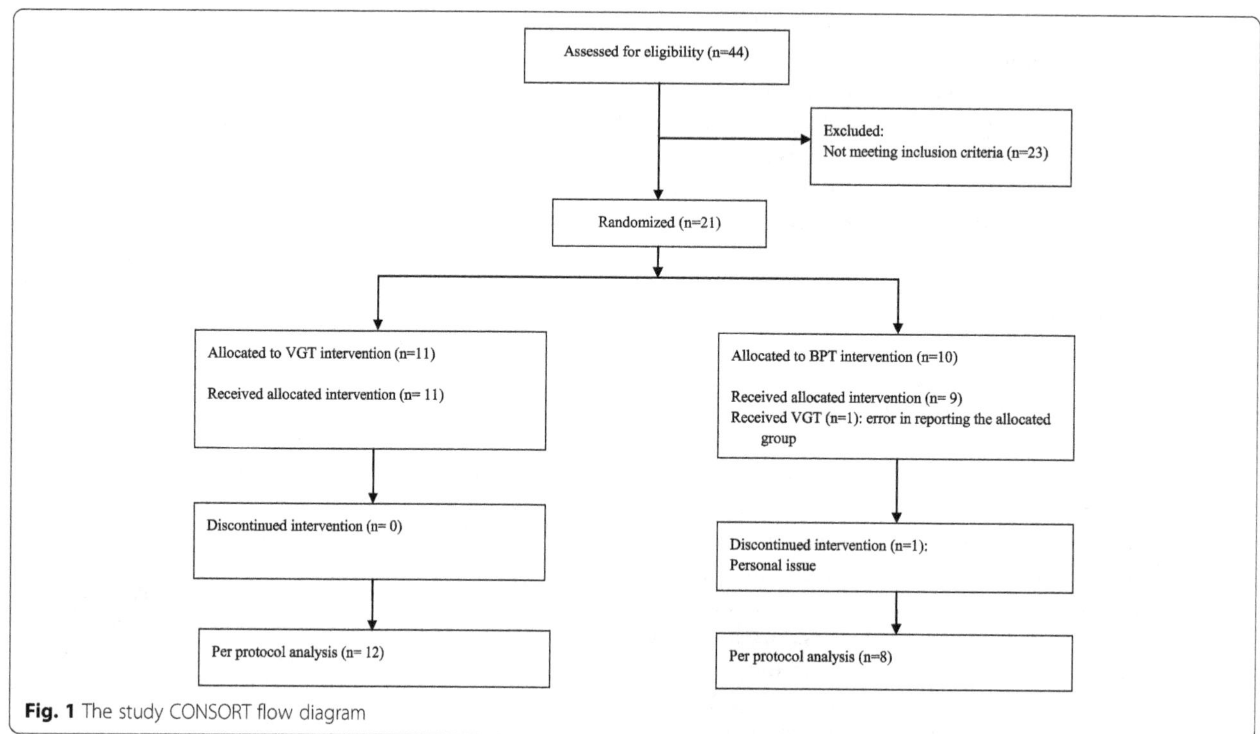

Fig. 1 The study CONSORT flow diagram

Balance and mobility clinical tests

For the CB&M, we found a significant treatment effect in both groups. Conversely, TUG and UBS outcomes improved only in the VGT group. Between-group differences were highlighted with respect to TUG and UBS improvements ($p < 0.05$).

Static balance

No significant effects after training in AP, ML and total path length or sway speed were found. However, a trend of improvement in the EO condition was noted in the VGT group.

Go/Nogo task

Selective attention improved significantly in VGT group ($p < 0.01$). Impulsivity was reduced after both treatments (−0.6 ± 1.2 false answers in the VGT group and −0.5 ± 1.5 false answers in the BPT group) but not significantly.

The results are summarized in Table 2.

No adverse effects were reported during the training periods.

Table 1 Sample characteristics (reported as median and IQR)

	VGT	BPT	All	*P* value*
Age (years)	30.5 (16)	37 (10)	36 (12)	0.14
Sex (M/F)	10/2	7/2	17/4	0.74
TBI onset (years)	2 (6)	8 (16)	4 (7)	0.02
Inpatient rehabilitation/ discharged at home	4/8	2/7	6/15	0.57

VGT video game therapy, *BPT* balance platform therapy, *TBI* traumatic brain injury; *Wilcoxon rank-sum test or Pearson's chi-squared

We performed a sample size calculation using the UBS improvements before and after the treatments. We estimated an effect size of 0.84 (d Cohen). Therefore, 48 patients (24 for group) would be required for a study with a power of 80% and an alpha of 5% (allocation ratio 1:1) in a future study.

Discussion

This exploratory study is the first to use the Xbox Kinect in chronic ambulatory TBI patients for balance and attention training. Chronic TBI patients are usually discharged to their homes when they reach a functional plateau; they accordingly do not receive any form of rehabilitation, even if postural instability and mobility deficits are often reported [34]. However, our results confirmed previous studies [21, 24, 35] that revealed how even in a chronic phase TBI survivors can improve their mobility and dynamic balance with a therapy based on use-dependent neuroplasticity principles [36].

Our primary findings are that dynamic balance and overall mobility improved after training; moreover, selective attention resulted increased, revealing a significant cognitive engagement during VGT.

We investigated balance using validated clinical tests and posturographic assessments. The CB&M scores, which evaluated each patient's ability to perform highly challenging balance and mobility tasks, were significantly improved after both treatments. However, only in VGT group were the gains clinically significant (8 vs 0.5 points). This finding is likely due to the fact that VGT

Table 2 Results (reported as median and IQR)

	VGT (n = 12)				BPT (n = 8)			
	Pre-treatment		Post-treatment		Pre-treatment		Post-treatment	
Clinical tests								
UBS	43 (20.5)		49.5 (20.5)**°°		49 (18.5)		51 (20.5)	
CB&M	17 (15)		25 (15.5)**		25 (32)		25.5 (31.5)*	
TUG (s)	18.7 (16.1)		16.4 (9.4)**°°		14.0 (20.3)		15.4 (16.2)	
Force platform	EO	EC	EO	EC	EO	EC	EO	EC
ML path length (mm)	154.9 (56.0)	161.2 (68.3)	140.7 (83.9)	188.1 (85.0)	169.5 (539.5)	218.8 (508.3)	201.0 (128.3)	233.5 (145.8)
AP path length (mm)	223.7 (80.9)	312.0 (141.1)	171.2 (137.6)	311.3 (147.9)	258.3 (127.6)	332.5 (419.6)	262.7 (226.1)	321.6 (480.4)
Sway speed (mm/s)	15.6 (6.9)	19.2 (4.3)	12.7 (8.6)	19.7 (10.1)	18.2 (24.4)	22.9 (35.8)	20.9 (9.8)	23.5 (22.8)
Tot path length (mm)	309.5 (137.0)	382.0 (85.6)	252.1 (170.7)	392.0 (201.6)	362.0 (486.4)	456.3 (714.3)	416.3 (194.8)	468.5 (454.5)
Go/Nogo task								
reaction time (ms)	569.5 (205)		557 (179)**		568 (146)		576 (166)	
False answers (n)	0 (2)		0 (0)		0 (0.5)		0 (0.5)	

VGT video game therapy, *BPT* balance platform therapy, *UBS* Unified Balance Scale, *CB&M* Community Balance & Mobility Scale, *TUG* Timed Up and Go, *ML* mediolateral, *AP* anteroposterior; $^{*}p < 0.05$; $^{**}p < 0.01$ Wilcoxon matched-pairs signed-rank test; $^{\circ\circ}p < 0.05$Wilcoxon rank-sum test

trains patients in more challenging and dynamic motor tasks, such as side stepping, reaching high and low, lateral weight shifting and jumping.

Mobility, measured by the TUG test, was significantly increased only in the VGT group. We noted differences in mobility between the groups. Moreover, 58% of patients exceeded the minimally detectable change (MDC) set at 2.9 s [37]. Similarly, the UBS that explored both static and dynamic balance was significantly improved in the VGT group, with differences between the groups. This new balance outcome measure covers all of the relevant aspects of balance, exhibits good psychometric properties and avoids the well-known ceiling effect characteristic of other balance scales [38]. Additionally, the UBS was more suitable for detecting differences among the groups compared with the CB&M.

In terms of postural sway, our sample swayed more in the EC condition, which is consistent with the visual deprivation that underlines these patients' sensory integration deficits [39]. After VGT, a slight but not statistically significant improvement was noted in the EO condition. The lack of improvement in static balance is consistent with the fact that it is not considered a predictor of mobility in TBI survivors measured as COP displacement in quiet standing [40]. Furthermore, VGT trains complex movements that require more acceleration, coordination and precision than standing tasks. For this reason, VGT, compared with BPT, appears to ameliorate dynamic rather than static balance domains. Examining other trials that use video games in TBI survivors [23, 24], Cutberth et al. found balance improvements after subacute TBI patients trained with a Nintendo Wii Fit balance board during multidisciplinary rehabilitation. These authors did not highlight any differences compared with standard therapy, which might be due to the fact that their sample was in a spontaneous phase of recovery or that multiple modes of therapy (VR + inpatient rehabilitation) were delivered [23]. In a subacute phase, it is logical that Nintendo Wii Fit—which permits more active guidance by physiotherapists—is more appropriate. In a chronic phase, training with Xbox Kinect can be introduced. Ustinova et al. proposed a Kinect-based customizable therapy for differing ranges of impairments that vary from mild to moderate in TBI severity [24].

In terms of attention assessment, our findings suggest that VGT can improve selective attention measured with the Go/Nogo task. This result is consistent with previous studies that highlighted how video game feedback is capable of improving visual selective attention in habitual players [41]. Video games increase information processing procedures to provide either an adequate response for stimulus processing (e.g., an increase in visual acuity [42] or contrast sensitivity [43] or to enhance top-down attentional control as an ability to strategically allocate one's attention [44]). Attentional control implies some skills related to executive functions such as goal-directed behavior, strategic allocation of one's attention, error monitoring and cognitive flexibility [45]. Game benefits might reflect shifts in strategy rather than changes in more basic cognitive capacities [46]. Our results confirm some previous studies [26] that showed that action video games resulted in different effects in a patient's selective attention compared with other "non-action" games (strategic or role-playing games). In our study, VGT was associated with a higher perception, higher attentional capture and a higher motor-load than BPT. In addition, video games had an influence on the reward system. Consequently, the involved reward system represents a key step in learning and cognitive processing [47]. Increased attention can help motor skill learning and functional recovery in TBI survivors and can partially explain the functional gains obtained by our cohort of patients who received VGT.

This exploratory study presents several limitations: our finding cannot be generalized to the entire TBI population. Specifically, Xbox Kinect, like other gaming devices, was developed for a healthy population and is not adjustable for people with cognitive and sensory-motor impairments. Furthermore, TBI survivors with extended frontal damage may not benefit from a reward-based learning delivered by VR. Additionally, the therapist was not blinded to the treatments received, which may represent a potential source of bias. Also, the VGT and BPT groups were significantly different at baseline with respect to the time since TBI (2 vs 8 years). We also have to consider that patients with an higher chronicity may have developed more compensatory strategies over time, rendering them less susceptible to modification with the rehabilitative interventions. Finally, five of the 20 patients were receiving multidisciplinary rehabilitation, even in a chronic phase, and the multiple interventions could mask specific effects of VGT or BPT. However, we decided to include chronic TBI patients even if they were undergoing rehabilitation given the preliminary nature of this trial and the difficulty of recruiting members of this particular population.

In future studies, it will be important to evaluate the effect of video games on other attention components (e.g., divided attention) and other executive functions such as working memory and flexibility, which are often impaired in people with TBI [48]. Such an evaluation can help to predict performance after VGT [49], either in the early or later phases of learning. It would also be helpful to use an adaptive video game characterized by a progressive increase in attentional and executive loads in order to make the intervention more effective, even for the most compromised patients.

Conclusions

Ambulatory chronic TBI patients appeared to benefit from 6 weeks of VGT in terms of dynamic balance, mobility and selective attention. However, these promising results were obtained from a small sample of convenience. Additional studies with more homogeneous and larger samples are required to confirm and better explore the role of video games on motor learning after TBI.

Abbreviations

AP: Anteroposterior; BPT: Balance platform therapy; CB&M: Community Balance & Mobility Scale; COP: Center of pressure; EC: Eyes closed; EO: Eyes opened; ML: Mediolateral; TBI: Traumatic brain injury; TUG: Timed Up and Go; UBS: Unified balance scale; VGT: Video game therapy; VR: Virtual reality

Acknowledgments

Thanks to: i) Sonia Ghilardelli, Silvia Milan and Giuseppe Lallo for their help during data collection; ii) Carlotta Martinuzzi, Marco Da Roit, Laura Di Marco Pizzongolo, Roberta Benasciutti and Antonella Bergonzoni for their support during the trial.

Funding

ASC and CP were supported by ER Grant 1786/2012.

Authors' contributions

SS, CP, AS and NB participated to the study design; CP, ASC and GG performed most of the clinical tests. SS, GS, AS and NB drafted the manuscript. SS performed the statistical analysis. All of the authors read and approved the final manuscript.

Competing interests

The authors declare that they have no competing interests.

Author details

[1]Neuroscience and Rehabilitation Department, Ferrara University Hospital, Ferrara, Italy. [2]School of Electrical and Electronic Engineering, University College Dublin, Dublin, Ireland.

References

1. Walker WC, Pickett TC. Motor impairment after severe traumatic brain injury: A longitudinal multicenter study. J Rehabil Res Dev. 2007;44:975–82.
2. Marsh NV, Ludbrook MR, Gaffaney LC. Cognitive functioning following traumatic brain injury: A five-year follow-up. NeuroRehabilitation. 2016;38:71–8.
3. Ponsford J, Kinsella G. Attentional deficits following closed head injury. J Clin Exp Neuropsychol. 1992;14:822–38.
4. Ustinova KI, Chernikova LA, Dull A, Perkins J. Physical therapy for correcting postural and coordination deficits in patients with mild-to-moderate traumatic brain injury. Physiother Theory Pract. 2015;31:1–7.
5. Brown TH, Mount J, Rouland BL, Kautz KA, Barnes RM, Kim J. Body weight-supported treadmill training versus conventional gait training for people with chronic traumatic brain injury. J Head Trauma Rehabil. 2005;20:402–15.
6. Esquenazi A, Lee S, Wikoff A, Packel A, Toczylowski T, Feeley J. A Comparison of Locomotor Therapy Interventions: Partial Body Weight-Supported Treadmill, Lokomat, and G-EO Training in People With Traumatic Brain Injury. PM R. 2017; Jan 16. pii: S1934-1482(17)30030-8. [Epub ahead of print].
7. Pilkar R, Arzouni N, Ramanujam A, Chervin K, Nolan KJ. Postural responses after utilization of a computerized biofeedback based intervention aimed at improving static and dynamic balance in traumatic brain injury: a case study. Conf Proc IEEE Eng Med Biol Soc. 2016;2016:25–8.
8. Kleffelgaard I, Soberg HL, Bruusgaard KA, Tamber AL, Langhammer B. Vestibular Rehabilitation After Traumatic Brain Injury: Case Series. Phys Ther. 2016;96:839–49.
9. Martino Cinnera A, Bonnì S, Iosa M, Ponzo V, Fusco A, Caltagirone C, Koch G. Clinical effects of noninvasive cerebellar magnetic stimulation treatment combined with neuromotor rehabilitation in traumatic brain injury. A single case study. Funct Neurol. 2016;31:117–20.
10. Bland DC, Zampieri C, Damiano DL. Effectiveness of physical therapy for improving gait and balance in individuals with traumatic brain injury: a systematic review. Brain Inj. 2011;25:664–79.
11. Rizzo AA. Virtual reality and disability: emergence and challenge. Disabil Rehabil. 2002;24:567–9.
12. Laver KE, George S, Thomas S, Deutsch JE, Crotty M. Virtual reality for stroke rehabilitation. Cochrane Database Syst Rev. 2015;12(2):CD008349.
13. Lauber B, Keller M. Improving motor performance: selected aspects of augmented feedback in exercise and health. Eur J Sport Sci. 2014;14:36–43.
14. Wulf G. Attentional focus and motor learning: a review of 15 years. Int Rev Sport Exer Psychol. 2013;6:77–104.
15. Tran DA, Pajaro-Blazquez M, Daneault JF, Gallegos JG, Pons J, Fregni F, Bonato P, Zafonte R. Combining dopaminergic facilitation with robot assisted upper limb therapy in stroke survivors: a focused review. Am J Phys Med Rehabil. 2016;95:459–74.

16. Bucker B, Theeuwes J. Pavlovian reward learning underlies value driven attentional capture. Atten Percept Psychophys. 2017;79:415-28.
17. Kiss M, Driver J, Eimer M: Reward priority of visual target singletons modulates event-related potential signatures of attentionalselection. Psychol Sci 2009, 20:245-251.
18. Russell C, Malhotra PA. Harnessing motivation to alleviate neglect. Front Hum Neurosci. 2013;7:230.
19. Dobkin BH. Behavioral self-management strategies for practice and exercise should be included in neurologic rehabilitation trials and care. Curr Opin Neurol. 2016;29:693–9.
20. Pietrzak E, Pullman S, McGuire A. Using virtual reality and videogames for traumatic brain injury rehabilitation: a structured literature review. Games Health J. 2014;3:202–14.
21. Sveistrup H, McComas J, Thornton M, Marshall S, Finestone H, McCormick A, Babulic K, Mayhew A. Experimental studies of virtual reality-delivered compared to conventional exercise programs for rehabilitation. Cyberpsychol Behav. 2003;6:245–9.
22. Thornton M, Marshall S, McComas J, Finestone H, McCormick A, Sveistrup H. Benefits of activity and virtual reality based balance exercise programmes for adults with traumatic brain injury: perceptions of participants and their caregivers. Brain Inj. 2005;19:989–1000.
23. Cuthbert JP, Staniszewski K, Hays K, Gerber D, Natale A, O'Dell D. Virtual reality-based therapy for the treatment of balance deficits in patients receiving inpatient rehabilitation for traumatic brain injury. Brain Inj. 2014;28:181–8.
24. Ustinova KI, Perkins J, Leonard WA, Hausbeck CJ. Virtual reality game-based therapy for treatment of postural and co-ordination abnormalities secondary to TBI: a pilot study. Brain Inj. 2014;28:486–95.
25. Chisholm JD, Hickey C, Theeuwes J, Kingstone A. Reduced attentional capture in action videogame players. Atten Percept Psychophys. 2010;72:667–71.
26. Green CS, Bavelier D. Learning, attentional control and action video games. Curr Biol. 2012;22:R197–206.
27. Eftekharsadat B, Babaei-Ghazani A, Mohammadzadeh M, Talebi M, Eslamian F, Azari E. Effect of virtual reality-based balance training in multiple sclerosis. Neurol Res. 2015;37:539–44.
28. Howe JA, Inness EL, Venturini A, Williams JI, Verrier MC. The Community Balance and Mobility Scale–a balance measure for individuals with traumatic brain injury. Clin Rehabil. 2006;20:885–95.
29. Inness EL, Howe JA, Niechwiej-Szwedo E, Jaglal SB, McIlroy WE, Verrier MC. Measuring balance and mobility after traumatic brain injury: validation of the community balance and mobility scale (CB&M). Physiother Can. 2011;63:199–208.
30. La Porta F, Franceschini M, Caselli S, Cavallini P, Susassi S, Tennant A. Unified Balance Scale: an activity-based, bed to community, and aetiology-independent measure of balance calibrated with Rasch analysis. J Rehabil Med. 2011;43:435–44.
31. Podsiadlo D, Richardson S. The timed "Up & Go": a test of basic functional mobility for frail elderly persons. J Am Geriatr Soc. 1991;32:142–8.
32. Zimmermann P, Fimm B. Testbatterie zur Aufmerksamkeitsprufung (TAP). Wurselen: Psytest; 1992.
33. Lehmann JF, Boswell S, Price R, Burleigh A, BJ DL, Jaffe KM, Hertling D. Quantitative evaluation of sway as an indicator of functional balance in post-traumatic brain injury. Arch Phys Med Rehabil. 1990;71:955–62.
34. Campbell M, Parry A. Balance disorder and traumatic brain injury: preliminary findings of a multi-factorial observational study. Brain Inj. 2005;19:1095–104.
35. Peters DM, Jain S, Liuzzo DM, Middleton A, Greene J, Blanck E, Sun S, Raman R, Fritz SL. Individuals with chronic traumatic brain injury improve walking speed and mobility with intensive mobility training. Arch Phys Med Rehabil. 2014;95:1454–60.
36. Kleim JA, Jones TA. Principles of experience–dependent neural plasticity: implications for rehabilitation after brain damage. J Speech Lang Hear Res. 2008;51:S225–39.
37. Flansbjer UB, Holmback AM, Downham D, Patten C, Lexell J. Reliability of gait performance tests in men and women with hemiparesis after stroke. J Rehabil Med. 2005;37:75–82.
38. La Porta F, Franceschini M, Caselli S, Susassi S, Cavallini P, Tennant A. Unified Balance Scale: classical psychometric and clinical properties. J Rehabil Med. 2011;43:445–53.
39. Geurts AC, Ribbers GM, Knoop JA, van Limbeek J. Identification of static and dynamic postural instability following traumatic brain injury. Arch Phys Med Rehabil. 1996;77:639–44.
40. Williams GP, Morris ME. Tests of static balance do not predict mobility performance following traumatic brain injury. Physiother Can. 2011;63:58–64.
41. Green CS, Bavelier D. Action video game modifies visual selective attention. Nature. 2003;423:534–7.
42. Green CS, Bavelier D. Action video game experience alters the spatial resolution of vision. Psychol Sci. 2007;18:88–94.
43. Caplovitz GP, Kastner S. Carrot sticks or joysticks: Video games improve vision. Nat Neurosci. 2009;12:527–8.
44. Clark K, Fleck MS, Mitroff SR. Enhanced change detection performance reveals improved strategy use in avid action video game players. Acta Psychol. 2011;136:67–72.
45. Colzato LS, van Leeuwen PJA, van den Wildenberg WPM, Hommel B. DOOM'd to switch: superior cognitive flexibility in players of first shooter games. Front Psychol. 2010;1:8.
46. Boot WR, Blakely DP, Simons DJ. Do action video games improve perception and cognition? Front Psychol. 2011;2:226.
47. Koepp MJ, Gunn RN, Lawrence AD, Cunningham VJ, Dagher A, Jones T, Brooks DJ, Bench CJ, Grasby PM. Evidence for striatal dopamine release during a video game. Nature. 1998;393:266–8.
48. Stuss DT, Levine B. Adult clinical neuropsychology: lessons from studies of the frontal lobes. Annu Rev Psychol. 2002;53:401–33.
49. O'Neil RL, Skeel RL, Ustinova KI. Cognitive ability predicts motor learning on a virtual reality game in patients with TBI. NeuroRehabilitation. 2013;33:667–80.

26

Clinical experience with transcutaneous supraorbital nerve stimulation in patients with refractory migraine or with migraine and intolerance to topiramate

Michail Vikelis[1,2,5], Emmanouil V. Dermitzakis[3], Konstantinos C. Spingos[4*], Georgios G. Vasiliadis[3], George S. Vlachos[1] and Evaggelia Kararizou[5]

Abstract

Background: Migraine is included in the top-ten disabling diseases and conditions among the Western populations. Non-invasive neurostimulation, including the Cefaly® device, for the treatment of various types of pain is a relatively new field of interest. The aim of the present study was to explore the clinical experience with Cefaly® in a cohort of migraine patients previously refractory or intolerant to topiramate prophylaxis.

Methods: A prospective, multi-center clinical study was performed in patients diagnosed with episodic or chronic migraine with a previous failure to topiramate treatment requiring prevention with Cefaly® according to the treating physician's suggestion. A 1-month period of baseline observation was followed by a 3-month period of observation during the use of transcutaneous supraorbital nerve stimulation (t-SNS) with Cefaly® as the only preventive treatment.

Results: A small but statistically significant decline was shown over time in the number of days with headache (HA), the number of days with HA with intensity ≥5/10, and the number of days with use of acute medication after 3 months ($p < 0.001$ for all of the three changes). Twenty-three patients (65.7%) expressed their satisfaction and intent to continue treatment with Cefaly®. Compliance was higher among satisfied subjects compared to non-satisfied subjects. None of the explored factors were significantly associated with the reason for the failure of topiramate.

Conclusion: Three-months of preventive treatment for episodic or chronic migraine with t-SNS proved to be an effective, safe and well tolerated option for the treatment of patients with migraine who were intolerant or did not respond to topiramate.

* Correspondence: kcspigos@gmail.com
[4]Corfu Headache Clinic, 13, Mitropolitou Methodiou str, 49100 Corfu, Greece
Full list of author information is available at the end of the article

Background

Migraine is ranked as the sixth most disabling condition, worldwide [1]. Presently, medications are the mainstream of migraine management; however, preventive treatment is often far from optimal [2]. Preventive treatment for migraine is usually considered when migraine pain is present more frequently than twice a week [3, 4].

Topiramate is currently the most commonly used first-line approved preventive medication for migraine [5]. With this being said, not all patients respond to preventive medications, due to either lack of efficacy or to adverse events. As a matter of fact, adherence to migraine preventive medications, including topiramate, may be insufficient. In a health insurance database based review, 70.2% of patients who initiated migraine prophylaxis with antiepileptics were reported to be non-adherent after 6 monhts [6]. Among preventive medication choices, patients are reported to adhere best, but not optimally to topiramate, with adverse events being the most common reason for topiramate discontinuation [7].

On the other hand, non-invasive neurostimulation is a relatively new field of interest for the treatment of various types of pain [8]. Clinical research in this field is active, as the recent technological advances allow for safe, convenient and ease by which to self-administer treatment sessions. Cefaly® electrically the supraorbital nerve in the forehead. The supraorbital nerve is a branch of the first trigeminal division. The trigeminovascular system has a well-known involvement in headache pain [9, 10]. Transcutaneous supraorbital nerve stimulation (t-SNS) with the Cefaly® (Cefaly® Technology sprl, Herstal, Belgium) device has proved to be a safe and efficient method for convenient self-delivered treatment sessions [11]. It has received approval for the prevention of episodic migraine by the American Food and Drug Administration and by the EU, including Greece, since early 2015 [12].

Although t-SNS use is spreading in Greece, it is not reimbursed by the social security system and in many cases it may be postponed until either a first line preventive medication fails to provide substantial relief or tolerability/safety issues ensue.

The aim of the present study was to explore and share the clinical experience with Cefaly® in a cohort of migraine patients previously refractory or intolerant to preventive treatment with topiramate, as this is a common situation in clinical practice. Additionally, we specifically explored whether the reason for the discontinuation of topiramate is correlated with the outcome of Cefaly® treatment. To the best of the authors' knowledge, no similar study has been published so far.

Methods

This was an exploratory prospective multicenter clinical study conducted in accordance with the principles of the Helsinki Declaration and approved by the principal investigator's (MV) Institutional Review Board. This study was done to explore the efficiency and safety of Cefaly® in migraine prevention in a population of patients previously refractory or intolerant to topiramate.

Participants to be treated with Cefaly® were enrolled from 2 private headache clinics, located in Athens (Glyfada area) and Thessaloniki, the first and second largest cities of Greece, respectively. Patients were diagnosed with episodic or chronic migraine, needed preventive treatment according to the treating physician's opinion, and they had not responded to previous topiramate treatment, either due to inefficacy or due to intolerability or safety issues. In order to consider topiramate as failed due to inefficacy, a dose of 100 mg/day for at least 3 months was required to have been received. Topiramate was considered as failed due to intolerability in any case a patient had decided to stop use of topiramate due to an adverse event regardless of its nature or severity. Patients had to have stopped topiramate at least 3 months prior to starting treatment with Cefaly®.

Both episodic and chronic (≥15 days of headache per month) migraine patients, according to the International Classification of Headache Disorders 3rd edition-beta version (ICHD IIIβ), were included [13]. Upon enrolment and after giving consent to participate in the study, demographics and clinical data were captured, including the reason for topiramate discontinuation. Patients were then provided with a headache (HA) diary to be self-completed over the course of the study including questions about occurrence of HA, peak intensity level on a 0–10 numerical scale, number of acute medication doses and any adverse event. A 1-month baseline observation period was followed by a 3-month active treatment period with Cefaly® as the only preventive treatment. During the active treatment period, compliance (days the device was used as recommended, e.g. 1 full session each day) was also recorded.

The European version of Cefaly® includes three stimulation programs; one for acute migraine relief and two programs to be implemented in daily 20-min sessions, one for migraine prevention and one for relaxation. In our study, Cefaly® was to be used based upon the protocol of the approval study of the device, in which it is used once every day on the migraine prevention program [14].

At their last evaluation, patients answered two additional questions regarding their total subjective satisfaction from treatment with t-SNS. The first question ("Are you satisfied with Cefaly® and wish to continue the treatment?") was aimed to access overall satisfaction from t-SNS treatment and the will to continue treatment, which was the primary evaluation of our study. The second question ("Did you encounter technical issues with the device?") was aimed to access any problems or technical difficulties arising from the use of the device.

Changes in total headache days, number of HA days with intensity ≥5/10 and days with acute medication use were analysed from baseline to the last observation or Month-3 of active treatment.

Additionally, the Fisher's Exact test and the Mann-Whitney test were performed to test the association between satisfaction from Cefaly® and all other factors, including the reason to discontinue topiramate. In order to evaluate longitudinal changes over time for the number of headache days, the number of medication doses or the number of adverse events (AEs), Linear Mixed Models were performed, with patients modelled as a random effect, time (study month), group (e.g. whether they were satisfied or not), and their interaction modelled as fixed effects.

Statistical significance was set to the observed level of 5%. All statistical analyses were performed using STATA v.13.

Results

From a total of 37 patients, 35 (F:31; age 22-62 yr.; median 45) were our intention-to-treat (ITT) population (2 dropped out before using Cefaly®), 32 were present for their last scheduled evaluation at 3 months and 27 (81.8%) had completed the 3-months of treatment with Cefaly®.

We recorded significant changes in headache days, headache days with pain intensity ≥5/10 and use of analgesics in patients under treatment with Cefaly® from 4 weeks baseline to the 4 weeks prior to last observation or at Month-3 (by a median of 2 days, $p < 0.001$; 2 days, $p < 0.001$; 4 doses, $p < 0.001$, respectively).

Twenty three patients out of 35 (65.7%) expressed their satisfaction and intent to continue treatment with Cefaly®. Trial completion was significantly higher among the satisfied subpopulation (21/27 [77.8%] vs. 6/27 [22.2%] in the non-satisfied subpopulation; $p = 0.001$). Compliance, expressed as the median [min-max] of total days the device was used as recommended, was 86/90 days, higher among satisfied subjects compared to non-satisfied (87 [78–90] days vs. 72.5 [30–90] days, respectively) (Table 1).

Table 1 Satisfaction and compliance at the end of 3-months trial of Cefaly®

	N (%)
Satisfaction-intent to continuation	
Yes	23 (65,7%)
No	12 (34,3%)
Completed 3 months trial	
Yes	27 (81,8%)
No	6 (18,2%)

The number of participants with a 50% or greater reduction in frequency of headaches at the end of the study vs. the baseline (responder rate) was 1/35, 0/32 and 1/31, for the 1st, 2nd and 3rd month of active treatment, respectively.

At baseline, mean (SD) number of days with HA was 8.9 (4.7) with a mean of 5.3 (2.4) showing peak intensity ≥5/10. Patients used acute medication for a mean of 8.2 (4.6) days (e.g. paracetamol, non-steroidal anti-inflammatories, triptanes etc.). On the last evaluation (the 3rd month of the trial), the respective means (SD) were 6.3 (3.5), 4.3 (1.8) and 4.4 (3.3). Results from longitudinal analysis with Linear Mixed Models showed significant decline over time in the number of days with HA and the number of days with HA with intensity ≥5/10 after 3 months ($p = 0.007$ and $p < 0.001$, respectively), the number of days with acute medication after 1 and 3 months ($p = 0.022$ and $p < 0.001$, respectively) and the days not used after 2 and 3 months ($p = 0.043$ and $p < 0.001$, respectively), for those who expressed satisfaction from Cefaly® in comparison to those who did not express satisfaction (Figs. 1 and 2).

The patients with chronic migraine (6 in our cohort) had similar percentages of satisfaction/intent to continue treatment compared to the patients with episodic migraine (66.7% vs. 65.5% respectively).

Four out of 35 patients (12.1%) experienced technical issues, which were easily resolved through on-call support. Twelve out of 35 (34.3%) patients reported an AE. All twelve reported AEs were unpleasant local paresthesias of mild intensity and they tended to decrease with time. No significant interaction of satisfaction with time was observed in regard to the number of AEs.

Among the intention-to-treat population, AEs were the primary reason of topiramate failure (57.1%). None of the explored factors was significantly associated with the reason for topiramate failure.

Discussion

In the present study we explored the efficiency and safety of Cefaly® used in episodic and chronic migraine prevention, after a failed trial of topiramate. Significant changes in headache days, headache days with headaches ≥5/10, use of analgesics, a high percentage of satisfaction and intent to continue treatment with Cefaly®, a poor responder rate and a very low percentage of AEs and technical issues were found in patients under active treatment with Cefaly from the 4 weeks of baseline period (Month-1) to the 4 weeks prior to the last observation or the 3rd month of active treatment.

A trial dose of 200 mg topiramate, as suggested by some experts but not all, was not offered to our patients. This was due to a recent meta-analysis of three studies that had included more than one dose of topiramate and suggested that the 200 mg dose is no more effective than

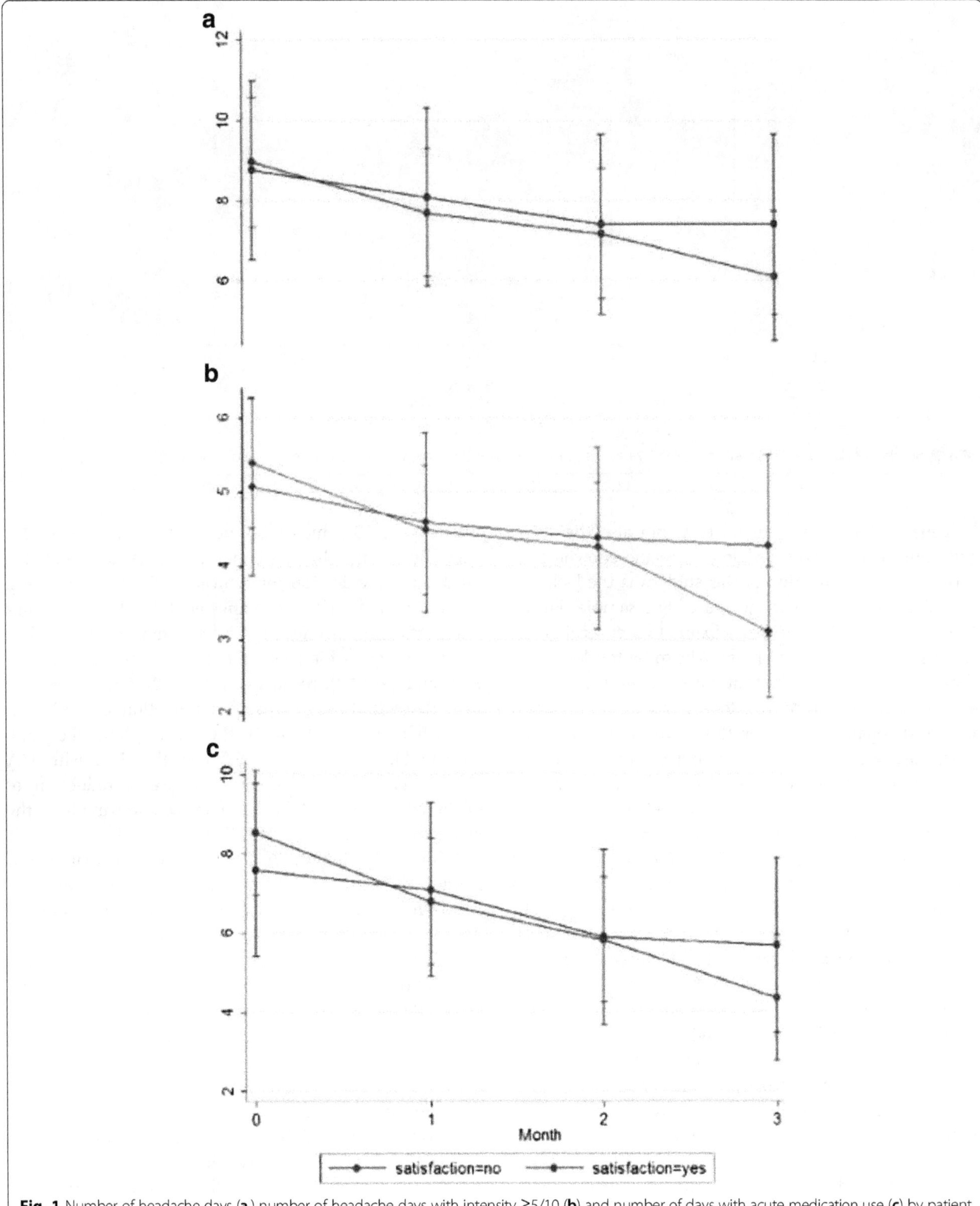

Fig. 1 Number of headache days (**a**,) number of headache days with intensity ≥5/10 (**b**) and number of days with acute medication use (**c**) by patient satisfaction over the 3-months active treatment period with Cefaly®

the 100 mg dose [15]. Up to the present (March 2017), Cefaly® is not reimbursed by insurance schedules as a migraine treatment in Greece though the recently approved (2015) device is frequently used after a failed trial of medical treatment - commonly topiramate. Therefore, this criterion for inclusion may represent not only

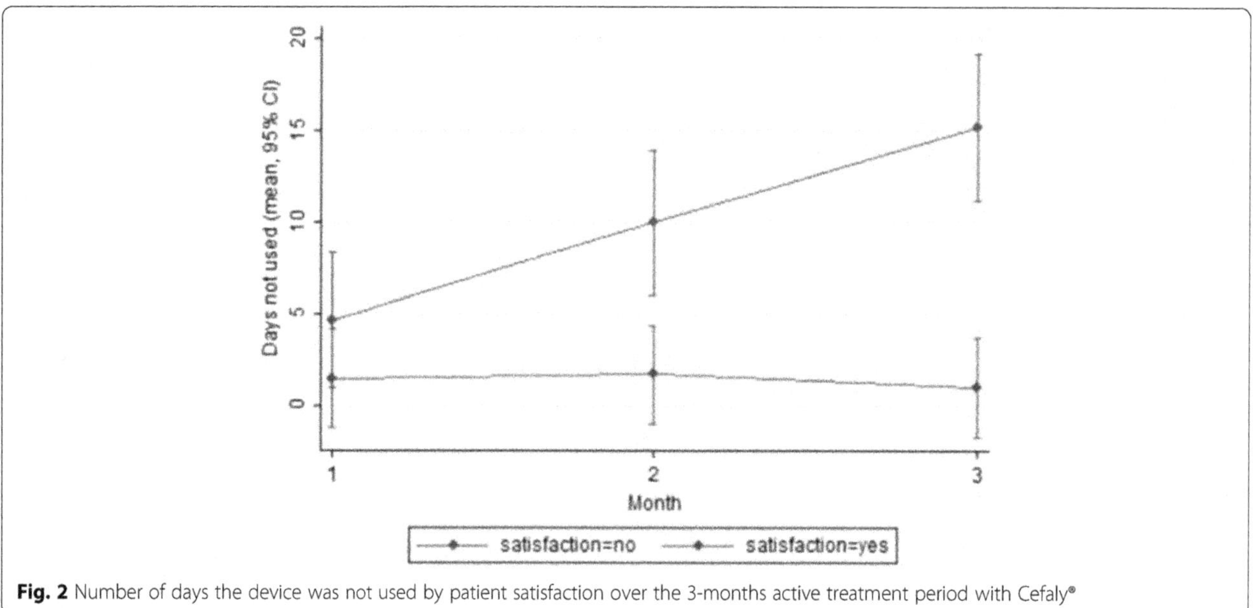

Fig. 2 Number of days the device was not used by patient satisfaction over the 3-months active treatment period with Cefaly®

the general clinical recommendations but also the actual clinical practice needs as well, in Greece and elsewhere.

An important limitation of this study was the lack of a control group and the small size of our sample. Future studies should randomise participants to a control group where stimulation current is thought to be too low to be efficacious vs. standard current. Or compare participants to 3 or 6 months receiving topiramate vs. stimulation use, in an open manner for those who have not tried topiramate. Headache location is not used as a criterion for management decisions in migraine and changes in location within the same attack or between attacks is common among migrainous patients. Because of this, data regarding location was not collected or analyzed in this small exploratory study [3]. However, future studies or meta-analyses might explore the response or the adverse events of Cefaly® in patients differentially grouped according to the usual location of their headache pain.

A comparable percentage (70.59%) of satisfied patients was found in the verum group of the prospective, multicentre, double-blinded, randomized and sham-controlled PREvention of MIgraine using CEfaly® (PREMICE) study, which enrolled migraine patients with at least 2 attacks per month [16]. In another recent survey, 46.6% of 2313 renters of Cefaly® chose to return the device, which implied that they were not satisfied [11]. That leaves a 53.4% of satisfied patients. The difference might be attributed, among other reasons, to the different selection criteria in the survey, where patients were included on the basis of their triptan use for their headaches [11].

At baseline, the mean (SD) number of days with HA, which was one of our measures of efficacy, was 8.9 (4.7) while a mean of 5.3 (2.4) of those HAs showed peak intensity ≥5/10, which was one of our measures of efficacy. Regarding our third measure of efficacy, patients used acute medication for a mean of 8.2 (4.6) days (e.g. paracetamol, NSAIDS, triptanes etc.). On the last evaluation (after the 3rd active treatment month of the trial), the means (SD) for those measures were 6.3 (3.5), 4.3 (1.8) and 4.4 (3.3), respectively. Regarding the days with HA, these findings represent a reduction of 29.2%. In PREMICE study, patients in the verum group showed a comparable reduction of 32.3% in the days with HA [16]. Regarding acute medication use, a reduction of 46.3% was noted in the present study, comparable to the respective 36.7% in the PREMICE study [16].

Results from longitudinal analysis with Linear Mixed Models showed statistically significant decline over time in the following: the number of days with HA and the number of days with HA with intensity ≥5/10 after 3 months (p = 0.007 and p < 0.001 respectively), the number of days with use of acute medication after 1 and 3 months (p = 0.022 and p < 0.001 respectively), the number of days the device was not used after 2 and 3 months (p = 0.043 and p < 0.001 respectively) and finally, for those who expressed satisfaction in comparison to those who did not express satisfaction (Figs. 1 and 2). This was an expected finding as it confirms that patients were satisfied when the device helped them. It also emphasizes the importance of a full 3-month trial of t-SNS before determining efficacy, as it has been suggested by the researchers of the PREMICE study, that the maximum reduction in migraine frequency occurred only after 3 months of treatment with Cefaly® [16].

The present study, due to the small size of our sample, does not qualify for any vigorous exploration of safety with Cefaly®. Nevertheless, around 1 in 3 patients mentioned an AE. This may seem contrasting to a much lower percentage of 4.3% for AEs in the aforementioned survey [11]. However, in our own definition for AEs we included any unpleasant local paresthesia of any intensity intending to explore the whole range of events during the Cefaly® trial.

Among our intention-to-treat population, AEs were the primary reason for topiramate failure (57.1%). In the present study, we specifically aimed to determine whether the primary reason for the failure of topiramate – lack of efficacy or AEs – might be related to the possible future response to Cefaly®. No factors of response to Cefaly® were significantly associated with the reason for topiramate failure. The absence of time correlation between satisfaction and AEs suggests that AEs of topiramate, as a reason for its discontinuation, could be a more organic and not individualised perceptional factor compared to the seemingly unaffected AEs and non-satisfaction from Cefaly®.

The subgroup of 6 patients with chronic migraine from our cohort showed a similar profile of satisfaction/ intent to continue treatment compared to the patients with episodic migraine (66.7% vs. 65.5% respectively). In an addendum to the PREMICE study [16], an increased effect size in relation to the frequency of HAs is reported, suggesting a possibly more favorable response in this subgroup with debilitating migraine, which is something that we were unable to confirm.

Conclusions

In conclusion, 3-months of preventive treatment for episodic and chronic migraine with t-SNS (Cefaly®) proved to be an effective, safe and well tolerated treatment option in patients having failed to respond to topiramate due to either lack of efficacy or tolerability/safety issues. Further studies are needed, leading eventually to a definitive phase-3 clinical trial, with a long-term follow-up of at least 1 year, as well as an economic evaluation, before treatment with Cefaly® is widely adopted.

Abbreviations

AE: Adverse events; EU: European Union; HA: Headache

Acknowledgements

The authors would like to thank Ms. Evie Delicha for performing the statistical analysis.

Funding

Cefaly-technology and Brain Therapeutics Greece have funded the article-processing fee for this publication.

Authors' contributions

MV, KS and ED designed the protocol. MV and ED recruited patients and performed the assessments. KS drafted the manuscript. MV, ED, GV, GSV and EK critically reviewed the final draft. All authors read and approved the final manuscript.

Competing interests

No author or any immediate family member has financial relationships with commercial organizations that might appear to present a potential conflict of interest with the material presented.

MV has received honoraria and travel grants from Allergan Greece, Brain Therapeutics Greece and is an investigator in Amgen-sponsored and Novartis-sponsored clinical trials on migraine prophylaxis. EVD has received honoraria and travel grants from Allergan, Greece and is an investigator in an Amgen-sponsored clinical trial on migraine prophylaxis. KS has received travel grants from Allergan, Greece. GV is an investigator in Amgen-sponsored and Novartis-sponsored clinical trials on migraine prophylaxis. EK has no competing interest.

Author details

[1]Mediterraneo Hospital, Headache Clinic, Glyfada, Greece. [2]Glyfada Headache Clinic, Glyfada, Greece. [3]Geniki Kliniki Euromedica, Department of Neurology, Thessaloniki, Greece. [4]Corfu Headache Clinic, 13, Mitropolitou Methodiou str, 49100 Corfu, Greece. [5]Headache Outpatient Clinic, 1st Department of Neurology, National and Kapodistrian University of Athens, Athens, Greece.

References

1. Global Burden of Disease Study 2013 Collaborators. Global, regional, and national incidence, prevalence, and years lived with disability for 301 acute and chronic diseases and injuries in 188 countries, 1990–2013: a systematic analysis for the Global burden of disease study 2013. Lancet. 2015;386(9995):743–800.
2. Malik SN, Hopkins M, Young WB, Silberstein SD. Acute migraine treatment: patterns of use and satisfaction in a clinical population. Headache. 2006;46(5):773–80.
3. Steiner TJ, Paemeleire K, Jensen R, et al. European principles of management of common headache disorders in primary care. J Headache Pain. 2007;8(Suppl 1):S3–47.
4. Vikelis M, Dermitzakis E, Spingos K. et al. Greek Headache Society guidelines for the treatment of migraine. http://www.kefalalgia.gr/images/PDF/KO_HMIKRANIA_2017.pdf. Accessed 10 May 2017.
5. Mulleners WM, McCrory DC, Linde M. Antiepileptics in migraine prophylaxis: an updated Cochrane review. Cephalalgia. 2015;35(1):51–62.
6. Berger A, Bloudek LM, Varon SF, Oster G. Adherence with migraine prophylaxis in clinicalpractice. Pain Pract. 2012;12:541–9.
7. Hepp Z, Bloudek LM, Varon SF. Systematic review of migraine prophylaxis adherence and persistence. J Manag Care Pharm. 2014;20(1):22–33.
8. Cruccu G, Aziz TZ, Garcia-Larrea L, et al. EFNS guidelines on neurostimulation therapy for neuropathic pain. Eur J Neurol. 2007;14:952–70.
9. Moskowitz MA. The neurobiology of vascular head pain. Ann Neurol. 1984;16(2):157–68.
10. Noseda R, Burstein R. Migraine pathophysiology: anatomy of the trigeminovascular pathway and associated neurological symptoms, cortical spreading depression, sensitization, and modulation of pain. Pain. 2013;154(Suppl 1):S44–53.
11. Magis D, Sava S. D' Elia TS et al. safety and patients' satisfaction of transcutaneous supraorbital neurostimulation (tSNS) with the Cefaly® device in headache treatment: a survey of 2313 headache sufferers in the general population. J Headache Pain. 2013;14:95.
12. Cefaly® Technology. http://www.cefalytechnology.com/. Accessed 11 May 2017.
13. Headache Classification Committee of the International Headache Society (IHS). The International Classification of headache disorders, 3rd edition (beta version). Cephalalgia 2013;33:629–808.
14. Riederer F, Penning S, Schoenen J. Transcutaneous Supraorbital nerve stimulation (t-SNS) with the Cefaly® device for migraine prevention: a review of the available data. Pain Ther December 2015, Volume 4, Issue 2, pp 135–147.
15. Linde M, Mulleners WM, Chronicle EP, et al. Topiramate for the prophylaxis of episodic migraine in adults. Cochrane Database Syst Rev. 2013;24(6):CD010610.

Health care cost associated with the use of enzyme-inducing and non-enzyme–active antiepileptic drugs in the UK

Simon Borghs[1*], Solène Thieffry[2], Matthias Noack-Rink[3], Peter Dedeken[2], Lai San Hong[4], Laura Byram[1], John Logan[5], Jane Chan[1] and Victor Kiri[6]

Abstract

Background: Some antiepileptic drugs (AEDs) induce expression of hepatic enzymes. This can contribute to comorbidities via interference with metabolic pathways and concomitant drug metabolization, thereby increasing the likelihood of health care interventions. Using medical records, we compared the direct health care cost in patients initiating epilepsy therapy with enzyme-inducing AEDs (EIAEDs) vs non-enzyme-active AEDs (nEAAEDs) over up to 12 years.

Methods: Patients with untreated epilepsy were indexed in the UK Clinical Practice Research Datalink and Hospital Episode Statistics database when prescribed a new EIAED or nEAAED between January 2001 and December 2010. Propensity score matching reduced confounding factors between cohorts. Patients were followed until cohort treatment failure or data cut-off. The primary outcome was the median standardized monthly direct health care cost during follow-up in 2014 £GBP, calculated using published reference costs and compared using a Mann–Whitney *U* test.

Results: The unmatched EIAED cohort ($n = 2752$) was older (54 vs 46 years), more likely to be male, had more comorbidities, and higher health care resource use/cost during the 1-year pre-index period (median £3014 vs £2516) than the nEAAED cohort ($n = 2{,}137$). The most common index EIAED and nEAAED were carbamazepine (63.3%) and lamotrigine (58.0%), respectively. After matching, cohorts had similar features ($n = 951$ each). Over up to 12 years of follow-up, the median standardized monthly direct health care cost was £229 for the EIAED and £188 for the nEAAED cohorts ($p = 0.0091$). The median cost was higher for the EIAED cohort in every year of follow-up. In the two cohorts, 25.1% and 20.1% of total mean cost during follow-up was epilepsy-related, with approximately 4.6% and 3.0% for AED acquisition, respectively. The median time to cohort treatment failure was shorter in the matched EIAED cohort (468 vs 1194 days).

Conclusions: Patients in the UK who initiated epilepsy therapy with an EIAED appeared to be at higher risk of complications associated with enzyme induction. In long-term matched cohort analyses, the median total direct health care cost associated with EIAED therapy was higher than with nEAAEDs. Changing current treatment practices could potentially improve patient outcomes and reduce costs.

Keywords: Epilepsy, Health care costs, Cytochrome P450 enzyme system, Drug-related side effects and adverse reactions, Comorbidity, Database, Hospital records

* Correspondence: simon.borghs@ucb.com
[1]UCB Pharma, Slough, UK
Full list of author information is available at the end of the article

Background

In 2010, the Joint Epilepsy Council of the UK and Ireland estimated that 0.97% of the UK population (~602,000 people) had epilepsy [1]. For many patients, epilepsy is a chronic disorder that requires long-term antiepileptic drug (AED) therapy. A broad array of AEDs is available, with varying mechanisms of action and pharmacokinetic profiles. Enzyme-inducing AEDs (EIAEDs), such as carbamazepine and phenytoin, stimulate the synthesis of endogenous cytochrome P450 (CYP450) enzymes as an off-target effect. Only a few CYP450 enzymes are responsible for approximately 80% of all oxidative drug metabolism [2]. Consequently, treatment with enzyme-inducing drugs can potentially lead to altered metabolization of some concomitant drugs, and requires a distinct set of treatment considerations [2–4]. Other AEDs, such as oxcarbazepine and topiramate (mild EIAEDs), induce only a few CYP450 enzymes, while valproate is a CYP450 inhibitor [2, 5].

Although non-enzyme-active AEDs (nEAAEDs) such as lamotrigine, zonisamide and levetiracetam are available [5], EIAEDs remain widely used in the treatment of epilepsy. No clear preference for EIAED or nEAAED prescribing is made in UK treatment guidelines, which are developed with consideration for the balance between clinical outcomes and cost [6].

It has previously been hypothesized that EIAED therapy could lead to higher long-term health care resource use and cost [2]. Firstly, patients prescribed EIAEDs may require higher dosages of concomitant drugs metabolized by the CYP450 system, with more frequent primary care appointments to monitor/titrate drug levels and manage potential side effects. Secondly, metabolic changes related to enzyme induction may contribute to the development of comorbidities such as osteoporosis, sexual dysfunction and vascular disease [2, 7, 8]. Additional investigation and treatment of these comorbidities may contribute to increased health care costs. Thirdly, discontinuation of EIAEDs may lead to increases in concomitant medication levels, requiring additional primary care appointments to monitor and manage any potential toxicity.

A recent literature review has shown that while costs associated with the use of specific AEDs have been reported, the costs associated with EIAED therapy vs other AED therapy have not previously been compared over a clinically meaningful time period [9]. Therefore, the objectives of this study were to compare the characteristics of patients prescribed EIAEDs and nEAAEDs, and to estimate and compare the all-cause direct health care cost associated with the use of EIAEDs vs nEAAEDs as epilepsy therapy in the UK over up to 12 years of follow-up.

Methods

Source data

This retrospective matched cohort study used primary care data included in the October 2014 update of Clinical Practice Research Datalink (CPRD-GOLD; The National Health Service National Institute for Health Research & The Medicines & Healthcare Products Regulatory Agency, London, UK), linked to admitted patient care data contained in the national Hospital Episode Statistics database (HES; Health and Social Care Information Centre, Leeds, UK). The study protocol was reviewed and approved by the Independent Scientific Advisory Committee (the scientific ethics committee concerned with the use of CPRD data).

Patient selection and follow-up

The study consisted of two cohorts: patients prescribed an index EIAED (carbamazepine, phenytoin, phenobarbital or primidone) and those prescribed an index nEAAED (gabapentin, lacosamide, lamotrigine, levetiracetam, perampanel, pregabalin, retigabine, vigabatrin or zonisamide). All other AEDs were not considered index AEDs. Mild EIAEDs (eslicarbazepine acetate, oxcarbazepine, rufinamide or topiramate) were not allowed during the pre-index or follow-up periods. Given these AEDs' mild enzyme induction profile, classifying them as either EIAEDs or nEAAEDs, or allowing their use in follow-up, would have potentially biased the comparison of cost outcomes between EIAEDs and nEAAEDs. Clonazepam and clobazam were not considered potential long-term therapies, and their use was permitted during the pre-index and follow-up periods.

Patients ≥ 16 years of age and diagnosed with epilepsy were selected from the CPRD database if they were first prescribed an EIAED or nEAAED (index AED) between January 1, 2001 and December 31, 2010 (the selection period). The index date was the time of first prescription of an index AED during the selection period. Patients could have been diagnosed on or at any time prior to the index date. For each selected patient, CPRD and HES data had to be available for the 1-year pre-index period. Patients had not previously used any index AED (i.e. any of the EIAEDs/nEAAEDs of interest) at any time during the available data coverage and had not received *any* AED treatment during the 1-year pre-index (i.e. baseline) period. Treatment with AEDs other than an index AED was permitted before the pre-index period, to avoid excluding patients who had used AEDs for non-epilepsy indications. At least 31 days of index AED exposure were required for inclusion, in order to include patients with short treatment durations, but at the same time exclude patients who might not have taken the index AED. Patients who were prescribed an index AED but remained registered in the CPRD for less than 31 days were nevertheless included, to avoid excluding patients who did take the index AED but for whom further prescription data to determine this is unavailable. Patients starting more than one AED on the index date were excluded.

Patients were followed until any of the following events occurred: end of primary care or HES data coverage, end of registration/death, cohort treatment failure (defined as addition of an AED belonging to the other cohort or discontinuation of all AED(s) belonging to the index cohort), or addition of a mild EIAED. Patients switching between/adding within-cohort AEDs (e.g. carbamazepine for phenytoin) remained in follow-up.

Exposure

Exposure was defined using primary care prescription data. We used an algorithm to impute the maximum duration of individual AED prescriptions. The most likely maximum duration of each AED prescription was calculated as twice the median duration for all prescriptions of that type (type defined based on generic name, dose and package size) in the entire study database. Each day of patient follow-up was then categorised as exposed or not exposed using the prescription dates and imputed maximum durations. The end of exposure to an AED was defined as the start date of an exposure gap longer than four times the imputed maximum duration of the last prescription.

Baseline characteristics

Patient demographics and clinical characteristics were identified using primary care data and read codes, and in HES, using the *International Classification of Disease (Tenth Revision)* codes. These were used to calculate a Germaine-Smith epilepsy comorbidity index score for each cohort [10]. Concomitant medications were identified through primary care prescription data.

Health care resource use and costs by type

The costs associated with each health care resource used were estimated, per type, in 2014 £GBP, including any prescriptions (AEDs or otherwise), primary care consultations (general practitioner [GP] consultations and patient-related activity at the GP practice), test procedures, accident and emergency (A&E) visits, hospitalizations and outpatient referrals and procedures. Our costing protocol was partly based on principles previously applied in the literature [9]. Further details on the costing procedure can be found in the Additional file 1.

Matching

Propensity score matching was used to reduce the effect of confounding factors between cohorts, a methodology commonly used in studies based on observational data [11]. EIAED and nEAAED patients were matched 1:1 on propensity score, where propensity score was defined as the probability of a patient being prescribed an EIAED. The propensity scores were derived using a multivariate logistic model. The choice of potential confounding variables used in the model was guided by the literature; variables were selected that were likely to influence treatment choice and affect the outcome. The estimation process used all available patient-level characteristics at baseline that had a minimum incidence of 1.0%, or were significantly different between the two unmatched cohorts when compared by either a two-sample *t* test, chi-square test or Fisher's exact test, as suitable. Table S1 shows variables that were found to be significantly different between the cohorts prior to propensity score matching. Patients were only included in the matched analysis if a suitable pairing was found.

Study outcomes and statistical analyses

To compare the characteristics of patients prescribed EIAEDs and nEAAEDs, baseline characteristics in the unmatched cohorts were compared using unpaired, two-sample *t* tests for continuous variables and chi-square tests for categorical variables. To assess propensity score matching success, baseline characteristics in the matched cohorts were compared using the same procedures.

To calculate the primary endpoint, the total health care cost per patient was summed over the follow-up period and divided by the number of months of patient follow-up, thus arriving at the standardized monthly direct health care cost during follow-up. Medians were compared between the matched cohorts using a Mann–Whitney *U* test. The median is preferred to the mean because of the highly skewed distribution of the health care cost variable. Standardized monthly cost per year was calculated in a similar manner, by summing costs for the year and dividing by the number of months of patient follow-up for that year. In addition, the cost and incidence of specific health care resources used during follow-up for the matched cohorts were split by type; the costs and incidence of epilepsy-related resource use were estimated; the incidence of new non-AED medication use and (non-epilepsy) comorbid diagnoses during follow-up were described for the matched cohorts; and the time to cohort treatment failure and to index AED treatment failure were compared between the matched cohorts using Kaplan-Meier methods, censoring patients reaching the end of follow-up. Index AED failure was defined as the end of exposure to the AED prescribed at index or addition of any other AED, whichever occurred earlier. Index AED failure differs from cohort treatment failure in that it does not allow within-cohort AED switching or add-on.

Analyses were performed using SAS 9.3 (SAS Institute, Cary, NC, USA). No formal power calculations for sample size were performed.

Results

Baseline characteristics in the 1-year pre-index period

In the overall population, 4889 unmatched patients were indexed. Patients in the EIAED cohort ($n = 2752$) were older, more likely to be male and had a higher mean baseline Germaine-Smith epilepsy comorbidity index score than those in the nEAAED cohort ($n = 2137$; $p < 0.0001$; Table 1). More patients with index EIAEDs had pre-index diagnoses of cardiovascular disease (EIAED 26.1% vs nEAAED 17.5%), hypertension (15.1% vs 11.3%) and neoplasms (11.4% vs 6.0%). A lower proportion of patients in the EIAED cohort received hormonal contraceptives (3.5% vs 11.9% in the nEAAED cohort) and antidepressant/antipsychotic drugs (27.4% vs 33.7%) in the 1-year pre-index period. The largest proportion of patients entered the EIAED cohort in 2004 (14.6%; Table 2), decreasing in subsequent years. Conversely, nEAAED cohort entry steadily increased over the selection period, peaking in 2010 (17.8%; Table 2). Carbamazepine was the most commonly prescribed index EIAED (63.3%), and lamotrigine the most common index nEAAED (58.0%) (Table 2).

During the 1-year pre-index period, patients in the unmatched EIAED cohort had a higher all-cause direct health care cost and a higher mean epilepsy-related health care cost than those in the unmatched nEAAED cohort (Table 3). Patients in the EIAED cohort had higher utilization of acute health care resources during the 1-year pre-index period; a reflection of higher mean numbers of A&E visits and inpatient hospitalizations per patient (Table 3). However, the mean numbers of GP consultations and outpatient hospitalizations were higher in the nEAAED cohort (Table 3).

After matching, each cohort consisted of 951 patients and baseline characteristics were similar for all available potential confounders (Tables 1–3).

Time to cohort treatment failure and index AED failure

In the matched populations, the proportion of patients remaining in follow-up after 1 year was smaller for the EIAED cohort than the nEAAED cohort (49.1% vs 60.6%). The median time to cohort treatment failure (allowing within-group AED switching) was 468 days in

Table 1 Baseline demographics and epilepsy characteristics in the 1-year pre-index period

Characteristic	Overall population			Matched population		
	EIAED ($n = 2752$)	nEAAED ($n = 2137$)	p value[a]	EIAED ($n = 951$)	nEAAED ($n = 951$)	p value[a]
Age, mean (SD), years	54.2 (19.8)	45.9 (19.9)	<0.0001	47.7 (19.9)	48.0 (20.0)	0.7969
Age group, n (%)			<0.0001			1.0000
16–20	116 (4.2)	239 (11.2)		75 (7.9)	75 (7.9)	
21–30	261 (9.5)	349 (16.3)		144 (15.1)	144 (15.1)	
31–40	404 (14.7)	344 (16.1)		167 (17.6)	167 (17.6)	
41–50	434 (15.8)	380 (17.8)		160 (16.8)	160 (16.8)	
51–60	406 (14.8)	285 (13.3)		133 (14.0)	133 (14.0)	
61–70	425 (15.4)	236 (11.0)		119 (12.5)	119 (12.5)	
71–80	434 (15.8)	191 (8.9)		94 (9.9)	94 (9.9)	
81–90	237 (8.6)	96 (4.5)		47 (4.9)	47 (4.9)	
Over 90	35 (1.3)	17 (0.8)		12 (1.3)	12 (1.3)	
Gender, n (%)			<0.0001			0.7130
Female	1243 (45.2)	1339 (62.7)		506 (53.2)	514 (54.0)	
Male	1509 (54.8)	798 (37.3)		445 (46.8)	437 (46.0)	
Germaine-Smith epilepsy-specific comorbidity index, mean score (SD)	1.0 (2.0)	0.6 (1.6)	<0.0001	0.7 (1.6)	0.7 (1.5)	0.8272
Time since first epilepsy diagnosis, years						
Mean (SD)	4.5 (10.3)	8.5 (13.5)	<0.0001	5.8 (11.1)	6.2 (12.0)	0.4604
Median (P25–P75)	0.2 (0.1–2.5)	1.3 (0.1–10.9)		0.4 (0.1–5.8)	0.6 (0.1–6.3)	
Epilepsy type, n (%)			0.0011			0.7202
Generalized	301 (10.9)	212 (9.9)		78 (8.2)	85 (8.9)	
Partial	470 (17.1)	291 (13.6)		148 (15.6)	138 (14.5)	
Unspecified	1981 (72.0)	1634 (76.5)		725 (76.2)	728 (76.6)	

Abbreviations: EIAED enzyme-inducing antiepileptic drug, *nEAAED* non-enzyme–active antiepileptic drug, *P25–P75* 25th to 75th percentile, *SD* standard deviation

[a] *t* test for continuous variables, chi-square test for categorical variables

Table 2 Index year and AED

	Overall population			Matched population		
	EIAED (*n* = 2752)	nEAAED (*n* = 2137)	*p* value[a]	EIAED (*n* = 951)	nEAAED (*n* = 951)	*p* value[a]
Year of index, *n* (%)			<0.0001			0.0669
2001	298 (10.8)	70 (3.3)		45 (4.7)	55 (5.8)	
2002	326 (11.8)	88 (4.1)		53 (5.6)	63 (6.6)	
2003	312 (11.3)	121 (5.7)		86 (9.0)	72 (7.6)	
2004	402 (14.6)	147 (6.9)		109 (11.5)	85 (8.9)	
2005	314 (11.4)	190 (8.9)		106 (11.1)	96 (10.1)	
2006	275 (10.0)	222 (10.4)		121 (12.7)	109 (11.5)	
2007	256 (9.3)	255 (11.9)		121 (12.7)	119 (12.5)	
2008	225 (8.2)	293 (13.7)		106 (11.1)	123 (12.9)	
2009	206 (7.5)	371 (17.4)		130 (13.7)	119 (12.5)	
2010	138 (5.0)	380 (17.8)		74 (7.8)	110 (11.6)	
Index AED, *n* (%)			<0.0001			<0.0001
EIAED cohort						
Carbamazepine	1742 (63.3)	—		690 (72.6)	—	
Phenytoin	971 (35.3)	—		245 (25.8)	—	
Phenobarbital	26 (0.9)	—		9 (0.9)	—	
Primidone	13 (0.5)	—		7 (0.7)	—	
nEAAED cohort						
Lamotrigine	—	1239 (58.0)		—	632 (66.5)	
Gabapentin	—	448 (21.0)		—	149 (15.7)	
Levetiracetam	—	261 (12.2)		—	126 (13.2)	
Pregabalin	—	185 (8.7)		—	41 (4.3)	
Zonisamide	—	2 (0.1)		—	2 (0.2)	
Vigabatrin	—	2 (0.1)		—	1 (0.1)	

Abbreviations: AED antiepileptic drug, *EIAED* enzyme-inducing antiepileptic drug, *nEAAED* non-enzyme–active antiepileptic drug
[a]Chi-square test

the EIAED cohort compared with 1194 days in the nEAAED cohort, with a total follow-up time of 2297 vs 2881 years, respectively (Fig. 1). Index AED failure (discontinuation of index AED, switch or addition of another) occurred in 68.3% of patients in the matched EIAED cohort and 62.7% of patients in the matched nEAAED cohort, with a median time to index AED failure of 452 days vs 869 days, respectively. Index AED failure owing to discontinuation of the index AED occurred in 41.3% of the EIAED cohort and 43.7% of the nEAAED cohort. Most discontinuations occurred during the first 3 months of treatment in both cohorts. Treatment failure owing to an addition of another AED occurred in 27.0% of the EIAED cohort and 18.9% of the nEAAED cohort.

All-cause direct health care cost

The median (range) standardized monthly direct health care cost over the entire follow-up period was £229 (£18–£18,613) for the EIAED cohort and £188 (£16–£33,880) for the nEAAED cohort ($p = 0.0091$; Table 4). Higher median monthly health care cost was observed in the EIAED cohort in every year post-index, for all patients who *started* the year in question (Fig. 2). The difference between the cohorts became consistently greater from year 3. When considering yearly cost for patients *completing* each year of follow-up, the median yearly direct health care cost was higher in the EIAED cohort than the nEAAED cohort in every year except year 2 (£53 difference). Similar findings were also observed when cost was calculated only for patients who still had an active match pairing at the start of the year.

Specific health care resource use and cost

Patients in the matched EIAED cohort had more GP practice consultations (mean standardized per month [standard deviation], 5.39 [5.87] vs 4.71 [4.62]) and outpatient referrals (0.12 [0.29] vs 0.07 [0.16]), than those in

Table 3 Health care costs and resource use in the 1-year pre-index period

	Overall population			Matched population		
	EIAED (n = 2752)	nEAAED (n = 2137)	p value[a]	EIAED (n = 951)	nEAAED (n = 951)	p value[a]
All-cause direct health care costs in the 1-year pre-index period, £						
Mean (SD)	5618 (7387)	4613 (6007)	<0.0001	4540 (6765)	4416 (5944)	0.6724
Median (P10–P90)	3014 (495–14,070)	2516 (568–11,657)		2333 (452–10,863)	2283 (448–11,180)	
Epilepsy-related direct health care costs in the 1-year pre-index period, £						
Mean (SD)	997 (2361)	633 (1965)	<0.0001	804 (2134)	726 (2201)	0.4314
Median (P10–P90)	42 (0–2797)	11 (0–2188)		23 (0–2599)	11 (0–2599)	
Health care resource use per patient in the 1-year pre-index period Mean (SD) number of:						
GP practice consultations	35.13 (29.55)	43.69 (36.33)	<0.0001	36.48 (31.92)	37.04 (31.15)	0.6973
A&E visits	0.83 (1.26)	0.70 (1.28)	0.0003	0.72 (1.41)	0.70 (1.15)	0.6173
Outpatient non-A&E referrals	0.96 (1.45)	1.27 (1.40)	<0.0001	1.08 (1.35)	1.08 (1.29)	0.9446
Inpatient hospitalizations	1.64 (5.63)	1.20 (2.70)	0.0004	1.44 (7.27)	1.22 (3.41)	0.4126
Hospitalization duration, mean (SD), days	6.96 (19.70)	3.64(11.89)	<0.0001	4.30 (11.32)	4.09 (11.48)	0.6873

Abbreviations: A&E accident and emergency, *EIAED* enzyme-inducing antiepileptic drug, *GP* general practitioner, *nEAAED* non-enzyme–active antiepileptic drug, *P10–P90* 10th to 90th percentile, *SD* standard deviation. [a]*t* test

the matched nEAAED cohort. Health care cost standardized by month were higher in the EIAED cohort for every resource category (costs of drugs [AEDs and other medications], GP consultations, test procedures, A&E visits, inpatient hospitalizations and outpatient referrals and procedures) (Table 4). The median standardized monthly cost of AED medication was £9 and £8 in the EIAED and nEAAED cohorts, respectively. The mean cost made up 4.6% and 3.0% of the total mean direct health care cost.

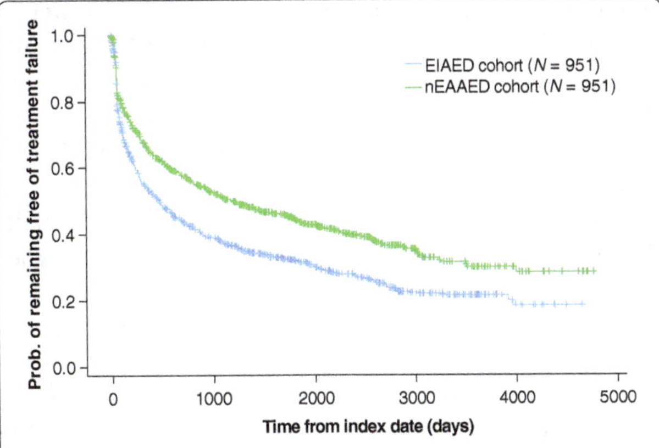

Fig. 1 Time to cohort treatment failure in the matched cohorts. *EIAED* enzyme-inducing antiepileptic drug, *nEAAED* non-enzyme–active antiepileptic drug

Epilepsy-related direct health care cost

The median standardized monthly direct epilepsy-related cost (range) was £27 (£3–£15781) for the matched EIAED cohort and £21 (£2–£3942) for the matched nEAAED cohort. Over the entire follow-up period, a larger percentage of the mean direct health care cost was epilepsy-related in the EIAED cohort than the nEAAED cohort (25.1% vs 20.1%; Table 4). The mean number of epilepsy-related visits per month over the follow-up period was numerically higher in the EIAED cohort in all categories except GP consultations. Over the entire follow-up period, the proportions of patients requiring epilepsy-related A&E visits, GP consultations and inpatient hospitalization were slightly higher in the nEAAED cohort compared with the EIAED cohort; however, these latter rates are not adjusted for differing follow-up time.

Incident comorbidities and concomitant medications

During the follow-up period, incident (new) comorbidities diagnosed in ≥ 5.0% of the patients in either cohort included soft tissue disorders, essential hypertension, respiratory infections, back pain, hypertension, joint disorders, urinary system disorders, convulsions, falls, disorders of skin and subcutaneous tissue, otitis externa, depression, abdominal and pelvic pain and conjunctivitis (Table S2).

Incidence rates were estimated using the number of patients with at least one new diagnosis during the post-

Table 4 Standardized monthly direct health care cost over the follow-up period

Costs are in 2014 £GBP		EIAED ($n = 951$)	nEAAED ($n = 951$)
Total direct all-cause health care costs	Median (range)	229 (18–18,613)	188* (16–33,880)
	Mean (SD)	495 (1016)	432 (1272)
A&E visits	Median (range)	0 (0–1740)	0 (0–316)
	Mean (SD)	9 (64)	6 (22)
AED medications	Median (range)	9 (2–1407)	8 (2–438)
	Mean (SD)	23 (58)	13 (22)
GP practice consultations	Median (range)	114 (12–2816)	102 (8–1591)
	Mean (SD)	161 (187)	143 (146)
Inpatient hospitalizations	Median (range)	0 (0–13,337)	0 (0–33,394)
	Mean (SD)	236 (830)	217 (1203)
Non-AED medications	Median (range)	7 (0–797)	6 (0–939)
	Mean (SD)	30 (69)	28 (71)
Outpatient, non-A&E referrals	Median (range)	1 (0–489)	2 (0–284)
	Mean (SD)	16 (43)	9 (22)
Test procedures	Median (range)	7 (0–761)	7 (0–518)
	Mean (SD)	20 (43)	16 (32)
Total epilepsy-related direct health care costs	Median (range)	27 (3–15,781)	21 (2–3942)
	Mean (SD)	124 (608)	87 (287)

Abbreviations: A&E accident and emergency, *AED* antiepileptic drug, *EIAED* enzyme-inducing antiepileptic drug, *GP* general practitioner, *nEAAED* non-enzyme-active antiepileptic drug, *SD* standard deviation
*$p = 0.0091$ vs EIAED, calculated by Mann-Whitney U test

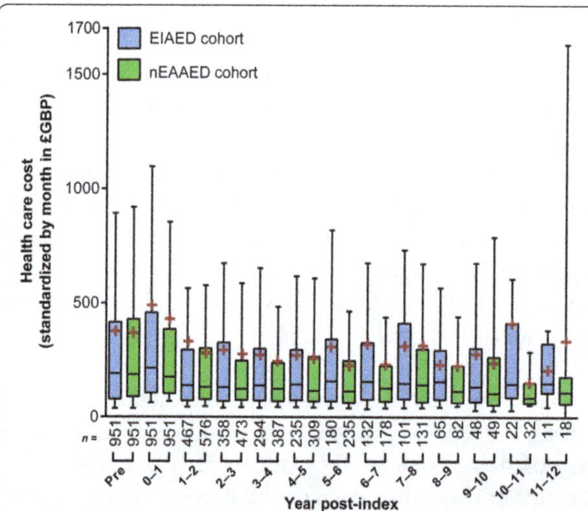

Fig. 2 Standardized monthly all-cause direct health care cost in each post-index year for the matched cohorts. Whiskers extend from the 10th to the 90th percentile; boxes extend from the 25th to the 75th percentile; center line is the median; red cross is the mean. *EIAED* enzyme-inducing antiepileptic drug, *nEAAED* non-enzyme-active antiepileptic drug

index period (and no diagnosis for the respective comorbidity during the pre-index period) divided by the total cohort follow-up time in years (Table S2). Rate ratios were calculated for the two cohorts. Differences between the cohorts were observed in both directions (higher and lower), and no relationship to exposure was observed. However, many of the common (≥5.0%) incident comorbidities were reported more frequently in the EIAED cohort than in the nEAAED cohort, including convulsions (1.43 times as frequently), otitis externa (1.61 times), essential hypertension (1.31 times), nonspecified fall (1.21 times), upper respiratory infections (1.20 times), other skin disorders (1.19 times) and abdominal and pelvic pain (1.05 times). Others were slightly more frequent in the nEAAED cohort: dorsalgia, joint disorders and injuries of unspecified body region (1.07, 1.11 and 1.22 times, respectively).

Among the less common (< 5.0%) incident comorbidities, the following were reported at a markedly higher frequency in the EIAED cohort: fracture of foot, forearm and lumbar spine (7.33, 4.64 and 4.40 times as frequently), other metabolic disorders and manic episode (4.33 and 4.33 times as frequently). Some other comorbidities were more frequently reported in the nEAAED cohort: complications and ill-defined descriptions of heart disease, and ulcerative colitis (9.75 and 4.25 times as often, respectively).

The profiles of new medications prescribed during post-index period (and not prescribed during the pre-index period) were generally similar in the matched cohorts. The most frequently prescribed drug classes (other than AEDs) were antibacterial drugs (39.0% in the EIAED cohort vs 43.8% in the n-EAAED cohort), analgesics (23.0% vs 31.0%), antisecretory drugs (16.5% vs 19.2%) and topical corticosteroids (22.5% vs 23.5%).

Among all drug classes, thyroid and anti-thyroid drugs, mucolytics, anti-diabetics and local anaesthetics/anti-pruritics had new prescription rates 3.73-, 2.26-, 2.14- and 2.13-fold more in the EIAED cohort than nEAAED cohort, respectively. Topical circulatory preparations, antiperspirants and preparations for warts/calluses had a new prescription rate 6.00-, 5.25- and 4.00-fold more in the nEAAED cohort than in the nEAAED cohort, respectively.

Discussion

This study evaluated up to 12 years of retrospective medical records from patients initiating AED therapy in the UK. Our unmatched data showed that during the study period (2001–2011), patients prescribed EIAEDs as initial AED therapy were older, more likely to be male and had more comorbidities than those prescribed nEAAEDs. These differences were, in turn, reflected in higher health care resource use and cost, comorbidity and concomitant medication use in the unmatched EIAED cohort for the pre-index year. The older age and lower proportion of female patients initiating therapy on an EIAED may be justified by the risks of reproductive hormone abnormalities and interactions with hormonal contraceptives associated with EIAED use [2, 12]. However, our findings remain somewhat surprising, as patients with pre-existing comorbidities and concomitant medications are generally less suited to receiving EIAEDs, owing to their potential for drug-drug interactions. This would suggest that EIAED prescribing was not optimally targeted during the assessed period.

Our findings suggest that after controlling for baseline differences between the cohorts by propensity score matching, the median total direct health care cost (standardized per month) associated with the use of EIAEDs was higher than with nEAAEDs. This study was the first to assess the relative direct cost of EIAED vs nEAAED therapy over a clinically relevant period of time. Our results suggest that the higher cost observed for the EIAED cohort was related to higher health care utilization in general. We were unable to identify any specific comorbidities linked to the higher observed costs, which might partly be due to limitations of the coded source data. The EIAED cohort showed higher AED costs, which might have been unexpected, as the acquisition cost of the newer nEAAEDs is usually higher. The larger AED costs could be related to the more frequent need for polytherapy observed in the EIAED cohort, demonstrated by the higher proportion of patients who added another AED and the shorter time on index AED monotherapy. Analyses of matched patient cohorts showed a shorter time to cohort treatment failure, and to index AED failure, for the EIAED cohort vs the nEAAED cohort. Although these findings might suggest poorer long-term clinical outcomes associated with EIAED therapy, the CPRD contains limited seizure frequency data, so we are unable to investigate these suggestions. Unfortunately, the reasons for AED failure are not readily available in the data source.

Cost analyses using CPRD data are uncommon. The major advantage of CPRD data over other patient record databases (such as US insurance claims databases) is that it offers a unique source of long-term, continuous patient data. The last estimate for the direct costs of epilepsy in the UK was published 22 years ago. Cockerell *et al.* [13] evaluated an average of 6.6 years of health care utilization data from up to 1195 UK patients, collected as part of the National General Practice Study of Epilepsy [14]. The cost of epilepsy to a newly diagnosed individual with epilepsy was estimated to be £611 in the first year, decreasing to £221 in year 2 and to £169 by year 8. Declining costs after the first year were also observed in other costing studies [15, 16]. These decreasing costs over time are dissimilar with our findings. A large part of the observed difference is likely to be due to methodology and study period, and results can therefore only be reliably compared within studies. The methodological challenges of costing epilepsy is discussed in detail by Cockerell et al. [13].

The profile of index AED prescription rates reflected the evolving treatment guidelines, AED availability and physician preferences over the 10-year selection period; nEAAEDs were increasingly preferred as the selection period progressed. In the UK, the National Institute for Health and Care Excellence (NICE) assesses the value of treatment options based on analyses of outcomes and costs, publishing treatment recommendation guidelines to actively influence the selection of interventions. The guidelines recommend that patients with epilepsy initiate AED treatment as monotherapy; however, a preference for EIAED or nEAAED has not been explicitly made. Later generation AEDs (mostly nEAAEDs) tend to gain market approval initially as adjunctive therapy, with a monotherapy indication added later. This leads to a lag in treatment availability for newly diagnosed patients [17]. The peak year for patient indexing in the EIAED cohort was 2004, which is consistent with the 2004 NICE guidelines supporting carbamazepine as a first-line epilepsy treatment (along with phenytoin, valproic acid and divalproex) [18]. For the nEAAED cohort, the peak year for patient indexing was 2010, which may be indicative of the changing prescribing attitudes following the publication of the 2007 SANAD study, which showed lamotrigine to be more clinically and cost-effective than carbamazepine [19]. Evidence from SANAD contributed to the 2012 update of the NICE guidelines [6], which recommend lamotrigine, alongside four other AEDs with differing enzyme induction properties (carbamazepine, levetiracetam, oxcarbazepine and sodium valproate), as a first-line treatment for patients with focal epilepsy. Mild enzyme inducing AEDs were not included in either cohort or allowed during follow-up. Given these AEDs' mild enzyme induction profile, classifying them as either EIAEDs or nEAAEDs, or allowing their use in follow-up, would have potentially biased conclusions regarding cost outcomes between EIAEDs and nEAAEDs. Based on our data it is therefore not possible to make inferences regarding the cost outcomes associated with mild enzyme inducers and how they compare with those of EIAEDs or nEAAEDs.

The nature of incident comorbidity diagnoses during the follow-up period was generally similar between matched cohorts. Differences between the cohorts were observed in both directions (higher and lower). New prescriptions for several types of drugs were less common in the EIAED cohort during the follow-up, and this may be indicative of the increased risk of drug interactions, leading to caution when selecting concomitant drug therapies. This is also potentially reflected in the shorter time to end of follow-up in the EIAED cohort, as patients may require relevant treatments that are not well suited for concomitant therapy with EIAEDs. Overall, findings relating to the incidence of new comorbidities or prescriptions were not clearly related to AED exposure or type. This may have been due to the limitations of using coded data.

A particular strength of our study was the patient matching by propensity score, which utilized several hundred available demographic and clinical characteristics. By eliminating known and observable confounding factors, patient matching allowed an accurate estimation of the cost and time to treatment failure associated with EIAED vs nEAAED therapy to be made in a generally representative population of previously untreated epilepsy patients. However, not all potential confounding factors could be controlled for in this analysis. For example, regional differences in the standard of epilepsy care have been noted in the UK [20, 21], and may relate to personal preferences of the GP, practice type, size, location and local formulary access to certain AEDs. There is also a known correlation between social deprivation and increased epilepsy prevalence [22]. Additional relevant factors may have been excluded from the propensity scoring owing to lack of information in CPRD data (e.g. seizure type and frequency). As such, there is the chance that the results are biased by residual, unmeasured confounding.

To obtain the most accurate costings, we attempted to match each health care resource used with the most up-to-date cost information in 2014 GBP. This approach was taken because of the long follow-up period in our study, and allowed comparison between the cohorts of patients entering the study longitudinally. Costs for each health care resource used were calculated from published unit costs and are as accurate as possible given the data available. The study's primary variable summed the value of every health care resource used over the entire follow-up period. When considering cost analyses over time, we chose to look at the standardized monthly cost per year for all patients starting the year in question. This had the benefit that cost data from patients who left follow-up during the year (following treatment success or failure) were reflected accurately in the analysis. Sensitivity analyses showed that the cost trends and cohort comparisons were similar when cost was only analysed for patients completing the year, and when considering only those patients with an active match at the start of the year. Cost analyses are nearly always estimates with inherent inaccuracies, and all electronic medical record and billing data are subject to some level of miscoding. The AED exposure in this study was based on sometimes incomplete prescription duration data. Initial assessments found structured duration information to be missing in over a quarter of individual AED prescriptions. Therefore, a novel algorithm was used to determine duration for each prescription, as described in the methods. The most likely maximum duration of each AED prescription was calculated as twice the median duration for all prescriptions of that type (type defined based on generic name, dose and package size) in the entire study database. Twice the median was chosen as the likely maximum duration in order to avoid underestimating a patient's exposure to an AED; since discontinuing an AED usually requires a slow down-titration, a longer treatment duration is typically associated with the last prescription. The end of exposure to an AED was defined as the start date of an exposure gap longer than four times the imputed maximum duration of the last prescription. This 'allowed gap' may appear liberal but was chosen to avoid ending exposure too soon in case of missing data – the assumption being that in case of a 'long' gap followed by a 'new' prescription of the same AED, it is clinically unlikely that there really was a gap. These miscoding issues and imputation assumptions are not expected to differ between cohorts and therefore do not lead to bias.

Our analyses are retrospective and descriptive in nature, and findings cannot be directly extrapolated to current clinical practice, as prescription behaviour may have changed according to guidelines. There were several other limitations in our study regarding information availability, such as the lack of seizure data, reasons for treatment discontinuation and adverse event reporting. While our results indicate increased health care resource use associated with the use of EIAEDs in epilepsy, the direct cause of this use, beyond its relation to epilepsy or otherwise, needs further investigation and will suffer from the lack of information noted above. Epilepsy comprises a diverse group of disorders and our analysis was conducted on a potentially diverse pool of patients; therefore, it might not accurately reflect patients with distinct subtypes of epilepsy (i.e. syndrome, localization or aetiology), which was found to be poorly coded in CPRD data. Furthermore, events occurring before the 1-year pre-index period were not included in the analysis. Taken together, there is a possibility that specific patient subgroups are erroneously included or omitted; for example, inclusion of those prescribed AEDs for indications other than epilepsy, and inclusion of patients misdiagnosed with epilepsy.

Conclusions

Our analysis of UK CPRD data suggests that during the studied period, EIAEDs were prescribed as an initial epilepsy therapy to older patients, who were more likely to be male and had higher baseline health care resource use and cost than patients prescribed nEAAEDs. Given the risks associated with enzyme induction, this prescribing pattern appears to be suboptimal. In long-term, matched cohort analyses, a higher average total direct health care cost and a shorter time to treatment failure were associated with EIAED vs nEAAED therapy. We conclude that changing current treatment practices could potentially improve patient outcomes and reduce health care costs.

Abbreviations

A&E: accident and emergency; AED: antiepileptic drug; CPRD: Clinical Practice Research Datalink; CYP450: cytochrome P450; EIAED: enzyme-inducing antiepileptic drug; GP: general practitioner; HES: Hospital Episode Statistics; nEAAED: non-enzyme-active antiepileptic drug; NICE: National Institute for Health and Care Excellence

Acknowledgements

This study is based on data from the General Practice Research Database obtained under licence from the UK Medicines and Healthcare products Regulatory Agency. However, the interpretation and conclusions contained in this report are those of the authors alone.
The authors acknowledge Shelley Fordred, (Savvy Stats Limited) for programming assistance, Jennifer Bodkin, PhD (Evidence Scientific Solutions, Horsham, UK) for writing assistance, which was funded by UCB Pharma, and Barbara Pelgrims, PhD (UCB Pharma, Brussels, Belgium) for overseeing the manuscript development.

Funding

This study was funded by UCB Pharma, who had a role in the design of the study, the collection, analysis and interpretation of data and in the decision to publish the manuscript. All authors were employees or paid consultants to UCB Pharma at the time of the study.

Authors' contributions

SB and ST had a role in the design of the study, the collection, analysis and interpretation of data and in the decision to publish the manuscript. MN-R, PD and LB had a role in the design of the study, the interpretation of data and in the decision to publish the manuscript. LSH, JL and VK had a role design of the study, the collection and analysis of data and in the decision to publish the manuscript. JC had a role in the design of the study, the collection and interpretation of data and in the decision to publish the manuscript.
All authors read and approved the final manuscript.

Competing interests

SB, ST, MNR, PD, LB and JC are employees of UCB Pharma. LSH worked for UCB Pharma at the time of the study, but is now employed by Redsen Limited. JL and VK are consultants, whose work on this study was funded by UCB Pharma.

Author details

[1]UCB Pharma, Slough, UK. [2]UCB Pharma, Brussels, Belgium. [3]UCB Pharma, Monheim Am Rhein, Germany. [4]Redsen Limited, Bournemouth, UK. [5]Stats4Pharma, Cork, Ireland. [6]FV & JK Consulting Ltd., Guildford, UK.

References

1. Joint Epilepsy Council of the UK and Ireland. Epilepsy prevalence, incidence and other statistics. http://www.epilepsyscotland.org.uk/pdf/Joint_Epilepsy_Council_Prevalence_and_Incidence_September_11_(3).pdf. Accessed 13 Sep 2016.
2. Brodie MJ, Mintzer S, Pack AM, Gidal BE, Vecht CJ, Schmidt D. Enzyme induction with antiepileptic drugs: cause for concern? Epilepsia. 2013;54:11–27.
3. Gunes A, Bilir E, Zengil H, Babaoglu MO, Bozkurt A, Yasar U. Inhibitory effect of valproic acid on cytochrome P450 2C9 activity in epilepsy patients. Basic Clin Pharmacol Toxicol. 2007;100:383–6.
4. Perucca E. Pharmacological and therapeutic properties of valproate: a summary after 35 years of clinical experience. CNS Drugs. 2002;16:695–714.
5. Perucca E. Clinically relevant drug interactions with antiepileptic drugs. Brit J Clin Pharmacol. 2006;61:246–55.
6. NICE National Institute for Health and Care. Epilepsies: diagnosis and management. NICE guidelines [CG137]. https://www.nice.org.uk/guidance/cg137?unlid=7842667020162363715. Accessed 17 Aug 2016.
7. Pack A. Bone health in people with epilepsy: is it impaired and what are the risk factors? Seizure. 2008;17:181–6.
8. Johannessen SI, Landmark CJ. Antiepileptic drug interactions - principles and clinical implications. Curr Neuropharmacol. 2010;8:254–67.
9. Xiong T, Gallagher E, MacGilchrist KS, Thieffry S. Costs associated with the use of enzyme-inducing anti-epileptic drugs versus non-enzyme-inducing anti-epileptic drugs: a systematic review. Value Health. 2014;17:A394–5.
10. St Germaine-Smith C, Liu M, Quan H, Wiebe S, Jette N. Development of an epilepsy-specific risk adjustment comorbidity index. Epilepsia. 2011;52:2161–7.
11. D'Agostino Jr RB. Propensity score methods for bias reduction in the comparison of a treatment to a non-randomized control group. Stat Med. 1998;17:2265–81.
12. Thomas SV. Controversies in contraception for women with epilepsy. Ann Indian Acad Neurol. 2015;18:278–83.
13. Cockerell OC, Hart YM, Sander JW, Shorvon SD. The cost of epilepsy in the United Kingdom: an estimation based on the results of two population-based studies. Epilepsy Res. 1994;18:249–60.
14. Sander JW, Hart YM, Johnson AL, Shorvon SD. National General Practice Study of Epilepsy: newly diagnosed epileptic seizures in a general population. Lancet. 1990;336:1267–71.
15. Begley CE, Famulari M, Annegers JF, Lairson DR, Reynolds TF, Coan S, et al. The cost of epilepsy in the United States: an estimate from population-based clinical and survey data. Epilepsia. 2000;41:342–51.
16. de Zélicourt M, Buteau L, Fagnani F, Jallon P. The contributing factors to medical cost of epilepsy: an estimation based on a French prospective cohort study of patients with newly diagnosed epileptic seizures (the CAROLE study). Seizure. 2000;9:88–95.
17. Mintzer S, French JA, Perucca E, Cramer JA, Messenheimer JA, Blum DE, et

al. Is a separate monotherapy indication warranted for antiepileptic drugs? Lancet Neurol. 2015;14:1229–40.

18. Payakachat N, Summers KH, Barbuto JP. A comparison of clinical practice guidelines in the initial pharmacological management of new-onset epilepsy in adults. J Manag Care Pharm. 2006;12:55–60.
19. Marson AG, Al-Kharusi AM, Alwaidh M, Appleton R, Baker GA, Chadwick DW, et al. The SANAD study of effectiveness of carbamazepine, gabapentin, lamotrigine, oxcarbazepine, or topiramate for treatment of partial epilepsy: an unblinded randomised controlled trial. Lancet. 2007;369:1000–15.
20. Dickson JM, Scott PA, Reuber M. Epilepsy service provision in the National Health Service in England in 2012. Seizure. 2015;30:26–31.
21. Dixon PA, Kirkham JJ, Marson AG, Pearson MG. National Audit of Seizure management in Hospitals (NASH): results of the national audit of adult epilepsy in the UK. BMJ Open. 2015;5:e007325.
22. Steer S, Pickrell WO, Kerr MP, Thomas RH. Epilepsy prevalence and socioeconomic deprivation in England. Epilepsia. 2014;55:1634–41.

Permissions

All chapters in this book were first published in NEUROLOGY, by BioMed Central; hereby published with permission under the Creative Commons Attribution License or equivalent. Every chapter published in this book has been scrutinized by our experts. Their significance has been extensively debated. The topics covered herein carry significant findings which will fuel the growth of the discipline. They may even be implemented as practical applications or may be referred to as a beginning point for another development.

The contributors of this book come from diverse backgrounds, making this book a truly international effort. This book will bring forth new frontiers with its revolutionizing research information and detailed analysis of the nascent developments around the world.

We would like to thank all the contributing authors for lending their expertise to make the book truly unique. They have played a crucial role in the development of this book. Without their invaluable contributions this book wouldn't have been possible. They have made vital efforts to compile up to date information on the varied aspects of this subject to make this book a valuable addition to the collection of many professionals and students.

This book was conceptualized with the vision of imparting up-to-date information and advanced data in this field. To ensure the same, a matchless editorial board was set up. Every individual on the board went through rigorous rounds of assessment to prove their worth. After which they invested a large part of their time researching and compiling the most relevant data for our readers.

The editorial board has been involved in producing this book since its inception. They have spent rigorous hours researching and exploring the diverse topics which have resulted in the successful publishing of this book. They have passed on their knowledge of decades through this book. To expedite this challenging task, the publisher supported the team at every step. A small team of assistant editors was also appointed to further simplify the editing procedure and attain best results for the readers.

Apart from the editorial board, the designing team has also invested a significant amount of their time in understanding the subject and creating the most relevant covers. They scrutinized every image to scout for the most suitable representation of the subject and create an appropriate cover for the book.

The publishing team has been an ardent support to the editorial, designing and production team. Their endless efforts to recruit the best for this project, has resulted in the accomplishment of this book. They are a veteran in the field of academics and their pool of knowledge is as vast as their experience in printing. Their expertise and guidance has proved useful at every step. Their uncompromising quality standards have made this book an exceptional effort. Their encouragement from time to time has been an inspiration for everyone.

The publisher and the editorial board hope that this book will prove to be a valuable piece of knowledge for researchers, students, practitioners and scholars across the globe.

List of Contributors

Andrea Ungar, Alice Ceccofiglio, Martina Rafanelli and Niccolò Marchionni
Department of Clinical and Experimental Medicine, Syncope Unit, Geriatric Cardiology and Medicine, University of Florence, Florence, Italy

Francesca Pescini
Department of Neurological and Psychiatric Sciences, Epilepsy Center, University of Florence, Florence, Italy

Chiara Mussi
Geriatric and Gerontology Institute, University of Modena, Modena, Italy

Gianni Tava
Geriatric Unit, Santa Chiara Hospital, Trento, Italy

Assunta Langellotto
Division of Geriatrics, Ospedale "S. Maria di Ca' Foncello", Treviso, Italy

J. Gert van Dijk
Department of Neurology, Leiden University Medical Centre, Leiden, The Netherlands

Gianlugi Galizia
Istituti Clinici Scientifici Maugeri- Syncope unit - UOC Cure sub-acute, Milan, Italy

Domenico Bonaduce and Pasquale Abete
Department of Translational Medical Sciences, University of Naples Federico II, Via S. Pansini, 80131 Naples, Italy

Gabriela Timarova
2nd Department of Neurology, Faculty of Medicine, Comenius University, Dérer's University Hospital, Limbova str.5, 83305 Bratislava, Slovak Republic

Andrej Šteňo
Department of Neurosurgery, Faculty of Medicine, Comenius University, Dérer's University Hospital, Bratislava, Slovak Republic

Amelia Smith
GKT School of Medicine, King's College London, London SE1 1UL, UK

Alison McKinlay, Gabriella Wojewodka and Leone Ridsdale
Institute of Psychiatry, Psychology & Neuroscience, Academic Neuroscience Centre, King's College London, SE5 8AF, UK

Xindi Li, Xiaoqing Gong, Heng Zhou, Anna Zhou, Yonghong Liu and Xinghu Zhang
Neuroinfection and Neuroimmunology Center, Department of Neurology, Beijing Tiantan Hospital, Capital Medical University, 6 TiantanXili, Dongcheng District, Beijing 100050, People's Republic of China
China National Clinical Research Center for Neurological Diseases, Beijing Tiantan Hospital, Capital Medical University, 6 TiantanXili, Dongcheng District, Beijing 100050, People's Republic of China

Shenghui Mei, Li Yang, Xingang Li and Zhigang Zhao
Department of Pharmacy, Beijing Tiantan Hospital, Capital Medical University, 6 TiantanXili, Dongcheng District, Beijing 100050, People's Republic of China

Orestes Santos-Morales, Yaisel Pomares-Iturralde, Carmen Viada-González, Patricia Piedra-Sierra and Daniel Amaro-González
NeuroEPO Research and Development Group, Center of Molecular Immunology, Havana, Cuba

Alina Díaz-Machado, Carlos A. González-Delgado, Sonia Pérez-Rodríguez and Eulalia Alfonso-Muñoz
National Center for Toxicology, "Carlos J. Finlay" University Hospital, Havana, Cuba

Daise Jiménez-Rodríguez, Idrian García-García and Tatiana Festary-Casanovas
Clinical Trials Group, Research Direction, Center for Drug Research and Development (CIDEM), Ave. 26 and Puentes Grandes, No. 1605, Nuevo Vedado, Havana, Cuba

Sung Ho Jang
Department of Physical Medicine and Rehabilitation, College of Medicine, Yeungnam University, Gyeongsan, South Korea

Hyeok Gyu Kwon
Department of Physical Therapy, College of Health Sciences, Catholic University of Pusan, 57 Oryundae-ro, Geumjeong-gu, Pusan 46252, Republic of Korea

Leonardo Lorente
Intensive Care Unit, Hospital Universitario de Canarias, Ofra s/n. La Laguna, 38320 Santa Cruz de Tenerife, Spain

María M. Martín
Intensive Care Unit, Hospital Universitario Nuestra Señora de Candelaria, Crta del Rosario s/n, 38010 Santa Cruz de Tenerife, Spain

Pedro Abreu-González
Deparment of Physiology, Faculty of Medicine, University of the La Laguna, Ofra s/n. La Laguna, 38320 Santa Cruz de Tenerife, Spain

Antonia Pérez-Cejas
Laboratory Deparment, Hospital Universitario de Canarias, Ofra, s/n. La Laguna, 38320 Tenerife, Spain

Luis Ramos
Intensive Care Unit, Hospital General La Palma, Buenavista de Arriba s/n, 38713 Breña Alta, La Palma, Spain

Mónica Argueso
Intensive Care Unit, Hospital Clínico Universitario de Valencia, Avda. Blasco Ibáñez n°17-19, 46004 Valencia, Spain

Jordi Solé-Violán
Intensive Care Unit, Hospital Universitario Dr. Negrín. CIBERES, Barranco de la Ballena s/n, 35010 Las Palmas de Gran Canaria, Spain

Juan J. Cáceres
Intensive Care Unit, Hospital Insular, Plaza Dr. Pasteur s/n, 35016 Las Palmas de Gran Canaria, Spain

Alejandro Jiménez
Research Unit, Hospital Universitario de Canarias, Ofra s/n. La Laguna, 38320 Santa Cruz de Tenerife, Spain

Victor García-Marín
Deparment of Neurosurgery, Hospital Universitario de Canarias, Ofra, s/n. La Laguna, 38320 Santa Cruz de Tenerife, Spain

Takashi Hosaka, Kazuhiro Ishii and Akira Tamaoka
Department of the Neurology, Division of Clinical Medicine, Faculty of Medicine, University of Tsukuba, 1-1-1 Ten'noudai, Tsukuba, Ibaraki 305-8575, Japan

Kensaku Kasuga and Takeshi Ikeuchi
Department of Molecular Genetics, Brain Research Institute, Niigata University, 1-757 Asahimachi, Niigata 951-8585, Japan

Takeshi Miura and Naomi Mezaki
Department of Molecular Genetics, Brain Research Institute, Niigata University, 1-757 Asahimachi, Niigata 951-8585, Japant
Department of Neurology, Brain Research Institute, Niigata University, 1-757 Asahimachi, Niigata 951-8585, Japan

Qisheng Tang, Zhifeng Shi and Liang Chen
Department of Neurosurgery, Huashan Hospital, Fudan University, Shanghai, China

Yuxi Lian, Jinhua Yu and Yuanyuan Wang
Department of Electronic Engineering, Fudan University, Shanghai, China

Jiawei Wang, Bingren Zhang, Chanchan Shen and Wei Wang
Department of Clinical Psychology and Psychiatry/ School of Public Health, Zhejiang University College of Medicine, Hangzhou, China

Jinhua Zhang
Department of Neurology, Zhejiang Provincial People's Hospital, Hangzhou, China

Shoko Ryu and Akshay Thontakudi
Department of Electrical and Systems Engineering, Washington University in St. Louis, 1 Brookings Dr. Campus St. Louis, MO 63130, USA

Osvaldo Laurido-Soto, Lawrence Eisenman and Terrance T. Kummer
Department of Neurology, Washington University School of Medicine, 660 S Euclid Ave. Campus St. Louis, MO 63110, USA

Yuko Hayashi, Gen Miura, Takayuki Baba and Shuichi Yamamoto
Department of Ophthalmology and Visual Science, Chiba University Graduate School of Medicine, Inohana 1-8-1, Chuo-ku, Chiba 260-8670, Japan

ShiNung Ching
Department of Electrical and Systems Engineering, Washington University in St. Louis, 1 Brookings Dr. Campus St. Louis, MO 63130, USA
Division of Biology and Biomedical Science, Washington University in St. Louis, St. Louis, MO 63110, USA

MohammadMehdi Kafashan
Department of Electrical and Systems Engineering, Washington University in St. Louis, 1 Brookings Dr. Campus St. Louis, MO 63130, USA
Harvard Medical School, Boston, USA

Mitchell J. Hargis
Department of Neurology, Washington University School of Medicine, 660 S Euclid Ave. Campus St. Louis, MO 63110, USA
Department of Neurology, Novant Health Forsyth Medical Center, Winston-Salem, USA

Debra E. Roberts
Department of Neurology, Washington University School of Medicine, 660 S Euclid Ave. Campus St. Louis, MO 63110, USA
Department of Neurology, University of Rochester, Rochester, USA

Akiyuki Uzawa
Department of Neurology, Graduate School of Medicine, Chiba University, Chiba, Japan

Jia Liu, Zhuo-lin Chen, Min Li, Huan Yi, Li Xu and Fu-hua Peng
Department of Neurology, the Third Affiliated Hospital of Sun Yat-Sen University, 600# Tianhe Road, Guangzhou 510630, Guangdong, China

Chuan Chen
Department of Neurosurgery, the Third Affiliated Hospital of Sun Yat-Sen University, Guangzhou 510630, Guangdong, China

Feng Tan
Department of Neurology, Foshan Chinese Medicine Hospital, Foshan 528000, Guangdong, China

Yujuan Jiao, Lei Cui, Weihe Zhang, Yeqiong Zhang, Xin Zhang and Jinsong Jiao
Department of Neurology, China-Japan Friendship Hospital, #2 Yinghuayuan East Street, Chaoyang District, Beijing 100029, China

Chunyu Zhang
Department of Health Reform and Development, China-Japan Friendship Hospital, Beijing, China

Nirmeen Kishk and Amany Ragab
Neurology Department, Faculty of Medicine, Kasr Alainy Hospital, Cairo University, Cairo, Egypt

Amani Nawito
Clinical Neurophysiology Unit, Faculty of Medicine, Kasr Alainy Hospital, Cairo University, Cairo, Egypt

Ahmed El-Damaty
Cardiovascular Department, Faculty of Medicine, Kasr Alainy Hospital, Cairo University, Cairo, Egypt

tP. Harmel and L. Harms
Klinik und Hochschulambulanz für Neurologie, Charité-Universitätsmedizin Berlin, Berlin, Germany

A.H. Nave
Klinik und Hochschulambulanz für Neurologie, Charité-Universitätsmedizin Berlin, Berlin, Germany
Berlin Institute of Health (BIH), Berlin, Germany

R. Buchert
Department of Diagnostic and Interventional Radiology and Nuclear Medicine, University Medical Centre Hamburg-Eppendorf, Hamburg, Germany

E. Devenney and J. R. Hodges
Brain and Mind Centre, University of Sydney, Sydney, NSW 2050, Australia
ARC Centre of Excellence in Cognition and its Disorders, Sydney, Australia

T. Swinn
Medical Research Council Cognition and Brain Sciences Unit, Cambridge, UK

E. Mioshi and M. Hornberger
Faculty of Medicine and Health Sciences, University of East Anglia, Norwich, UK

K. E. Dawson and J. B. Rowe
Department of Clinical Neurosciences, University of Cambridge, Cambridge, UK

S. Mead
MRC Prion Unit, Department of Neurodegenerative Disease, UCL Institute of Neurology, Queen Square, London, UK

Tongtao Zhao, Gang Wang, Jiaman Dai, Yong Liu and Shiying Li
Department of Ophthalmology, Southwest Hospital, The Third Military Medical University (Army Medical University), Chongqing, China

Yi Wang
Aier Eye Hospital, Chongqing, China

M. Jonsson
Department of Psychiatry and Neurochemistry, Institute of Neuroscience and Physiology, Sahlgrenska Academy at the University of Gothenburg, Mölndal, Sweden

E. Kapaki and G. P. Paraskevas
1st Department of Neurology, Eginition Hospital, Medical School, National and Kapodistrian University of Athens, Athens, Greece

M. Boban and B. Malojcic
Department of Neurology, University Hospital Centre Zagreb, Medical School, University of Zagreb, Zagreb, Croatia

S. Engelborghs
Memory Clinic and Department of Neurology, Hospital Network Antwerp (ZNA) Middelheim and HogeBeuken, Antwerp, Belgium
Reference Center for Biological Markers of Dementia, Department of Biomedical Sciences, Institute Born-Bunge, University of Antwerp, Antwerp, Belgium

M. Bjerke
Reference Center for Biological Markers of Dementia, Department of Biomedical Sciences, Institute Born-Bunge, University of Antwerp, Antwerp, Belgium

G. Weinstein
School of Public Health, University of Haifa, Haifa, Israel

A. Korczyn
Department of Neurology, Sackler School of Medicine, Tel Aviv University, Tel Aviv, Israel

G. Rosenberg
University of New Mexico Health Sciences Center, Albuquerque, NM 87131, USA

A.Wallin
Department of Psychiatry and Neurochemistry, Institute of Neuroscience and Physiology, Sahlgrenska Academy at the University of Gothenburg, Mölndal, Sweden
Memory Clinic at Department of Neuropsychiatry, Sahlgrenska University Hospital, Institute of Neuroscience and Physiology at Sahlgrenska Academy, University of Gothenburg, Wallinsgatan 6, SE-431 41 Mölndal, Sweden

Sushil Khanal and Subhash Prasad Acharya
Department of Critical Care, Grande International Hospital (GIH), Kathmandu, Nepal

Matthias Wawra
Department of Neurology, Charité - Universitätsmedizin Berlin, Freie Universität Berlin, Humboldt-Universität zu Berlin, Berlin Institute of Health, Berlin, Germany

Viktor Horst
Center for Stroke Research Berlin, Charité - Universitätsmedizin Berlin, Freie Universität Berlin, Humboldt-Universität zu Berlin, Berlin Institute of Health, Berlin, Germany

Christian Schinke
Department of Neurology, Charité - Universitätsmedizin Berlin, Freie Universität Berlin, Humboldt-Universität zu Berlin, Berlin Institute of Health, Berlin, Germany
Department of Experimental Neurology, Charité - Universitätsmedizin Berlin, Freie Universität Berlin, Humboldt-Universität zu Berlin, Berlin Institute of Health, Berlin, Germany

Ludwig Schlemm
Department of Neurology, Charité - Universitätsmedizin Berlin, Freie Universität Berlin, Humboldt-Universität zu Berlin, Berlin Institute of Health, Berlin, Germany
Center for Stroke Research Berlin, Charité - Universitätsmedizin Berlin, Freie Universität Berlin, Humboldt-Universität zu Berlin, Berlin Institute of Health, Berlin, Germany
Berlin Institute of Health (BIH), Berlin, Germany
London School of Economics and Political Science, London, UK

Michael Scheel
Department of Neuroradiology, Charité - Universitätsmedizin Berlin, Freie Universität Berlin, Humboldt-Universität zu Berlin, Berlin Institute of Health, Berlin, Germany

Jed A. Hartings
Department of Neurosurgery, University of Cincinnati (UC) College of Medicine, Cincinnati, OH, USA

Jens P. Dreier
Department of Neurology, Charité - Universitätsmedizin Berlin, Freie Universität Berlin, Humboldt-Universität zu Berlin, Berlin Institute of Health, Berlin, Germany
Center for Stroke Research Berlin, Charité - Universitätsmedizin Berlin, Freie Universität Berlin, Humboldt-Universität zu Berlin, Berlin Institute of Health, Berlin, Germany
Department of Experimental Neurology, Charité - Universitätsmedizin Berlin, Freie Universität Berlin, Humboldt-Universität zu Berlin, Berlin Institute of Health, Berlin, Germany
Bernstein Center for Computational Neuroscience Berlin, Berlin, Germany
Einstein Center for Neurosciences Berlin, Berlin, Germany

Yonghui Liu and Tianlu Wei
Department of Encephalopathy, The First Affiliated Hospital of Guangxi University of Chinese Medicine, Nanning 530023, China

Liena Elsayed and Mutaz Amin
Department of Biochemistry, Faculty of Medicine, University of Khartoum, Khartoum, Sudan

Arwa Babai, Rayan Abubakr and Razaz Idris
Institute of Endemic Diseases, University of Khartoum, Khartoum, Sudan

Mustafa A. Salih
Division of Pediatric Neurology, Department of Pediatrics, College of Medicine, King Saud University, Riyadh, Saudi Arabia

Sarah Misbah El-Sadig
Department of Medicine, Faculty of Medicine, University of Khartoum, Khartoum, Sudan
Department of Neurology, Soba University Hospital, Khartoum, Sudan

Mahmoud Koko
Department of Neurology & Epileptology, Hertie Institute for Clinical Brain Research, University of Tübingen, Tübingen, Germany

Shaimaa Omer M.A. Taha
Department of Radiology, Dar Al Elaj specialized hospital, Khartoum, Sudan

Ammar Eltahir Ahmed
Department of Physiology, Faculty of Medicine, University of Khartoum, Khartoum, Sudan
Department of Neurology, Soba University Hospital, Khartoum, Sudan

Ashraf Yahia
Department of Biochemistry, Faculty of Medicine, University of Khartoum, Khartoum, Sudan
Department of Biochemistry, Faculty of Medicine, National University, Khartoum, Sudan
Institut du Cerveau et de la Moelle épinière, INSERM U1127, CNRS UMR7225, Sorbonne Universités UMR_S1127, 75013 Paris, France

Giovanni Stevanin
Ecole Pratique des Hautes Etudes, EPHE, PSL Research University, Paris, France
Institut du Cerveau et de la Moelle épinière, INSERM U1127, CNRS UMR7225, Sorbonne Universités UMR_S1127, 75013 Paris, France

Alexis Brice
Department of Genetics, APHP, Pitié-Salpêtrière Hospital, Paris, France
Institut du Cerveau et de la Moelle épinière, INSERM U1127, CNRS UMR7225, Sorbonne Universités UMR_S1127, 75013 Paris, France

Salah A. Elmalik
Department of Physiology, College of Medicine, King Saud University, Riyadh, Saudi Arabia

Thor Jensen
Center for Neuroscience, Section for Integrative Neuroscience, University of Copenhagen, Panum Institute, Building 33.3, Nørre Allé 20, DK-2200 Copenhagen N, Denmark

Jens Bo Nielsen and Jakob Lorentzen
Center for Neuroscience, Section for Integrative Neuroscience, University of Copenhagen, Panum Institute, Building 33.3, Nørre Allé 20, DK-2200 Copenhagen N, Denmark
Elsass Instituttet, Holmegårdsvej 28, DK-2920 Charlottenlund, Denmark

Camilla B. Voigt
Elsass Instituttet, Holmegårdsvej 28, DK-2920 Charlottenlund, Denmark

Mark Schram Christensen
Center for Neuroscience, Section for Integrative Neuroscience, University of Copenhagen, Panum Institute, Building 33.3, Nørre Allé 20, DK-2200 Copenhagen N, Denmark
DTU Compute, Department of Applied Mathematics and Computer Science, Technical University of Denmark, Richard Petersens Plads, Building 324, DK-2800 Kgs. Lyngby, Denmark

Sofia Straudi, Amira Sabbagh Charabati, Claudia Pavarelli, Giulia Gamberini Anna Scotti and Nino Basaglia
Neuroscience and Rehabilitation Department, Ferrara University Hospital, Ferrara, Italy

Giacomo Severini
School of Electrical and Electronic Engineering, University College Dublin, Dublin, Ireland

George S. Vlachos
Mediterraneo Hospital, Headache Clinic, Glyfada, Greece

Michail Vikelis
Mediterraneo Hospital, Headache Clinic, Glyfada, Greece
Glyfada Headache Clinic, Glyfada, Greece
Headache Outpatient Clinic, 1st Department of Neurology, National and Kapodistrian University of Athens, Athens, Greece

Emmanouil V. Dermitzakis and Georgios G. Vasiliadis
Geniki Kliniki Euromedica, Department of Neurology, Thessaloniki, Greece

Konstantinos C. Spingos
Corfu Headache Clinic, 13, Mitropolitou Methodiou str, 49100 Corfu, Greece

Evaggelia Kararizou
Headache Outpatient Clinic, 1st Department of Neurology, National and Kapodistrian University of Athens, Athens, Greece

Simon Borghs, Laura Byram and Jane Chan
UCB Pharma, Slough, UK

Solène Thieffry and Peter Dedeken
UCB Pharma, Brussels, Belgium

Matthias Noack-Rink
UCB Pharma, Monheim Am Rhein, Germany

Lai San Hong
Redsen Limited, Bournemouth, UK

John Logan
Stats4Pharma, Cork, Ireland

Victor Kiri
FV & JK Consulting Ltd., Guildford, UK

Index

www.ingramcontent.com/pod-product-compliance
Lightning Source LLC
Chambersburg PA
CBHW082026190326
41458CB00010B/3288

* 9 7 8 1 6 3 9 2 7 3 0 8 9 *